DATE DUE

Demco, Inc. 38-293

Pain Updated
Mechanisms and Effects

Edited by
Rashmi Mathur
Department of Physiology
All India Institute of Medical Sciences
New Delhi - 110 029, India

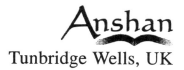
Tunbridge Wells, UK

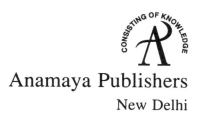
Anamaya Publishers
New Delhi

A catalogue record for the book is available from the British Library

ISBN 1-904798-60-8

Copublished by
Anshan Limited
6 Newlands Road
Tunbridge Wells
Kent, TN4 9 AT
UK
Tel/Fax: +44 (0) 1892 557767
E-mail: info@anshan.co.uk
Website: www.anshan.co.uk

Sold and distributed in all the countries, except
India, Pakistan, Sri Lanka, Bangladesh and Nepal,
by Anshan Limited, 6 Newlands Road, Tunbridge Wells
Kent, TN4 9 AT UK

In India, Pakistan, Sri Lanka, Bangladesh and Nepal by
Anamaya Publishers, F-154/2, Lado Sarai, New Delhi-110 030, India
E-mail: anamayapub@vsnl.net

Printed in India.

Preface

Recent studies in the field of pain have highlighted the vital pain control neural sites, their mechanisms and some neuro-chemicals involved in their modulation of pain. The widespread use of recent techniques for identification of neural connections, chemical configuration, neuronal activity in either animal model or human volunteers; in health or in abnormal pain conditions have significantly contributed towards it. However, in the process it has opened up new vistas. Suffice it to say that it has given a new direction for pain research. The principles of physiology have been applied to develop novel ways of assessing pain status besides utilizing it as a marker for diagnosis of disease condition.

The physiological maturation of concepts related to pain modulation from Gate Control Theory of Wall and Melzack to the recent Neuromatrix Theory has been elaborated in this book. The status of pain modulation depends heavily on the opioidergic system. The techniques to assess them are not reported *per se* in the literature. Nevertheless, one such novel technique, the Naloxone Challenge Test has been discussed here in the context of health and disease including Syndrome X, Trigeminal neuralgia and Chronic tension type headache. The aberration in central processing of nociceptive information is believed to be the prime reason for the chest pain in Syndrome X, which has been intentionally included to emphasize the need for understanding the interaction amongst central processing units. This has further support from the chapters discussing the pain modulation mechanisms exerted by several such brain units, e.g. hypothalamus and amygdala. Needless to say, these higher influences exert through the spinal cord, which has an inherent complex processing system per se.

A section has been included about the ageing brain, and Alzheimer's disease for a better understanding of pain status in them, while the status of pain in neonates has been included to highlight the specific pain mechanisms present at birth, which is contrary to the belief that the neonates do not feel pain.

Recently, there is an upsurge in the information about interaction amongst environmental time dependent magnetic fields, the brain opioidergic and serotonergic systems. The former system is predominantly implicated in nociception while the latter in aggressive behaviour. Their mechanism of interaction is far from clear. However, an attempt has been made to hypothesize mechanism of magnetic fields bio-interaction.

The above information will remain irrelevant until and unless they are utilized for the relief of pain. Principles of some of the unconventional global approaches, namely yoga vis-à-vis life style or stress management or behavioural management of pain and herbal preparations are included.

Recently, pain has been defined in a wider perspective, which should go hand in hand with the understanding of pain. Therefore, it is implied that we are not only concerned with the effective treatment of the cause *per se* but also envisage a pain free society, which has been also dealt with in this book.

The book has a great reference value for the students of pain physiology, biochemistry, endocrinology and pharmacology, besides, the clinicians who try to figure out the waxing and waning of pain in their patients and have a roving eye for a suitable, safe, and reliable method to assess and treat pain. It will strengthen the pain instructors, too. I hope they will find this book handy.

Developing a book coalescing into a theme is not an easy task particularly those who have been involved in widely different activities. It would simply never have been completed if it were not for the efforts of the contributors who have met the deadlines as well as have agreed to share their research work.

I am thankful to Mrs. Nidhi and Mrs. Mamta Sharma who worked most closely and have been very patient and encouraging.

RASHMI MATHUR

Contents

Pain Updated: Mechanisms and Effects
Edited by R. Mathur
Copyright © 2006 Anamaya Publishers, New Delhi, India

1. Animal Experiments on Pain: Ethical Guidelines

V.M. Kumar

Department of Physiology, All India Institute of Medical Sciences,
New Delhi-110029, India

Introduction

The greatest contribution to the understanding of human biology has come from experimental research on animals. Some of the most spectacular progress in modern physiology was dependent on the right choice of animal for experimental research. A careful search can always find an animal that is designed by nature for the investigations to be carried out by the researchers. It is necessary to select an animal in which the physiological functions have been developed to an extreme, for example, renal responses in desert rodents, two very large nerve cells in the central nervous system of the squid Loligo etc. The choice of the animal for any experiment should be based on valid scientific and practical considerations like availability, knowledge of their anatomy and ability to maintain them in captivity. However, lately the choice of animals is greatly influenced by the animal welfare acts. Cats, dogs, rabbits, hamster and all wild, warm-blooded animals except birds are included under the purview of the 'Animal Welfare Act', which became law in the United States in 1966. The Act exempted rats, mice and humans while the Indian Parliament, passed a legislation called "Prevention of Cruelty to Animals Act" in 1960 which included the crucial words of wisdom: "nothing contained in this Act shall render unlawful the performance of experiments (including experiments involving operations) on animals for the purpose of advancement by new discovery of physiological knowledge or of knowledge which will be useful for saving or for prolonging life or alleviating suffering or for combating any disease, whether of human beings, animals or plants".

The research work undertaken by the staff should be in conformity with the rules laid down by the Committee for the Purpose of Control and Supervision of Experiments on Animals (CPCSEA), Ministry of Environment and Forest, and other rules laid down by the government, from time to time. No research project involving the use of animals should be conducted without the prior approval of the Ethics Committee constituted by the institute/laboratory. Besides any study on pain is strictly guided by the report of the Committee for Research and Ethical Issues of the International Association for the Study of Pain (IASP) headed by Professor M. Zimmermann, II Physiologisches Insitüt, Universität Heidelberg, 69120 Heidelberg, Germany. The committee is concerned with the ethical aspects of studies producing experimental pain and any suffering it may cause to animals. Such studies are essential if new and clinically relevant knowledge about the mechanisms of pain is to be acquired. Investigations in conscious animals intended to stimulate chronic pain in man are being performed. Such experiments require careful planning to avoid or at least minimize pain in the animals.

Investigators of animal models for chronic pain, as well as those applying acute painful stimuli to animals, should be aware of the problems pertinent to such studies and should make every effort to minimize pain. They should accept a general attitude in which the animal is regarded not as an object for exploitation, but as a living individual.

In practice, investigators engaged in research on pain in animals should consider the following guidelines aimed at minimizing pain in animals and, when submitting a manuscript, state explicitly that they have been followed. The guidelines are concerned with the importance of the investigation, the severity and the duration of the pain.

1. It is essential that the intended experiments on pain in conscious animals be reviewed beforehand by scientists and lay-persons. The potential benefit of such experiments to our understanding of pain mechanisms and pain therapy needs to be shown. The investigator should be aware of the ethical need for a continuing justification of his investigations.

2. If possible, the investigator should try the pain stimulus on himself; this principle applies for most non-invasive stimuli causing acute pain.

3. To make possible the evaluation of the levels of pain, the investigator should give a careful assessment of the animal's deviation from normal behavior. To this end, physiological and behavioral parameters should be measured. The outcome of this assessment should be included in the manuscript.

4. In studies of acute or chronic pain in animals measures should be taken to provide a reasonable assurance that the animal is exposed to the minimal pain necessary for the purpose of the experiment.

5. An animal presumable experiencing chronic pain should be treated for relief of pain, or should be allowed to self-administer analgesic agents or procedures, as long as this will not interfere with the aim of the investigation.

6. Studies of pain in animals paralyzed with a neuromuscular blocking agents should not be performed without a general anesthetic or an appropriate surgical procedure that eliminates sensory awareness.

7. The duration of the experiment must be as short as possible and the number of animals involved kept to a minimum.

The above guidelines have been approved by the Council of IASP in December 1982. They replace a previously published version [2] and account for comments and suggestions of scientists as solicited in a Newsletter of IASP (Pain, 13/2 (1982)).

References

1. Bowd, A.D. Ethics and animal experimentation. *Amer. Psychol.* 1980; **35**: 224–225.
2. Covino, B.G., Dubner, R., Gybels, J., Kosterlitz, H.W., Liebeskind, J.C., Sternbach, R.A., Vyklicky, L., Yammamura, H. and Zimmermann, M. Ethical Standards for Investigations of Experimental Pain in Animals. *Pain* 1980; **9**: 141–143.
3. Halsbury. The Earl of, Ethics and the exploitation of animals. *Conquest* 1973; **164**: 2–11.
4. Hoff C. Immoral and moral uses of animals. *New Engl. J. Med.* 1980; **302**: 115–118.
5. Iggo A. Experimental study of pain in animals—Ethical aspects. In : Bonica, J.J., Liebeskind, J.C. and Albe-Fessard D.G. (Eds). Advances in Pain Research and Therapy, Vol. 3, Raven Press, New York, 1979, pp. 773–778.
6. Smyth, D.H.Y. Alternatives to Animal Experiments, Scolar-RDS, London, 1978.
7. Sternbach, R.A. The need for an animal model of chronic pain. *Pain* 1976; **2**: 2–4.
8. Wall, P.D. Editorial. *Pain* 1975; **1**: 1–2.
9. Wall, P.D. Editorial. *Pain* 1976; **2**: 1.

Pain Updated: Mechanisms and Effects
Edited by R. Mathur
Copyright © 2006 Anamaya Publishers, New Delhi, India

2. Central Mechanisms of Pain: From Gate Control to Neuronal Maze

Solomon S. Senok and Usha Nayar

Department of Physiology, College of Medicine and Medical Sciences,
The Arabian Gulf University, P.O. Box 22979, Manama, Kingdom of Bahrain

Abstract. Melzack and Wall [5] proposed the gate control theory of pain, emphasizing the CNS mechanisms that control the perception of pain. They suggested that the brain actively filters, selects and modulates inputs received from pain receptors in the periphery as well as dorsal horns. This theory generated vigorous debate and research. However, the phenomenon of phantom limb pain could not be fully explained. Melzack [20] then proposed the neuromatrix theory, which proposes that the brain is made up of an array of widely distributed neural networks (the neuromatrix), based on the genetic make up of the individual. These neural networks create an image of the self, based on past experience. The perception and reporting of pain are therefore determined by a complex interaction of the afferent inputs on the neuromatrix. While stress and learned experiences modulate the perception of pain, they are themselves strongly impacted upon by pain. Our understanding of pain has ascended from the purely psychophysical description of pain to the gate control theory to now pain as a damaging or potential threat to the individual's imprinted self-image. This has implications for a multidimensional approach to the management of pain and suffering.

Introduction

Pain is a vital sensory modality. It alerts the organism of the presence of a damaging or potentially deleterious situation, thereby, proving the truth of Sherrington's description of pain as 'the physical adjunct of an imperative protective reflex'. Such a physiological pain is relatively short-lived with two clearly identifiable components: a fast pain (sharp or first pain), which is carried by small (2-5 μm) myelinated Aδ afferents, and a slow (dull) pain carried by the thin (0.4-1.2 μm) unmyelinated C fibres (Fig. 1). The latter projection is known to play a role in the affective components of pain [1-3].

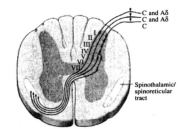

Fig. 1 A simplified representation of the termination and connections of the C and myelinated Aδ afferents in the dorsal horn. Projection neurons from laminae I and V ascend in the contralateral spinothalamic tracts.

The International Association for the Study of Pain defines pain as 'an unpleasant sensory and emotional experience associated with actual or potential tissue damage, or described in terms of such damage' [4]. The sensation of pain therefore depends on the nature and physical parameters of the evoking agent/stimulus, besides the perceived threat to the organism's biological integrity.

The spinal cord was considered as a relay station for pain signals on their way to the brain until Melzack and Wall [5] proposed their Gate Control Theory (Fig. 2). They proposed that the spinal cord integrates both the input and output pain signals and the pain felt is the resultant of interactions between large and small diameter sensory fibres, dorsal horn interneurons and projection neurons. Both groups of fibres are excitatory to the projection neurons (Fig. 1). The non-nociceptive large fibres also make excitatory connections with the tonically active inhibitory interneurons (lamina II). Therefore, strong stimulation of the touch receptors in the skin will have the effect of reducing the transmission of pain signals from the same region because excitation of the inhibitory interneurons will make the projection neurones less excitable. The nociceptive fibers on the other hand are inhibitory to the same interneurons and their stimulation is to block the (tonically active) interneurons simultaneously with activation of the projection neurons. Thereby, interneurons in lamina II (substantia gelatinosa) are the primary site for control [6]. Furthermore, the 'gate' is under efferent control from the brain mainly from descending fibres from the periaqueductal grey (PAG), which modulate the interneurons and projection neurons (post-synaptically) as well as the primary fiber input to the superficial dorsal horn (pre-synaptically).

As a framework for inquiry, the gate control theory generated a lot of interest and research, which accelerated our understanding of many of the processes involved in the perception of pain (e.g. mechanical allodynia, hyperalgesia,

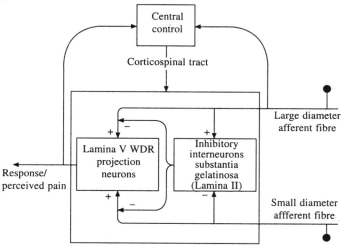

Fig. 2 The sensory 'gate' mechanism as originally proposed by Melzack and Wall [5]. See text for a discussion of the effects of an imbalance in the sensory inflow along the large and small diameter afferent fibres. For comprehensive reappraisal of the evidence and subsequent re-statement of the theory, refer to Wall [29].

referred pain). In particular, the brain was understood as actively filtering, selecting and modulating pain; with the dorsal horns acting as dynamic modulators of the sensory input and not merely as passive transit stations. The gate control theory does not however explain all aspects of pain perception e.g. pain in the absence of tissue pathology in phantom limb phenomena [7, 8].

It is a common observation that amputee patients experience distressing sensations of pain from the amputated part of the limb. In many instances of phantom limb pain, the Cartesian model of pain as a sensation produced by injury, inflammation or other tissue pathology, cannot apply. While phantom limb theories like neuroma formation [9], reorganisation of cerebral cortical maps [10] and corollary discharge from motor commands to the limbs might approximate the Cartesian model. The fact that phantom limb phenomena are reported in patients who have congenital absence of limbs [11,12], would suggest something beyond the basic premise of the gate control theory.

Cortical Center Monitoring Incongruence of Sensation (CIS)

Based on the studies in patients with 'left neglect' Ramachandran [8, 13, 14] had proposed a hypothetical center in the right cerebral cortex that monitors consistency between motor intention, proprioception and vision which was later demonstrated by Fink and co-workers [15] using functional imaging studies to be located in the right dorsolateral prefrontal cortex. Harris [16] hypothesized that the CIS is the cortical substrate for pain in the absence of tissue pathology. When one or more of our senses present information that is incongruent with that of other senses an unpleasant sensation results. For example, when our eyes present the brain with information that is incongruent with that about our body position, balance and equilibrium, we experience nausea. Similarly, the effect of discordance between awareness of motor intention, muscle-joint proprioception and vision might be an unpleasant sensation i.e. pain [16]. In an amputee, there is a lack of proprioceptive and visual information from the missing limb congruent with motor intention. Presumably, since the brain cannot tell that a limb has been removed, it continues to plan and 'execute' movements. This would be expected to activate CIS, and result in pain, since there is no sensory feedback. This has been supported by the elegant work of Ramachandran and Hirstein [17] using a mirror box that allowed the amputee to see a mirror image of the normal hand while performing motor tasks which provided a virtual image of the phantom limb. Surprisingly, such a visual illusory feedback was found to relieve phantom pain [18].

Taking incongruence between motor intention and visual and proprioceptive feedback as the common factor, it is reasonable to infer that the affective sensation of nausea when vision is not congruent with vestibular sensation approximates with the affective sensation of pain when feedback is either lacking (as in phantom limb), or inappropriate (as in a frustrated golfer trying to learn a new motor skill, where intention and outcome can be highly incongruent).

Beyond Gate Control: The Neuromatrix Theory

The limitations of the gate control theory became more obvious with the progress in pain research. It became necessary to distinguish acute pain from non-acute pain of the 'suffering' type. While the former finds adequate explanation in the gate control theory, the latter called for a more all-encompassing hypothesis. The primary problem was, and still is, a rather poor understanding of brain function. While a large volume of data has been generated on the cellular connections and functions of neurons in the CNS, broad conceptual models that explain complex issues like cognition and memory are still relatively rudimentary. The neuromatrix hypothesis [19] was suggested as a conceptual model of brain function to accommodate the mystifying findings surrounding phantom limb pain and the chronic pain. The theory, proposes that there is a pattern generating mechanism in the CNS (the neuromatrix), which though genetically determined, is a cumulative embodiment of our body's sensory experiences. It forms the body-self, distinct from other people and the surrounding world, and serves as a fulcrum or reference point around which the rest of our reality revolves. At a cognitive level, the experience of pain is therefore dependent on the synaptic architecture of the neuromatrix and the multiple modulating influences from without and within the brain itself [20].

The basic premises upon which the hypothesis is predicted are [20]; (i) if phantom limbs feel so real, they must be subserved by the same brain processes that allow us to feel our normal body; (ii) that the brain processes that underlie our normal sensations are capable of being generated in the absence of the requisite inputs, in other words, the qualities of experience pre-exist in a neural network in the brain and are triggered by the sensory inputs rather than being produced by them; (iii) there is a unitary self which is not the product of spinal cord or peripheral nervous system input; and (iv) that the body-self has a genetically imprinted substrate, which is subject to experiential modification. Some of these premises are not in themselves novel. The concept of a 'body image' or 'self' has intrigued neurologists, psychologists and philosophers for a long time [17]. The idea of a unitary self built into a diffuse, genetically programmed neuromatrix is however novel and might explain some of the phenomenology of phantom limbs. The notion that the body-self is predetermined and evolving on the basis of cumulative experience however implies a certain persistence and coherence of the 'image' which is at variance with the results of illusion experiments where body parts can be so easily extended or translocated. If the brain can so easily accept or believe such illusionary drastic changes to the 'image' (cultured over so many years), in favour of a few minutes of trickery, the body image may not be circumscribed or permanent. Ramachandran and Hirstein [17] has gone as far as to posit that the body image is no more durable than a transitory internal construct which is subject to profound alterations by varied stimulus contingencies.

The neuromatrix theory does not seek to replace the gate control theory but to extend. Instead of treating pain as an experience associated with actual or potential tissue damage, the theory extends the sphere of actual or potential damage to a theorized 'body image', of which the body's tissues constitute a concrete and tangible component. The concept of pattern generation in CNS function is not new. Learnt complex motor movements are encoded as patterns rather than a compendium of discrete hierarchical movements requiring conscious instructions to each muscle. Movement patterns are generated and stored as programs that are called upon and executed when the particular motor skill is required [21,22]. Perhaps, the pattern generating mechanism of the neuromatrix envisaged for pain perception is a program for sensory response that is generated and encoded, ready to be executed when the appropriate sensation arrives. The execution of this 'response' program, of a necessity, involves multiple areas of the brain sub serving the pain experience and behaviour. One might argue that what happens in pathological pain is that the program or pattern is inappropriately triggered. The experience and behaviour is therefore not different from the one with actual tissue damage.

Melzack and Loeser [23] postulated that synaptic areas along the transmission routes of the major sensory projection systems (from the dorsal horns to the somatosensory projection areas in the thalamus and cortex), could become pattern generating mechanisms. Activities in these pathways that exceed a critical threshold (frequency coding), or fit a predetermined pattern are then able to project to other areas that subserve the pain experience and localization of the sensation. Assuming frequency modulation and coincidence detection as substrates for pattern generation in the neuromatrix, one would expect that situations associated with high firing levels, including tissue injury, loss of input to central structures by deafferentation after amputation or cord transection as well as input to hyperactive central cells, may produce severe persistent pains [20]. The pattern generating mechanism is in turn dynamically modulated by multiple inputs and the internal milieu.

In addition to producing pain, partly as a result of activation of the body's interoceptive mechanisms (i.e. the brain's monitor of the physiological condition of all tissues in the body [24]), injury also disrupts the brain's homeostatic regulatory systems, thereby producing stress. Stress arises from the complex programs that are initiated to reinstate homeostasis and occurs beneficial physiological adaptation. It however becomes maladaptive when the stimulus persists (e.g. in chronic pain conditions), and the stress response becomes destructive to the individual [25]. The interplay between a negative physical stressor like tissue trauma/pain and the central pain pathways, the immune and the endocrine (hypothalamo-pituitary-adrenocortical-axis) systems, is illustrated in Fig. 3. Tissue damage resulting from trauma or infection/inflammation leads to the activation of neural and humoural mediators, which may produce an extended stress response which is manifested as fatigue, dysphoria,

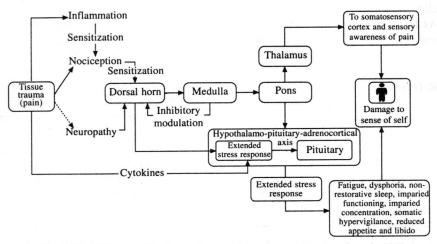

Fig. 3 Mechanisms and effects of stress in patients with chronic pain [25]

poor sleep etc. which the patient may associate with the pain. This results in suffering—a perception of damage to the integrity of the self [25]. Suffering is thus a natural consequence of chronic pain. The disability engendered by the extended stress response produces a conflict between what is expected of one's self and what one is or does [26], thereby causing pain by impinging on the neuronal maze that constitutes the neuromatrix.

The corollary is also true; stress can manifest as pain. Stressful conditions and suffering arising from other causes, including social deprivation, can produce a sense of helplessness and inability to resolve life's conflicts. The incongruence between expectation and performance feedback may be associated with pain [27], which are resistant to usual treatments that are developed primarily to manage pains triggered by sensory inputs. The prolonged cortisol output associated with the stress response also causes destruction of muscle, bone and neural tissue, which may cause myopathy, fatigue and chronic pain [28].

Conclusion

Pain is clearly not the passive consequence of the transfer of a defined peripheral input to a single/simple pain centre in the brain. The gate control theory, which underlined the non-passive role of the spinal cord in the processing of noxious impulses, was a step forward from the psychophysical concept that sought a direct translation between injury and pain. We have moved further, in the light of the inability of gate control to explain pain in the absence of tissue pathology, to a theoretical framework that considers pain as a response to real or potential damage to a genetically imprinted body-self, which is modulated by the stress system and cognitive functions.

How may this be applied to the treatment of pain? Analgesics and anti inflammatory agents may not be the appropriate therapy in conditions of pain without tissue pathology. Instead, treatments targeted at restoring the integrity of cortical information processing might be more appropriate. To this end, several antidepressants have already found use in pain therapy. Interdisciplinary pain clinics ought to expand to include specialists in endocrinology and immunology. As far as pain research goes, more attention should be paid to stress, suffering and immune function, when studying pain.

References

1. Casey KL. Neural mechanisms of pain: an overview. *Acta Anaesthesiol Scand Suppl* 1982; **74**: 13–20.
2. Hunt SP, Mantyh PW. The molecular dynamics of pain control. Nat Rev *Neurosci* 2001; **2(2)**: 83–91.
3. Lorenz J, Casey KL. Imaging of acute versus pathological pain in humans. *European Journal of Pain* 2005; **9(2)**: 163–165.
4. Merskey H. Pain terms: a list with definitions and a note on usage. Recommended by the International Association for the Study of Pain (IASP) Subcommittee on Taxonomy. *Pain* 1979; **6**: 249–252.
5. Melzack R, Wall PD. Pain mechanisms: a new theory. *Science* 1965; **150(699)**: 971–979.

6. Gebhart GF. Descending modulation of pain. *Neurosci Biobehav Rev* 2004; **27(8)**: 729–737.
7. Katz J, Melzack R. Pain 'memories' in phantom limbs: review and clinical observations. *Pain* 1990; **43(3)**: 319–336.
8. Ramachandran VS. Phantom limbs, neglect syndromes, repressed memories, and Freudian psychology. *Int Rev Neurobiol* 1994; **37**: 291–333; discussion 369–72.
9. Schott GD. Mechanisms of causalgia and related clinical conditions. The role of the central and of the sympathetic nervous systems. *Brain* 1986; **109(Pt 4)**: 717–738.
10. Merzenich MM, Nelson RJ, Stryker MP, Cynader MS, Schoppmann A, Zook JM. Somatosensory cortical map changes following digit amputation in adult monkeys. *J Comp Neurol* 1984; **224(4)**: 591–605.
11. Melzack R, Israel R, Lacroix R, Schultz G. Phantom limbs in people with congenital limb deficiency or amputation in early childhood. Brain 1997; **120(Pt 9)**: 1603–1620.
12. Saadah ES, Melzack R. Phantom limb experiences in congenital limb–deficient adults. *Cortex* 1994; **30(3)**: 479–485.
13. Ramachandran VS, Rogers–Ramachandran D, Cobb S. Touching the phantom limb. *Nature* 1995; **377(6549)**: 489–490.
14. Ramachandran VS. Anosognosia in parietal lobe syndrome. *Conscious Cogn* 1995; **4(1)**: 22–51.
15. Fink GR, Marshall JC, Halligan PW, Frith CD, Driver J, Frackowiak RS et al. The neural consequences of conflict between intention and the senses. *Brain* 1999; **122(Pt 3)**: 497–512.
16. Harris AJ. Cortical origin of pathological pain. *Lancet* 1999; **354(9188)**: 1464–1466.
17. Ramachandran VS, Hirstein W. The perception of phantom limbs. The D. O. Hebb lecture. *Brain* 1998; **121(Pt 9)**: 1603–1630.
18. Ramachandran VS, Rogers-Ramachandran D. Synaesthesia in phantom limbs induced with mirrors. *Proc Biol Sci* 1996; **263(1369)**: 377–386.
19. Melzack R. Phantom limbs and the concept of a neuromatrix. *Trends Neurosci* 1990; **13(3)**: 88–92.
20 Melzack R. From the gate to the neuromatrix. *Pain* 1999; Suppl 6:S121–6:S121–S126.
21 Thompson S, Watson WH, III. Central pattern generator for swimming in Melibe. *J Exp Biol* 2005; **208(Pt 7)**: 1347–1361.
22 Yuste R, MacLean JN, Smith J, Lansner A. The cortex as a central pattern generator. *Nature Reviews Neuroscience* 2005; **6(6)**: 477–483.
23 Melzack R, Loeser JD. Phantom body pain in paraplegics: evidence for a central "pattern generating mechanism" for pain. *Pain* 1978; **4(3)**: 195–210.
24 Craig AD. Interoception: the sense of the physiological condition of the body. *Curr Opin Neurobiol* 2003; **13(4)**: 500–505.
25 Chapman CR, Gavrin J. Suffering: the contributions of persistent pain. *Lancet* 1999; **353(9171)**: 2233–2237.
26 Higgins ET. Self-discrepancy: a theory relating self and affect. *Psychol Rev* 1987; **94(3)**: 319–340.
27 McEwen BS. The neurobiology of stress: from serendipity to clinical relevance. *Brain Research* 2000; **886(1-2)**: 172–189.
28 Clauw DJ, Chrousos GP. Chronic pain and fatigue syndromes: overlapping clinical and neuroendocrine features and potential pathogenic mechanisms. *Neuroimmunomodulation* 1997; **4(3)**: 134–153.
29 Wall PD. The gate control theory of pain mechanisms. A re-examination and re-statement. *Brain* 1978; **101(1)**: 1–18.

3. Endogenous Opioid System: A Novel Method to Assess Healthy Volunteers

M. Bhattacharjee, R. Bhatia, N. Gupta* and R. Mathur

Department of Physiology, *Department of Endocrinology,
All India Institute of Medical Sciences, New Delhi-110029, India

Abstract. The endogenous opioid system significantly modulates pain perception. It is hypothesized to be aberrant in abnormal pain perception. The aberration may play a causal role in certain chronic pain syndromes. Hence, its evaluation is pertinent in understanding and management of these pain syndromes. A neuro endocrine approach (naloxone challenge test) has been introduced for its evaluation. However, the sensitivity of this method to detect subtle changes in endogenous opioid levels is not known. Besides, it is also not reported whether it can be manipulated in health. In the present study the endogenous opioid tone was assessed using this test following sucrose (a palatable substance) ingestion in healthy volunteers. Our results indicate that the fine changes in this neuro endocrine axis induced by sucrose ingestion could be detected by the naloxone challenge test. This test so far has been applied in chronic pain syndromes. We suggest that it has a wider application—both as a diagnostic and research tool.

Introduction

The endogenous opioids significantly contribute towards pain modulation [1]. Recently, it has been extensively reviewed and its role in descending control of pain has been identified [2, 3]. Pain modulation is a dynamic process which involves continuous interaction between complex ascending and descending systems [4]. The pain impulses are modulated at the level of the dorsal horn [5, 6]. Modulation of the descending inhibitory system largely depends on opioids. This mechanism has a wide implication since it can be manipulated clinically to alleviate suffering. It is, therefore, pertinent to evaluate the endogenous opioid system in vivo. The system can be evaluated directly by estimating either plasma or cerebrospinal fluid (CSF) concentration of β-endorphins although the relationship between plasma, CSF and pituitary compartments is not clear [7]. The former may or may not truly reflect endogenous opioid system (EOS), as the plasma concentrations do not truly correlate with the central nervous system activity. Moreover, the temporal and metabolic factors corrupt the concentration [8]. While CSF withdrawal per se is an invasive procedure, it cannot be repeated frequently and is not acceptable to many patients. Therefore, there is a need for an indirect, simpler albeit reliable technique to assess EOS. Any aberration in the EOS activity may significantly contribute towards deviation in the nociceptive behaviour such as chronic pain in syndrome X [9], slipped disc [10] and headache [11].

Recently, neuroendocrine approach to evaluate the EOS activity has been proposed by Fedele et al. [9]. This is based on the reports that the endogenous opioids exert a tonic inhibition on the gonadotropin releasing hormone (GnRH) neurons in the hypothalamus [12]. Withdrawal of this inhibition by an opioid antagonist (naloxone) is accompanied by a release of luteinizing hormone releasing hormone (LH-RH) mediated luteinizing hormone (LH) release into the plasma [13]. The LH release is proportional to the tonic inhibition exerted by central endogenous opioid, which is unmasked by the naloxone challenge test. It has been applied in some chronic pain syndromes, namely, chronic headache [11] and chest pain in syndrome X [9]. Primary headache patients with characteristically different temporal patterns (episodic or chronic) and severity were subjected to naloxone challenge test. The endogenous opiate activity was blunted in patients with severe pain, namely, common migraine and migraine with interparoxysmal headache. Therefore, opioid deficiency could have a causal role in development or aggravation of the headache syndromes. Similarly, the pattern of LH concentration post-naloxone injection is reported to be different for the chest pain due to coronary insufficiency or syndrome X.

Therefore, the tone of the EOS in cases of chronic pain can be utilised to differentiate as well as manage various pain syndromes. However, these conditions are associated with a long-term derangement of the EOS. Whether or not this technique is valid and sensitive in healthy individuals to non-noxious stimuli is not known. An aberrant response to non-noxious stimuli may possibly be in pari passu with that of noxious stimuli. The system may be insensitive or hypersensitive thereby significantly contributing towards chronic disturbances in perception of pain. It may then assist in typing the individuals. Besides, it will be of interest to determine EOS modulating factors. The endogenous opioids are reportedly modulated by a number of factors including diet, ovulation and cold water swim [14-16]. Acute changes in the opioid levels can be induced experimentally by ingestion of palatable food such as sucrose [14].

Incidentally, sucrose ingestion is known to produce analgesia both in animals [17-19] and humans [20-23]. Several researchers have reported that sucrose induced analgesia is opioid peptide mediated activation of descending inhibitory system triggered by the "palatable" information in ventromedial hypothalamic nucleus [14, 17, 19, 23]. The sucrose ingestion leads to a feeling of pleasure, and reduces pain via release of opioids. It, therefore, alleviates stress, including stress-induced analgesia. Sucrose induced analgesia is a pre-absorptive phenomenon as intra-gastric administration of sucrose fails to produce analgesia [24].

Therefore, in this study oral sucrose was used as a trigger to activate opioid peptide from the ventromedial hypothalamus (VMH), induce analgesia behaviourally while concomitantly inhibiting the LH secretion. Simultaneous with these happening, the antiopioid (naloxone) was injected intravenously which disinhibited the opioid action on LH release, thereby stimulating its secretion. Temporal effects of these two opposing manipulations were tested. It was hypothesized that if the abovementioned antagonistic interventions, introduced at strategic time intervals are reflected in LH secretion, the system is very sensitive, quick, finely regulated and liable to manipulations. On the contrary if it did not reflect, the neuro endocrine circuitry is hard-wired.

Sucrose has been studied for its analgesic efficacy by several authors in both animals [19] and humans [23]. However, in humans most of the studies have been conducted in infants and only a few studies have reported sucrose induced analgesia (SIA) in children and adults [25, 26]. Therefore, the fine regulation of opioid modulated LH secretion by sucrose ingestion was explored in normal adult volunteers.

Materials and Methods

Twelve male volunteers (age 19-40 years) were enrolled into the study. They were divided randomly into control and sucrose-fed groups. The sucrose-fed group received a 25% sucrose solution to drink whereas the controls received tap water. All volunteers were subjected to the naloxone challenge test wherein serial blood samples were collected. The volunteers suffering from either a chronic pain condition or were on analgesic, morphinomimetics and hormonal therapy or having a history of allergy to drugs were excluded from the study. The Institutional Ethical Committee for human studies approved the protocol.

Experimental Design

The subjects were asked to report to the laboratory at 08:30 h after an overnight fast. An informed consent was obtained. The blood pressure of the subject was recorded. An intravenous cannula was placed in the antecubital vein under aseptic conditions. Ten samples of blood (2 ml each) were withdrawn at 15 min interval. After withdrawal of the third sample (basal) the subject received either a freshly prepared sucrose solution (25%, 100 ml) or tap water (control group) to drink. The volunteers remained in the laboratory till the collection of the last (10th) blood sample. Naloxone (4 mg, Samarth Pharma Pvt. Ltd., Mumbai, India) was injected intravenously slowly 14 min post-drink. Serum was separated and the samples were stored at 20°C, for estimation of plasma LH concentration by radioimmunometric method utilizing LH estimation kit (Medicorp, Canada). The inter- and intra-assay variation for the procedure was < 5%.

Results

Effect of Sucrose Ingestion on LH Response of Naloxone Challenge Test

Control group : The mean basal LH level in the blood was 3.27 ± 0.96U/L. After 30 min of naloxone injection the plasma LH concentration increased (Table 1, Fig. 1). The peak concentration (6.61 ± 2.27 U/L) was attained at 60 min post naloxone injection. The increase in the plasma LH concentration as a function of time after naloxone injection was highly significant ($P < 0.000$). After attaining the maximal concentration, the LH concentration gradually decreased to basal values at 120 min post-naloxone injection.

Table 1   LH levels (mean ± SD U/L) in volunteers of both the control and sucrose fed groups.

Time (min)	Control	Sucrose fed
0	3.51 ±2.27	3.28 ± 1.09
15	3.43 ± 2.38	3.60 ± 1.36
30	2.93 ± 2.15	3.20 ± 1.33
45	Naloxone injection	Naloxone injection
60	3.55 ± 1.86	5.67 ± 4.06
75	6.16 ± 2.17	7.88 ± 6.65
90	6.61 ± 2.27	6.81 ± 4.23
105	5.78 ± 1.35	7.15 ±4.65
120	5.15 ± 1.36	4.40 ± 1.92
135	5.25 ± 1.18	4.51 ± 2.62
150	3.73 ± 0.88	4.78 ± 2.86

A univariate and multivariate repeated measure analysis was done to analyse the changes in LH levels over a period of time. The increase in LH concentration as compared to the pre-naloxone level is statistically highly significant as a function of time post-naloxone in both the groups. $P<0.000$ and 0.005 in control and sucrose fed groups of volunteers, respectively.

Sucrose fed group: The basal LH level in the blood was 3.36 ± 1.25 U/L. After 30 min of naloxone injection, the LH level increased (Table 1, Fig. 1). The peak level (7.88 ± 6.65 U/L) was attained at 45 min post-naloxone injection. The increase in the LH concentration as a function of time after naloxone injection was highly significant ($P < 0.005$). The LH concentration gradually decreased, although they were higher than the basal values at 120 min post-naloxone injection.

Discussion

The objective of this study was to evaluate the opioidergic status of an individual using a neuro endocrine technique. This method had so far been

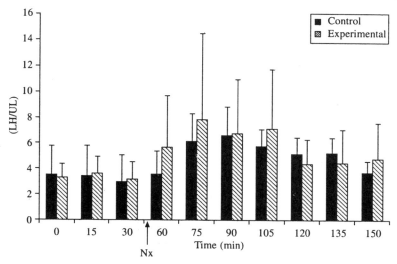

Fig. 1. Concentrations of luteinizing hormone (mean ± SD) pre- and post-naloxone injection in control and sucrose fed volunteers.

utilized in chronic pain conditions wherein a long-term derangement of the EOS is expected. In the present study, a novel paradigm was designed to assess whether this neuro endocrine approach can detect acute changes in opioid levels. The naloxone challenge test was done following sucrose ingestion in healthy adults. Sucrose induced analgesia is mediated via an opioidergic mechanism; hence any changes in opioid levels following sucrose ingestion should be detected by the naloxone challenge test thereby reflecting its sensitivity.

Assessment of EOS Status by Naloxone Challenge Test
Early studies have demonstrated that morphine can inhibit LH secretion. These observations suggested that the endogenous opioid peptides might regulate LH-RH secretion. On the other hand, naloxone, an opioid antagonist, stimulates LH release. Naloxone appears to act by increasing the frequency of LH-RH secretion [13]. This action is most marked in the late luteal and follicular phases of the menstrual cycle. The amplitude of LH release is small when LH-RH pulse frequency is high and vice-versa. Naloxone is ineffective in increasing LH levels in post-menopausal women [27].

Assessment of EOS Status by Naloxone Challenge Test in Sucrose-fed Volunteers
The LH levels increased immediately after ingestion of sucrose in the volunteers. The study was specially designed to evaluate the sensitivity of the test. Sucrose solution was given to the volunteers immediately after collection of the 3rd sample. Volunteers were exposed to a naloxone challenge 14 min after ingestion of sucrose. The design of the study was chosen for

two reasons. First, if naloxone was injected immediately after ingestion of sucrose it would have interfered with the sucrose induced analgesic mechanism both by its central and peripheral actions [17]. Secondly, it would have also interfered with the release of β-endorphins from the hypothalamus. Therefore, an interval of 14 min was chosen because a highly significant analgesic effect of sucrose persists upto 20 to 30 min [28]. Therefore, once the peak analgesic effect of sucrose was attained, a systemic naloxone injection was planned so that the β-endorphin release is inhibited, thereby, a sequential stimulation and inhibition of opioid peptide secretion was achieved. Besides, the data also can be interpreted in support of the hypothesis of opioidergic involvement in sucrose-induced analgesia. In our volunteers, there was no statistically significant difference in the peak values of control and sucrose fed groups, since sucrose facilitates the β-endorphin secretion, the naloxone is inhibitory. However, because of the temporal differences in these interventions there are subtle differences in the LH levels between the control and the experimental group of subjects. This is of greater interest to us. The probable effect of sucrose alone on the LH levels is shown in Fig. 2. Sucrose by way of enhancing the EOS facilitates further inhibition of the LH-RH neurons, which decreases the LH levels. However, this predicted fall in the LH levels could not be detected by our study paradigm since we did not collect a blood sample 15 min post-sucrose ingestion. In fact those values would have been more informative. Presuming that the predicted effect of sucrose on the LH levels did occur, let us further discuss the effect of naloxone on LH levels in these studies (Fig. 2). Naloxone injection was given 14 min after sucrose ingestion. By this time, the predicted fall in the LH levels could have possibly stimulated LH-RH release by a negative feedback loop. But

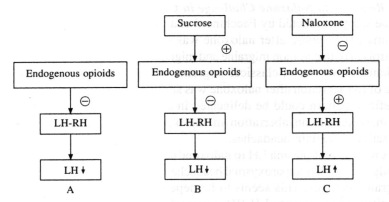

Fig. 2.   Principle of naloxone challenge test. Panel A depicts role of opioids in the secretion of LH. Opioid peptide tonicaly inhibit GnRH neurons in the hypothalamus which attenuates LH concentration in the plasma. Panel B depicts the possible sucrose mediated changes in plasma LH concentration. Sucrose ingestion potentiates the effect of opioids as sucrose ingestion acts through opioid secretion. Panel C shows the effect of naloxone, an antiopioid substance.

contrary to this, the facilitatory effect of sucrose on opioids is challenged by the antiopioid injection (naloxone). Thereby the opioid inhibition is removed by the naloxone, which may enhance the stimulatory signal for LH-RH release, ultimately leading to an increase in the LH levels. This may be the underlying mechanism for an observed greater increase in the LH levels of the experimental group of volunteers. It is, therefore, obvious that the differences between the groups were not statistically significant. Therefore, it appears that sucrose has possibly influenced the LH levels by acting upon the opioid-LHRH-LH axis. It was felt that it is crucial to collect frequent blood samples.

The study, in addition to revealing sucrose-induced analgesia in human adults, also indicates towards an involvement of opioids for the same. At the same time the neuroendocrine naloxone challenge test seems to be a highly sensitive and reliable method to detect endogenous opioid tone because it truly reflects both long term [9, 11] and acute changes in opioid levels. Since the effect of opioids on LH-RH is a tonic one, this test truly reflects the EOS status of an individual.

Assessment of EOS by Naloxone Challenge Test in Chronic Pain Conditions

In the literature, similar tests have been conducted to detect dysfunction in the endogenous opioid system in some chronic pain conditions [11], or abnormal pain perception as in syndrome X [29]. These studies have yielded promising results in evaluating central opiate activity in primary headache disorders too [11]. Although the method is indirect, it is efficient for assessment of EOS in vivo as suggested by our study.

LH Response to Naloxone Challenge in Chronic Headache Syndromes

In the study conducted by Facchinetti et al. [11] the areas under the curve of plasma LH response after naloxone was significantly lower with respect to controls in both common migraine and migraine with interparoxysmal headache patients. However, in classical migraine and cluster headache patients the area of LH secretion after naloxone was similar to that of controls. Therefore, a definite pattern could be delineated in different headache patients. Based on these results an aberration in the opiate activity is implicated in the causation of certain headaches.

A response of plasma LH to naloxone challenge was lacking in two-thirds of migraine with interparoxysmal headache sufferers and in half of the common migraine patients. This seems to be dependent on the hypothalamus, since the pituitary response to LH-RH is normally maintained in the same patients. Interparoxysmal headache and a subgroup of common migraine patients have impaired secretion of β-endorphins into CSF [30, 31]. Whereas almost every patient of classical migraine displayed a normal response of plasma LH to naloxone suggesting a well functioning opioid system, which is further supported by a normal concentration of CSF β-endorphins. Cluster headache patients also showed a normal response to naloxone and they also have a normal or even slightly elevated plasma β-endorphin levels [32-34] while their met-enkephalin levels in CSF are pathologically decreased [33, 35]. To sum up, it appears that the naloxone response is impaired in those subgroups of patients showing a specific reduction of their CSF β-endorphin levels. It is worth noting that this response does not depend on the temporal pattern of head pain, which was episodic in the case of common migraine and classical migraine and chronic in the case of interparoxysmal headache and cluster headache. However, within migraine syndromes, the lower percentage of responders to the naloxone challenge test (33.3 < 54.5 < 77.8) was found in the groups with the most severe forms of head pain (interparoxysmal headache > common migraine > classical migraine) [11].

LH Response to Naloxone in Patients with Abnormal Chest Pain Perception

Fedele et al. [9] used the naloxone challenge test to evaluate the opioidergic system in long lasting chest pain of syndrome X patients. Syndrome X patients have normal coronary angiogram although ST segment depression and angina (more pain than coronary artery disease patients) on exercise testing are noted. A significantly lower LH response was found in syndrome X patients as compared to coronary artery disease patients and controls. This suggests a lower central opiate activity in syndrome X, which may be related to their higher anginal pain perception. Further, these patients are hypersensitive (chest pain) to catheter manipulations or electrical stimulation during right heart catheterization and to endogenously produced adenosine [36].

It is suggested that there are trigger mechanisms in these patients other than ischemia such as ectopic beats, changes in heart rate or minor reductions in myocardial blood flow that may lead to the release of algogenic mediators [37]. This finding has been interpreted as indicative of hypersensitive cardiac afferents. After naloxone injection, integral LH increase was lower in patients with syndrome X than in patients with coronary artery disease. Such a result supports the hypothesis that the EOS plays a role in anginal pain perception. The ST segment changes may be possibly because of microvascular dysfunction [38, 39]. A simultaneous analysis of the pain perception and the presence of ischemic marker during the same provocative maximal stress tests were done. Patients with syndrome X showed no difference in ECG modification compared with patients with coronary artery disease but did show an increased pain perception, a low response to naloxone challenge and the minor echocardiographic ischemic changes.

It appears that naloxone challenge test is a sensitive test for evaluation of the status of endogenous opioid system. The endogenous opioid system responds quickly and significantly to the modulators. It can, therefore, be utilised to type apparently healthy individuals and explain certain poorly understood pain syndromes besides serving as a tool for research on opioids.

Acknowledgement

The Institute Research Grant 2002-2003 supported this research. We thank Mrs. Mamta Sharma, Ms. Nidhi Mathur for secretarial assistance and Mr. Sadhu Ram, Mr. Karam Chand and Mr. Sanjeev for technical assistance.

References

1. Akil, H., Watson, S.J., Young, E., Lewis M.E., Khachaturian, H., Walker, J.M., Endogenous opioids : Biology and Function. *Ann. Rev. Neurosci.* 1984; **7**: 223–55.
2. Millan, M.J., Desending control of pain. *Progress in Neurobiology*, 2002; **66**: 355–474.
3. Narita, M. Tseng, L.F. Evidence for the existence of the β-endorphin-sensitive "ε-opioid receptor" in the brain : The Mechanisms of ε-mediated Antinociception. *Jpn. J. Pharmacology*, 1998; **76**: 233–253.
4. Melzack, R., Dennis, S.G. Neuro physiological foundation of pain. In: Psychology of pain (ed. Sternback RP.) pp 1–26, Raven Press, New York, 1978.
5. Besson, J.M. and Chaouch, A. Peripheral and spinal mechanism of nociception. *Physiol. Rev.* 1987; **67**: 67–186.
6. Boess, F.G. and Martin I.L. Molecular Biology of 5 H-T Receptors. *Neuropharmacology* 1994; **33**: 275–317.
7. Pert, A. Mechanism of opiate analgesia and role of β-endorphins in pain suppression. In : M. Critchley et al (Eds.), Advances in Neurology, Vol. 33, Raven Press, New York 1982; 107–122.
8. Oliver, C., Micol, R.S., Porter, R.S. and Porter, J.C. Hypothalamic pituitary vasculature. Evidence for retrograde flow in the pituitary stalk. *Endocrinology*, 1977; **101**: 598–602.
9. Fedele, F., Agati, L., Pugliese, M., Cervellini, P., Benedetti, G., Magni, G. and Vitarelli, A. Role of the central endogenous opiate system in patients with syndrome X. *Am. Heart J.* 1998; **136**: 1003–9.
10. Cleeland, C., Sacham, S., Dahl, J.L. and Orrison, W. CSF β-endorphin and the severity of pain. *Neurology* , 1984; **34**: 378–380.
11. Facchinetti, F., Martignoni, E., Gallai, V., Micielli, G., Petraglia, F., Nappi, G. and Gennazani, A.R. Neuroendocrine evaluation of central opiate activity in primary headache disorders. *Pain* 1988; **34**: 29–33.
12. Grossman, A., Moult, P.J.A. and Gaillard, R.C. et al. The opioid control of LH and FSH release : Effects of a met-enkephalin analogue and naloxone. *Clin. Endocrinology* 1981; **14**: 41–47.
13. Quigley, M.E. and Yen, S.S.C. The role endogenous opiates on LH secretion during the menstrual cycle. *J. Clin. Endocrinol Metab.* 1980; **51**: 179–181.
14. Dum, J., Gramsch, C. and Herz, A. Activation of hypothalamic β-endorphin pools by reward induced by highly palatable foods. *Pharmacol. Biochem. Behav.* 1983; **18**: 443–447.
15. Saad, E.A., Bromham, D.R., Bhabra, K. and Ambrose, C.L. Peripheral plasma met-enkephalin levels in ovulatory and anovulatory human menstrual cycles. *Fertility and Sterility* 1992; **58**: 307–313.

16. The pharmacology of opioid peptides. Edited by Leon, F. Tseng. Medical College of Wisconsin, Wisconsin, USA, Harwood Academic Publishers, 1995; p. 288.

17. Blass, E.M., Fitzgerald, E., Kehoe, P. Interaction between sucrose, pain and isolation distress. *Pharmacol, Biochem. Behav.* 1987; **26**: 483–489.

18. D. Anci, KE, Kanarek, R.B. and Kaufman, R.M. Duration of sucrose availability differentially alters morphine induced analgesia in rats. *Pharmacol. Biochem. and Behav.* 1996; **54**: 693–697.

19. Dutta, R., Mookherjee, K., Mathur, R., Effect of VMH lesion on sucrose fed analgesia in formalin pain. *Jpn. J. of Physiol.* 2001; **51**; (1) 63–69.

20. Blass, E.M., Lisa, B., Hoffmeyer, M.A. Sucrose as an analgesic for newborn infants. *Paediatrics* 1991; **87**: 215–218.

21. Ramenghi, L.A., Griffith, C.G., Wood, C.M. and Levene, M.I. Effect of non-sucrose sweet tasting solution on neonatal heel prick responses. *Arch Dis Childhood*, 1996; **74**: 129–131.

22. Stevens, B., Taddio, A., Ohlsson, A. and Einarson, T. The efficacy of sucrose for relieving procedural pain in neonates-A systematic review and metanalysis. *Acta Paediatrics*, 1997; **86**: 837–842.

23. Haourari, N., Christophar, W., Gillian, G. and Malcolm, C. The analgesic effects of sucrose in full term infants : a randomised control trial. *Bri. Med. J,* 1995; **310**: 1498–1500.

24. Ramenghi, L.A., Evans, D.J. and Levene, M.I. "Sucrose analgesia" : Absorptive mechanisms or taste perception? *Arch. Dis Child Fetal.* Neonatal edition 1999; **80**: 146–147.

25. Miller, A., Barr, R.G. and Young, S.N. The cold pressor test in children : methodological aspects and the analgesic effect of intraoral sucrose. *Pain* 1994; 56 L 175–183.

26. Mercer, E.M. and Holder, M.D. Antinociceptive effects of palatable sweet ingesta on human responsivity to pressure pain. *Physiol. Behaviour* 1997; 61, No. **2**: 311–318.

27. Reid, R.C., Quigley, M.E. and Yen, S.S.C. The disappearance of opioidergic regulation of gonadotropin secretion in post-menopausal women. *J. Clin. Endocrinol Metab* 1983; **57**: 1107–1110.

28. Taddio, A. Pain management for neo-natal circumcision. *Pediatric Drug,* 2001; **3** (2): 101–11.

29. Fedele, F., Vizza, C.D., Benedetti, G., Dagianti, A.I., Penco, M. and Agati, L. et al. A endogenous opioid system modulation in anginal pain : demonstration of its central activity. *Am Heart J* 1992; **124**: 589–595.

30. Genazzani, A.R., Nappi, G., Facchinetti, F., Micieli, G., Petraglia, F., Bono, G., Monittola, C. and Savoldi, F. Progressive impairment of CSF β-endorphins levels in migraine sufferers. *Pain* 1984; **18**:127–133.

31. Nappi, G., Facchinetti, F., Bono, G., Petraglia, F., Micieli, G., Volpe, A. and Genazzani, A.R. Failure of central opioid tonus in migraine : modulation of steroid milieu. In : Clifford Rose (Ed.), Migraine, Karger, Basel, 1985: 72–78.

32 Appenzeller, O., Atkinson, R.A., Standefer, J.C. Serum β-endorphin in cluster headache and common migraine. In: Clifford Rose and Zilkha (eds.) Vol. 1, Pitman, London 1981; 106–109.

33. Hardebo, J.E., Ekman, M., Eriksson, M., Holgersson, S. and Ryberg, B. CSF opioid levels in cluster headache. In : Clifford Rose (Ed.), Migraine, Karger, Basel, 1985: 79–85.

34. Nappi, G., Facchinetti, F., Martignoni, E., Petraglia, F., Bono, G., Micieli, G., Rosaschino, C., Manzoni, G.C. and Genazzani, A.R. Plasma and CSF endorphin levels in primary and symptomatic headaches. *Headache,* 1985; **25**: 141–144.

35. Anselmi, B., Baldi, E., Casacci, F. and Salmon, S. Endogenous opioids in cerebrospinal fluid and blood in idiopathic headache sufferers. *Headache* 1980; **20**: 249–299.

36. Shapiro, L.M., Crake, T. and Poole-Wilson, P.A. Is altered cardiac sensation responsible for chest pain in patients with normal coronary arteries? Clinical observation during catheterization. *Bri. Med. J.*, 1988; **296**: 170–171.

37. Cannon, R.O., Quyyumi, A.A., Schenki, W.H. et al. Abnormal cardiac sensitivity in patients with chest pain and normal coronary arteries. *J. Am Coll Cardiol* 1990; **16**: 1359–1366.

38. Maseri, A., Crea, F. and Cianflone, D. Myocardial ischemia caused by distal coronary vasoconstriction. *Am J Cardiol*, 1992; **70**: 1602–1605.

39. Asbury, E.A. and Collins, P. Cardiac syndrome X. *Int. J. Clin. Pract*, 2005; **59**: 1063–1069.

4. Pain Assessment: Patient Diagnosis, Role of Functional and Behavioral Evaluations, Measuring Pain and Understanding Treatment Outcomes

Manjari Tripathi

Department of Neurology, All India Institute of Medical Sciences,
New Delhi-110029, India

Introduction

For every clinical trial there are two primary statistics, viz. an estimate of the difference that is found between the treatment and comparison groups, which is known as the effect size, and the statistical test for the probability of finding an association by chance alone, i.e. statistical significance. While it is necessary that a trial result be statistically significant, it is not sufficient to make the outcome of a trial useful or of any benefit to patient care. Much more important is the clinical importance of the effect size which is the only indication of whether or not the study treatment works well.

In addition, it is a mathematical truism that the statistical significance is primarily a matter of sample size. Specifically, the sample size required for a given clinical trial is determined by the power of the study to detect that difference (beta: usually set arbitrarily to 80 or 90%), the percentage risk of getting the wrong answer (alpha: set arbitrarily by convention at 5%, i.e. $p < 0.05$), the level of variability that is observed or expected in the general population to be studied (the normal variance of the measured outcome without any treatment), and the size of the difference that the investigator wants to detect. Therefore, even very small effects, that are larger than the normal population variance, can be demonstrated to be statistically significant at $p < 0.05$ value if the sample size is large enough.

As an example, consider the following report which was presented at the national meeting of the American Association for the Study of Headache [1]. "The multicenter trial, known as ZOMCO, involved 1,455 patients from 61 research centers. A total of 6,187 migraine attacks were treated with ZOMIG (TM-Zeneca Pharmaceuticals-zolmitriptan) and sumatriptan. The percentage of patients responding at 2 h post-dose significantly favored ZOMIG 2.5 mg against sumatriptan 25.0 mg ($p < 0.001$) and 50 mg ($p = 0.017$), (67.1%

agains 59.6% and 63.8%, respectively, percentages obtained from raw data) and the statistical difference over sumatriptan 50.0 mg was maintained at 4 h (84% vs 81% with pain relief $p = 0.039$)". The author then concluded that "the data presented show that there was a statistically significant difference between treatment groups, favoring ZOMIG 2.5-mg tablets versus both sumatriptan 25.0 mg and 50.0 mg" [1]. Note that the difference in the effect between equivalent doses of the two drugs (i.e. 2.5 mg of zolmitriptan and 50 mg of sumatriptan) is only 3% at both 2 and 4 h. It took almost 1500 patients to reach statistical significance. However, it is hard to attribute any clinical importance to a 3% difference in the response rates for migraine headache pain.

Issues in the Determination of a Clinically Important Difference

What is much harder to determine is what constitutes a real clinically important difference (CID). Some clear outcomes are survival, death, hospitalization, use of a particular drug, etc. However, in general, many outcomes are on a continuum with no obvious cut-off point. Establishing a fixed cut-off is difficult because there is no distinct difference between 29%, 30% and 31%. However, attributing a clinical importance to a specific level of change in the central tendency (mean, median, or mode) is equally difficult, if not harder for the reasons outlined above. Therefore, it is useful to examine the methods that have been utilized in an effort to establish a clinically important difference. Factors involved in this decision include:

- (a) severity of the disease process (self limited to fatal).
- (b) effect we hope to achieve with treatment (amelioration of symptoms to cure).
- (c) potential side-effects (none to severe).
- (d) tools utilized for assessment of outcome of the trial.
- (e) whose opinion is important (patient, family, care giver or society).
- (f) what clinical or scientific question are we trying to answer.

In considering what constitutes a clinically important outcome for clinical trials of pain therapies, we must take into consideration that pain is a symptom, which can be severely distressing to the patient, but is not by itself a fatal process. Although a ubiquitous phenomenon, pain is inherently subjective and pain measures, no matter how quantitative they may appear, reflect the subjective response of the patient. Our goal in treating pain is to ameliorate or stop the symptom, while trying to avoid the substantial side-effects, albeit occasional.

A better understanding of the interaction between central and peripheral nervous systems has led us to the conclusion that the nociceptive input from the nerve endings (somatic pain) or damaged nervous system (neuropathic pain) are not the sole determinants of the pain experience. Rather the perception of the level of pain by the individual is influenced by a number of other cognitive processes including their affective state, previous experience, level of expectation and coping ability. Besides these factors, the patients report about their perception of the nociceptive experience often varies with the duration of pain condition especially chronic pain. The extended nociceptive input in chronic pain often leads to a more complex interaction between these 'other factors' [2]. However, in both cases the external manifestation of the pain response will vary from individual to individual, making it difficult for external observers to accurately assess the patients experience. This is borne out by a number of studies that have demonstrated that external observers do not truly reflect the report of pain level by the patient himself [3]. Measures of function are sometimes applicable, and potentially more objective, but are also influenced by many of the same central nervous system factors as well. As such, the only person who can provide information about the level of pain and/or suffering is the patient. Therefore, it is only the patient who can be the final arbitrator of how well or how poor a particular therapy is for him.

All of these potential problems have made it very difficult for clinicians and pain researchers to decide the optimum level of pain relief. In the realm of clinical care, the usual procedure is to ask the patient about the patient's own assessment of pain relief and improvement with the prescribed treatment. As long as the caregiver is willing to believe the answer, it is a good method of determining the effectiveness of a treatment. However, if the patient's subjective complaints do not fit with a known scientific medical model or are otherwise poorly understood (i.e. a clear etiology leading to a clear disease state), then the observing care giver may become uncomfortable with the purely subjective report of the patient. Thus, it is not uncommon to revert to judging improvement on the basis of the patient's ability to perform the basic functions of day-to-day life, including activities of daily living, the ability to move and get around, the ability to interact with others in a normal fashion, and ultimately the ability to be a productive member of society. These are the major components of the current concept of a general measure of quality of life, which is again highly individualistic and subjective [4].

While selecting the outcomes for a clinical trial, its important determination of benefit must be standardized in such a way that the collection of data is not biased by the observer. A variety of pain measurement scales have been developed over the years in an attempt to minimize this bias. Such scales usually result in a numeric score [5-8]. One convention is to measure the level of pain intensity reported by the subject before and after the treatment. In addition it is common to measure the level of pain relief vis-à-vis the level of benefit or global performance the subject ascribes to the pain therapy being tested. Often additional factors such as level of function, degree of depression and more recently an assessment of the subjects quality of life have also been assessed to further investigate the factors that are affected by the treatment of interest [9].

Since the data collected often appears to be normal or can be transformed to a normal distribution, a common method of analyzing the pain data is to determine the central tendency (namely, mean, median or mode) as a summary statistic for the group along with the corresponding probability statistic. The most common statistical test is the Student's-*t* (or the more general Z statistic) or a regression variation of this test, which determines the probability that the difference found in the central tendency between two groups could have occurred by chance more often than in one out of 20 clinical trials (i.e. $p < 0.05$). If the differences in the central tendency are large then the clinical importance may be obvious, but with smaller changes it has been difficult to determine what should be considered clinically important. This has to do in part with the ambiguous nature of the central tendency statistic, especially when the result is applied to an individual patient in a clinical setting. Instead the key clinical question is "What is the probability that a treatment will be of sufficient benefit to the patient to warrant the risk of side effects or toxicity?" However, what happens to a group on average does not adequately answer this clinical question. For example, consider a clinical trial in which the mean value for the change in pain intensity from baseline to after treatment is an improvement of 10% in the treatment group compared to the placebo group. Assuming that there was no change in the placebo group, the same result would be observed (except for the confidence interval) if (a) every patient in the treatment group improved by 10%, or (b) if 50% of the treatment group got better by 20 and 50% had no improvement, or (c) if 50% of the treatment group got better by 40 and 50% got worse by 20%. Thus the difference in means between the groups provides an ambiguous answer to the most relevant clinical question. These different situations could lead to strikingly different clinical decisions, since a 10% improvement might not be sufficiently important to consider trying a new medication (especially if it has risks or side effects), whereas if 50% of the patients would get substantially better, even though 50% might get moderately worse, the medication would be worth trying, provided the worsening was not permanent. Any unresponsive patient could then be switched to an alternative therapy. A more clinically relevant way to express these data would be as a comparison of the proportion of patients who improved by a clinically important amount.

A second reason why a central tendency analysis may not be aｰ ｊropriate for pain intensity data is that there are many instances when the population represents a mixture of potential responders and non-responders, such that the central tendency is an inappropriate summary value. There are a number of medications, which are effective in some patients and not in others due to genetic or environmental factors such as differences in absorption (e.g. gabapentin), metabolism (e.g. amitriptyline), or a multitude of other factors. If there are adequate criteria to separate the groups prior to enrollment in the clinical trial, the trial should be conducted only in the group of potential responders. However, given the large number of factors that can influence a specific patient's response, it is often difficult to predict the potential for response in advance. As such, the study subjects will actually be drawn from a population, which is bimodal, i.e. containing both high probability responders and low probability responders. In such situations, the analysis of the central tendency for the combined groups will not give an appropriate summary of the treatment efficacy. Examples include trials in cancer-related pain, when it is often hard to determine the type of pain which is predominant, i.e. somatic vs. visceral vs. neuropathic pain.

If only one type of pain is likely to be responsive to a particular therapy, then the population should be considered to be bimodal. In the clinical trial of gabapentin for treatment of post-herpetic neuralgia [10], only 37% of the active treatment group got moderate or better relief, but this was much better than the 15% in the placebo group. In this study, the number of patients was high enough to demonstrate a statistically significant 1.6/10 change in the mean values for the two groups as well, but greater than 2 times larger number of moderate or better improvement subjects in the treated group is a much more meaningful and useful statistic.

Other syndromes that exemplify this concept are headaches where it is difficult to be sure of the exact underlying etiology [11]. In facial neuralgia [12], anticonvulsant medications [13], and in neuropathic pain tricyclic antidepressants are effective in some patients but ineffective in others [14].

Methods to Calculate a Clinically Important Difference

It is important to acknowledge that there is wide disagreement on the choice of the best outcome measure for pain clinical trials [15-17]. If we assume that there are times when it would be important to define a cut-off point for a clinically important difference, how should this be done for pain. Measures of pain include pain intensity, pain relief, global assessment, and time to rescue. First consider the commonly used pain intensity (PI) scored on a 0-10 likert scale or 100 mm visual analogue scale (VAS). By its nature the PI-scale often produces data with a near normal distribution. However, Scott and Huskisson, one of the originators of the VAS-PI scale, has noted that the distribution of data collected on such a scale may not be normal, and that non-parametric statistical analysis, which does not assume normality, may be more appropriate [18]. To adjust for the inter-subject variability in initial pain scores, the changeover time in the PI score is usually used. Price et al. [19] carried this one step further and have recommended that the scale be considered as a ratio scale, with change represented as a percentage. This is consistent with a common form of the pain relief scale, which asks patients to rate their relief as a percentage of improvement. In addition, clinical experience suggests that patients frequently describe their improvement in pain as a percentage change. Percent change has been used as the definition of a clinically important difference outcome in a number of analgesic studies [20, 21], but using a range of values from 25 to 75% without any clear data based justification. Another interpretation of change was proposed by Serlin et al. [22] who presented data to suggest that users of the 0-10 point scale tend to interpret the regions of the scale unequally and demonstrated an association between the numbers 1-4 and 'mild' pain, 5-6 and 'moderate' pain, 7-10 and 'severe' pain and suggested that a change in category represent a possible definition of a clinically important benefit [22]. Since the various formats of the PI-scale are all closely correlated [6], it is highly possible that this is also true of other types of PI scales including the VAS-PI and 1-10 numeric rating scale (NRS).

Others have looked at the difference in patient reported pain that is perceived as real by an observer. Another example is a study in which the authors defined a minimally important clinical difference by using the patients' reports of a global improvement of a moderate degree or more as the reference standard to which they compare pain relief scores [23]. However, it is unclear how valid the overall question may be because the patients' response to a single question can be biased by the patients' sense of what the interviewer wanted to hear or what they thought the answer ought to be. In addition, the timing and order of the questions asked could affect the results [24, 25]. In their pioneering work in the use of meta-analysis to combine outcomes from smaller trials, Moore and McQuay et al. [26, 27] have pointed out the importance of a common outcome that can be combined and have pushed the concept of the number needed to treat. In their initial paper, they chose 50% as the cut-off for the %Maximum of the Total Pain Relief (%Max TOTPAR) reasoning that "it is a simple clinical endpoint of pain half relieved, easily understood by professionals and patients."

They also pointed out that this proportion is highly correlated with the mean of the continuous analysis of the %Max TOTPAR, which demonstrates consistency. While this value has been successfully applied to a number of subsequent studies, its importance to the patients to whom it has been applied has never been established. There have been several other attempts to calculate or use expert opinion to select the change necessary to claim a clinically important difference for use in clinical trials. Some outstanding work has also been carried out to develop the Outcome Measures in Rheumatology Clinical Trials [28], which make a clear distinction between a clinically important and a statistically significant difference. However, because of the nature of arthritis, this measure in another study, which evaluated the pain experienced by patients in an emergency department, a change of 18 mm/100 mm in the physician's assessment of the patient was found to correlate with the patient's assessment of being a 'little bit better' [29]. Although the authors concluded that this is the minimum level of clinical importance that should be considered in clinical trials, several studies have shown that the use of external observers to judge subjective outcomes of patients is unlikely to provide a valid measure of a patient's pain [3].

In a recent study of oral transmucosal fentanyl citrate to treat individual episodes of breakthrough pain [30], the investigators allowed subjects to use a second rescue medication, if the study medication did not work in a physiologically appropriate time frame. The patients decision to take additional medication at the time of the peak blood level was used as one of the outcomes. This measure is clearly different from the more standard time-to-next-rescue dose response, which incorporates both initial efficacy and length of effect. This combination can introduce a level of ambiguity into the analysis. In contrast, the measurement of the action (yes or no) of taking an additional dose of rescue medication is relatively objective and specific, that is does the study treatment work well enough not to require additional treatment at the time of maximal pharmacologic activity. This outcome allows the patient to integrate his or her perception of the amount of relief and any potential side effects experienced.

As such, it is likely to be a better estimate of the patients integrated assessment of the efficacy of the study medication. Although, it is only applicable to trials of rapidly acting medications for treatment of intermittent pain syndromes, it should be considered for future trials of medications that have rapid onset and potential efficacy in the treatment of breakthrough or acute pain. Other features of this study include a titration run-in period which is intended to clearly define a potentially responsive group of patients while also providing valuable information about patients who may not benefit as much from the therapy. The use of a group of 10 randomly-ordered active and placebo medications for the trial portion of the study, along with a short waiting period (30 min) before the use of additional rescue medication if needed, provides an ethical way to incorporate placebo controls into an efficacy clinical trial. Given the significant advantages of a placebo control and the clear ethical issues surrounding the administration of a placebo to sick patients, this feature is important.

The primary limitation of this definition of a clinically important difference is the issue of generalizability to other pain syndromes, especially chronic pain. The rapid onset of action of the OTFC allowed patients to make an early judgment about efficacy and the design allowed early re-medication if the dose was ineffective. However, the response to pain and its meaning in cancer patients may affect the way in which the patients respond to painful situations. For example, the use of opioid medications is more acceptable in cancer patients, so they may have made a bigger effort to treat their pain aggressively, which would result in an underestimated size of the clinically important difference. Therefore, similar studies are needed in patients with acute pain from other causes.

Since acute and chronic pains are substantially different constructs, there are concerns as to the applicability of this model to clinical trials of chronic pain and that require chronic slow onset treatments. Clearly, there are factors other than strict anti-nociceptive effects that have been shown to influence a patient's use of pain medication. While these may not vary substantially between episodes of acute pain treated with active and placebo medication, they are likely to influence the response in longer-term studies and with medications that are less effective than opioids.

Therefore, the 'use of rescue' outcome is not applicable to the evaluation of treatments that require long period of time to achieve their maximal effect. As such, methodological innovations will be necessary to develop this type of outcome for chronic pain studies.

However, because the 'use of rescue' outcome requires a definitive action, and may offer a more objective measure of the patient's perspective on what represents clinically important analgesia, this outcome represents a logical choice as a gold standard for the clinical importance of the effect (i.e. did the treatment work well enough and does NOT require supplements). Using this measure to standardize the cut-off point for the other pain scales (0-10 intensity, 0-4 pain relief and 0-4 global medication performance have provided a cut-off value that can be used as a starting point for the analysis of other studies. The values best associated with the gold standard were ≥ 33% for scales calculated as the percentage and ≥ 2 (moderate) for the relief and global performance.

Although beyond the scope of this article, a recent paper describes this analysis and the implications in greater detail [31]. The similarities to values used in other clinical trials is reassuring [14, 26, 32, 33]. In addition to providing a more clinically interpretable result, the use of a standard outcome across different pain studies will increase the potential for direct comparison of results between treatments and across different patient populations.

Conclusion

The definition of what constitutes a clinically important difference plays an important role in the interpretation of all clinical trials, including those using central tendency analyses. The determination of the proportion of subjects that obtain a clinically important improvement is most relevant to studies in which the goal is to evaluate whether or not a medication provides a clinically important effect, especially Phase III efficacy trials. At some of the earlier stages of drug development, the study objective may be to identify the presence of any analgesic effect at all, no matter how small. In such cases, it may be appropriate to use a lower cut-off point or even to consider use of the group mean or median analysis using ordinary parametric statistics. However, it is important that the investigator be aware that the question being addressed in such cases is very different from the practical clinical efficacy question.

The decision about the appropriate value for a cut-off point is often difficult and is sometimes considered arbitrary, but it is vital nonetheless in assessing treatment efficacy. When possible, using the behavior of taking or not taking an additional dose of medication is an easily measured indicator of the efficacy of a treatment for acute pain, which is clinically relevant and objectively measurable. For studies where this outcome is not possible the use of a cut-off point for other pain measurement scale that has been shown to be best associated to the 'use of rescue outcome' should be considered.

Although the choice of the measurement scale and analysis will depend on the study question and design, the use of cut-off points will also lead to a more standardized approach to the design of clinical trials for pain treatments and better validity, comparability, and clinical utility of the results of future clinical trials.

References

1. Gallagher, M.A. Multicenter, Double-Blind, Randomized Comparison of Zolmitriptan (311C90 Zomig) and Sumatriptan in the Acute Treatment of Multiple Migraine Headaches. American Association for the Study of Headache (AASH) 1998.
2. Sternbach, R.A., Pain Patients: Traits and Treatment, Academic Press, New York, 1974.
3. Grossman, S.A., Sheidler, V.R., Swedeen, K., Mucenski, J. and Piantadosi, S. Correlation of patient and caregiver ratings of cancer pain. *Journal of Pain Symptom Management*, 1991; **6**: 53–57.
4. Ware, J.E., Jr., Kosinski, M., Bayliss, M.S., McHorney, C.A., Rogers, W.H. and Raczek, A. Comparison of methods for the scoring and statistical analysis of SF-36 health profile and summary measures: summary of results from the medical outcomes study. *Medical Care*, 1995; **33**: AS264–279.
5. Choiniere, M. and Amsel, R. A visual analogue thermometer for measuring pain intensity. *Journal of Pain Symptom Management* 1996; **11**: 299–311.
6. De Conno, F., Caraceni, A., Gamba, A., Mariani, L., Abbattista, A., Brunelli, C., La Mura, A. and Ventafridda, V. Pain measurement in cancer patients: A comparison of six methods. *Pain*, 1994; **57**: 161–166.
7. Gracely, R.H., McGrath, F. and Dubner. R. Ratio scales of sensory and affective verbal pain descriptors. *Pain*, 1978; **5**: 5–18.
8. Paice, J.A. and Cohen, F.L. Validity of a verbally administered numeric rating scale to measure cancer pain intensity. *Cancer Nursing* 1997; **20**: 88–93.
9. Ahmedzai, S. Recent clinical trials of pain control: impact on quality of life. *European Journal of Cancer*, 1995; **31A**: S2–7.
10. Rowbotham, M., Harden, N., Stacey, B., Bernstein, P. and Magnus-Miller, L. Gabapentin for the treatment of postherpetic neuralgia: A randomized controlled trial. *JAMA*, 1998; **280**: 1837–1842.
11. ter Kuile, M.M., Spinhoven, P. and Linssen, A.C. Responders and nonresponders to autogenic training and cognitive self-hypnosis: prediction of short- and long-term success in tension-type headache patients. *Headache*, 1995; **35**: 630–636.
12. Loeser, J.D. Tic douloureux and atypical facial pain. In: P.D. Wall and R. Melzack (Eds.), Textbook of Pain, Churchil Livingstone, London, 1994, 699–710.
13. McQuay, H., Carroll, D., Jadad, A.R., Wiffen, P. and Moore, A. Anticonvulsant drugs for management of pain: a systematic review. *BMJ*, 1995; **311**: 1047–1052.
14. Max, M.B., Lynch, S.A., Muir, J., Shoaf, S.E., Smoller, B. and Dubner, R. Effects of desipramine, amitriptyline and fluoxetine on pain in diabetic neuropathy. *New England Journal of Medicine*, 1992; **326**: 1250–1256.
15. Houde, R.W. Methods for measuring clinical pain in humans. *Acta Anaesthesiologica Scandinavica*. Supplementum 1982; **74**: 25–29.

16. LeResche, L. Assessment of physical and behavioral outcomes of treatment. *Oral Surgery Oral Medicine Pathology Radiology Endodontics*, 1997; **83**: 82–86.
17. Max, M.B. and Portenoy, R.K. Methodological Challenges for Clinical Trials of Cancer Pain Treatments. In: C.R. Chapman and K.M. Foley (Eds.), Current and Emerging Issues in Cancer Pain: Research and Practice, Raven Press, New York, 1993, pp. 283–299.
18. Scott, J. and Huskisson, E.C. Graphic representation of pain. *Pain*, 1976; **2**: 175–184.
19. Price, D.D., McGrath, P.A., Rafii, A. and Buckingham, B. The validation of visual analogue scales as ratio scale measures for chronic and experimental pain. *Pain*, 1983; **17**: 45–56.
20. Goldsmith, C.H., Boers, M., Bombardier, C. and Tugwell, P. Criteria for clinically important changes in outcomes: development, scoring and evaluation of rheumatoid arthritis patient and trial profiles. OMERACT Committee. *Journal of Rheumatology*, 1993; **20**: 561–565.
21. Max, M.B. Antidepressants as analgesics, Pharmacological Approaches to the Treatment of Chronic Pain. The Fourth Annual Bristol-Meyers Squibb Symposium on Pain Research, Seattle, 1994.
22. Serlin, R.C., Mendoza, T.R., Nakamura, Y., Edwards, K.R. and Cleeland, C.S. When is cancer pain mild, moderate or severe? Grading pain severity by its interference with function. *Pain*, 1995; **61**: 277–284.
23. Juniper, E.F., Guyatt, G.H., Willan, A. and Griffith, L.E. Determining a minimal important change in a disease-specific quality of life questionnaire. *Journal of Clinical Epidemiology*, 1994; **47**: 81–87.
24. Grootendorst, P.V., Feeny, D.H. and Furlong, W. Does it matter whom and how you ask? Inter- and intra-rater agreement in the Ontario Health Survey. *Journal of Clinical Epidemiology*, 1997; **50**: 127–135.
25. Ware, J.E. Jr. Effects of acquiescent response set on patient satisfaction ratings. *Medical Care*, 1978; **16**: 327–336.
26. Moore, A., McQuay, H. and Gavaghan, D. Deriving dichotomous outcome measures from continuous data in RCT of analgesics. *Pain*, 1996; **66**: 229–237.
27. Moore, A., Moore, O., McQuay, H. and Gavaghan, D. Deriving dichotomous outcome measures from continuous data in randomised controlled trials of analgesics: use of pain intensity and visual analogue scales. *Pain*, 1997; **69**: 311–315.
28. Cranney, A., Welch, V., Tugwell, P., Wells, G., Adachi, J.D., McGowan, J. and Shea, B. Responsiveness of endpoints in osteoporosis clinical trials—an update. *Journal of Rheumatology*, 1999; **26**: 222–8.
29. Todd, K.H. and Funk, J.P. The minimum clinically important difference in physician-assigned visual analog pain scores. *Acad Emergency Medicine*, 1996; **3**: 142–146.
30. Farrar, J.T., Cleary, J., Rauck, R., Busch, M. and Nordbrock, E. Oral transmucosal fentanyl citrate: randomized, double-blinded, placebo-controlled trial for treatment of breakthrough pain in cancer patients. *Journal of the National Cancer Institute*, 1998; **90**: 611–616.
31. Farrar, J.T., Portenoy, R.K., Berlin, J.A., Kinman, J., Strom, B..L. Defining the Clinically Important Difference in Pain Outcome Measures. *Pain*, 2000; **88**: 287–294.
32. Leijonm, G. and Boivie, J. Central post-stroke pain—a controlled trial of amitriptyline and carbamazepine. *Pain*, 1989; **36**: 27–36.
33. Sheiner, L.B. A new approach to the analysis of analgesic drug trials, illustrated with bromfenac data. *Clinical Pharmacology & Therapeutics*, 1994; **56**: 309–322.

Pain Updated: Mechanisms and Effects
Edited by R. Mathur
Copyright © 2006 Anamaya Publishers, New Delhi, India

5. Role of Ventromedial Hypothalamus in Pain Modulation

R. Mathur[1] and Usha Nayar[2]

[1]Neurophysiology Laboratory, Department of Physiology,
All India Institute of Medical Sciences, New Delhi-110029, India

[2]Department of Physiology, College of Medicine and Medical Sciences,
The Arabian Gulf University, P.O. Box 22979, Manama, Kingdom of Bahrain

Abstract. Pain is an alerting protective symptom that is modulated by several noxious or non-noxious, endogenous or exogenous factors including previous exposure to pain itself. However, in favour of the physiological processes of the individual to continue, it is modulated. Several neural sites have been identified utilizing different animal and experimental models, parameters and noxious stimuli. Nonetheless, there is a lack of information regarding the relative status of each one of them. Therefore, we are ignorant regarding the specific role of any such neural site besides their interaction amongst themselves. The precise function of ventromedial hypothalamus (VMN) in pain modulation is analyzed and presented here. The place of VMN as a site modulating pain is evaluated on the basis of the criterion set by Dafny et al. [1]. The data presented satisfies these criterion, namely, a response evoked by noxious stimuli should arrive at the site; focal electrical stimulation in a remote "pain modulation" site should modulate the noxious evoked responses arriving at the investigated site; systemic and/or local application of opioid should modulate the arriving responses evoked by noxious stimuli at the investigated site; focal electrical stimulation of the site under investigation should produce behavioural analgesia; and local opioid application in this site should produce behavioral analgesia. It is felt that these criterion are essential to generally identify the modulation site but are insufficient to provide them an independent identity. It is suggested that the modulation of pain is characteristic to the neural site and is very closely linked to its function. This aspect of the modulation will be discussed for VMN. The modulation by VMN is in pari passu with its primary function, namely, satiety having control components of meal size, food preference, diurnal rhythm and secretion of releasing hormones. The studies conclude that the pattern of pain modulation by VMN has all these attributes and interacts with food related cues to modulate nociceptive behaviour.

Introduction

The actions of hypothalamus in pain modulation are manifested individually as well as an integrated part of the hypothalamo-hypophyseal system in modulating pain, combating stress and a multitude of other functions encompassing the maintenance of the hormonal milieu of the body. It has an integrative role in the manifestation of the complex pain behaviour, including its sensory-discriminative and emotional-affective components. Hypothalamotomy or injection of alcohol have been reported to be successful in the treatment of severe pain patients, while stimulation of either hypothalamus or periventricular gray (PVG) in analgesia [2]. The effects are opioidergic since the former had a concomitant elevation of beta-endorphin level and the latter was naloxone reversible. It is speculated that since the fibers from the hypothalamus to the periaqueductal gray area (PAG) have a periventricular course, they are probably stimulated by PAG/PVG electrodes and may contribute to stimulation produced analgesia (SPA) in human patients.

Pain modulation is a dynamic process, which involves continuous interactions between complex ascending and descending systems. Several supraspinal sites have been implicated in pain modulation; the PAG and the raphe nuclei are the initial sites to be implicated in pain modulation processes [3]. Different criteria have been used [3-7] to identify the site as a putative pain modulation site. However, to establish its relative status and precise function as a pain modulator, standard criterion should be utilised. Dafny and colleagues [1] have suggested that the following physiological criteria are essential for the endorsement of a site(s) involved in pain modulation: [i] a response evoked by noxious stimuli should arrive at the site, (ii) focal electrical stimulation in a remote "pain modulation" site should modulate the noxious evoked responses arriving at the investigated site, (iii) systemic and/or local application of opioid should modulate the arriving responses evoked by noxious stimuli at the investigated site, (iv) focal electrical stimulation of the site under investigation should produce behavioral analgesia; and (v) local opioid application in this site should produce behavioral analgesia.

Although, several areas are reported to be involved in pain modulation, the possibility of redundancy is bleak. We believe that each of them should be subserving a specific function. However, there is no information regarding this in the literature. We hypothesized that a given site should exert modulation unique to it, which is intertwined with its primary function. For example, ventromedial hypothalamic nucleus (VMN) is reported to modulate pain while it primarily mediates "satiety" on the basis of certain neuro-chemical information received via neural, blood and cerebrospinal fluid routes. Besides, VMN is involved in the reproductive functions through its control on respective hormones. Therefore, it is logical to conjecture that VMN should be modulating pain responses in relation to various nutrients and fed states of the individual. We investigated these aspects utilising various animal models (rat and monkey), states (anesthetised/conscious), food status (sucrose or normal fed) neuro physiological and behavioural techniques and a variety of noxious stimuli. The modulation by VMN was hypothesised to be in response to food intake, circadian rhythm; and reproductive cues.

Pain Modulation by VMN in Relation to Various Hypothalamic and Extra Hypothalamic Structures

In elaboration of the role of VMN pain related evoked responses were recorded from ipsilateral muscle digastricus (dEMG) after tooth pulp stimulation of left lower incisor tooth (TP- JOR) while any area belonging to pain modulation circuit, viz. hypothalamus (anterior or lateral hypothalamic area or VMN), hippocampus and amygdala were electrically stimulated (Fig. 1 a, b, c). The analgesic effects were observed from these pain modulating areas including anterior, posterior, lateral and medial hypothalamus. However, the latter areas were found to be more effective which is in line with earlier reports (Fig. 1 d) [5, 8]. These results support a significant contribution of VMN in comparison to other neighbouring areas also implicated in pain modulation.

Stimulation of lateral hypothalamic area (LHA) also causes antinociception besides thirst, eating and increase in the general level of activity of the animal.

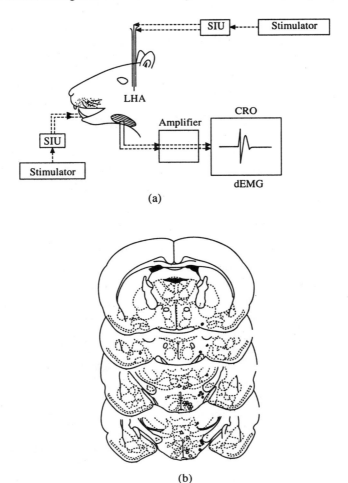

(a)

(b)

However, there is evidence that LHA influence varies with the type of pain [4]. Electrical stimulation of LHA when delivered concurrently with a peripheral pain stimulus (tail shock) selectively inhibits post-stimulus vocalization response that is integrated rostral to hindbrain, while vocalization during pain stimulus and motor response of tail are not affectected since they are integrated caudal to hind brain. On the other hand, bilateral lesion of LHA produces a significant increase in the thresholds for vocalization during and after stimulus which are indicative of analgesia while motor response of tail was unaffected (Fig. 2 a, b). Besides, there was a shorter tail flick latency and higher pain rating in formalin model indicative of hyperalgesia in the same rat (Fig. 2c).

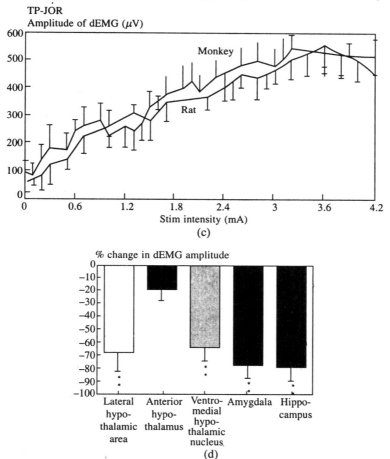

Fig. 1 (a) Experimental set-up for stimulation (0.5Hz, 0.3 ms duration and 1.5-3.0 times the threshold) of the lower incisor tooth pulp (TP) of rat and recording of EMG from m. digastricus (anterior belly, dEMG). (b, d) post-LHA or VMN or amygdala or hippocampus stimulation is plotted, (c) amplitude of EMG at 1.5-3.0 times the threshold was taken as basal. The dEMG amplitude is plotted against gradual increase in the strength of TP stimulation in rats and monkeys, (d) the % change in amplitude of dEMG as compared to basal, only during the initial 37 sec.

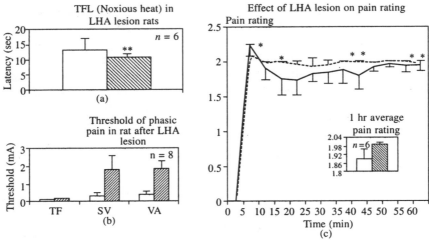

Fig. 2   Effect of LHA lesion (electrolytic) on latency, threshold of phasic pain and tonic pain responses of rats. Open bars/continuous line shows control and hatched bars/interrupted line shows post-LHA lesion data.

On the contrary, there was analgesia when the LHA was repeatedly stimulated (square wave pulses of 20 Hz, 0.2 msec duration, 600 μA intensity) for 2 min after every 10 min during 60 min duration of the experiment (formalin test) on behaving monkeys [9]. After 20 min (late phase of formalin pain) of algogen injection there was a significant analgesia, which is possibly mediated through PAG because naloxone pre-treatment at PAG partially blocked the analgesia (Fig. 3).

Despite the differences in our experimental paradigm for tonic pain behaviour (after 4-5 days of electrolytic lesion of LHA) in rats and monkeys (repeated LHA stimulation during tonic pain) there was hyperalgesia and analgesia respectively. The results of these experiments suggest that tonic pain is reduced when LHA is activated while phasic pain such as threshold of motor response of tail is not affected. The latency is indicative of hyperalgesia while the thresholds of vocalization during and after stimulus are inconclusive. Nonetheless, LHA modulates responses to both phasic and tonic noxious stimuli that are modulated at different levels of neuraxis namely, spinal and limbic levels. Moreover, LHA has been reported to fulfil all the pre-set criterion for a neural site involved in pain modulation utilising thermal noxious stimulus [1, 10]. The LHA projects to the midbrain periaqueductal grey (PAG), area of mesenchyme and upper pons surrounding the Aqueduct of Sylvius. Stimulation of PAG also like LHA inhibits tail flick reflex which is suggested to be mediated via the descending connections in the nucleus raphe magnus, a thin midline nucleus located in the lower pons and upper medulla and thence to the dorsal horn of spinal cord [4, 5]. LHA also projects to the mid brain reticular formation, which are implicated in the inhibition of the response of the dorsal horn neurons to noxious heating of skin. Results

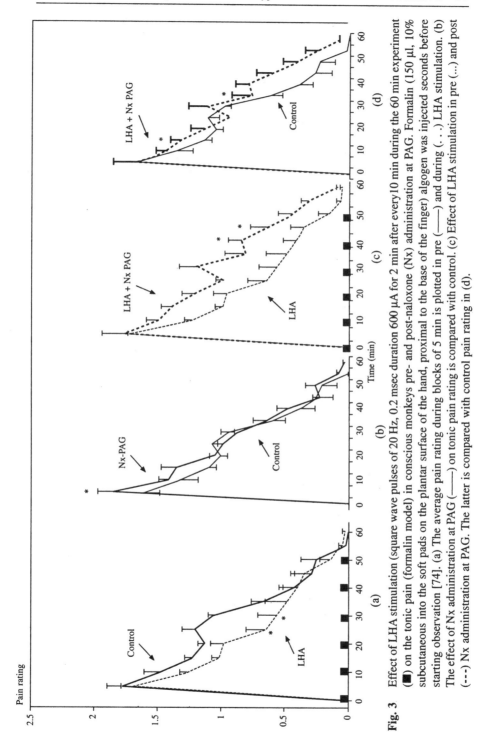

Fig. 3 Effect of LHA stimulation (square wave pulses of 20 Hz, 0.2 msec duration 600 µA for 2 min after every 10 min during the 60 min experiment (■) on the tonic pain (formalin model) in conscious monkeys pre- and post-naloxone (Nx) administration at PAG. Formalin (150 µl, 10% subcutaneous into the soft pads on the plantar surface of the hand, proximal to the base of the finger) algogen was injected seconds before starting observation [74]. (a) The average pain rating during blocks of 5 min is plotted in pre (——) and during (. . .) LHA stimulation. (b) The effect of Nx administration at PAG (——) on tonic pain rating is compared with control. (c) Effect of LHA stimulation in pre (...) and post (- - -) Nx administration at PAG. The latter is compared with control pain rating in (d).

also indicate that a stimulus specific modulation by LHA is probably governed by the mediating site, its neuro-chemical profile and connections with LHA [11].

Stimulation of wide spread areas of the ventromedial hypothalamus, which include the periventricular nucleus (PVN), medial mammillary nucleus (MMN), AH and arcuate nucleus produces the inhibition of tail flick response [12]. The role of PVN in analgesic modulation of pain has been documented [13] because of its activation of the pain inhibitory system. In rats the PVN stimulation causes analgesia (tail flick, cold water swim tests), which is mediated without the involvement of opioids and vasopressin [14]. The inhibitory effects may be mediated by direct uncrossed hypothalamospinal projections originating in the PVN and posterior hypothalamus, containing neurophysin to the spinal cord dorsal horn, including lamina 1 and to the intermediolateral horn [15]. The PVN on the other hand is recognised as a major integrating site for stress response activating the endogenous pain inhibitory system [16].

Preoptic stimulation has been shown to raise pain threshold in primates [17]. In awake rats, localized stimulation of arcuate nucleus elevates TFL [18]. The effect has been attributed to a robust distribution of β-endorphin in these areas [19].

Pattern of Pain Modulation by VMN Hypothalamus
The recent evidences extend the role of VMN in pain control besides its function in feeding and hormonal secretion [20]. In the chemical (gold

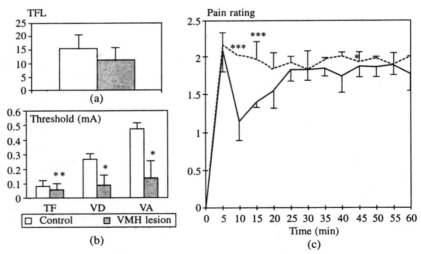

Fig. 4   Effect of VMN lesion on (a) latency, (b) threshold of phasic pain and (c) tonic pain in rats. Tonic pain was recorded by formalin model (50 µl, 5% subcutaneous plantar region of right or left paw). Both types of pain are increased post-VMN injection of formalin in lesion (. . . ./▦).

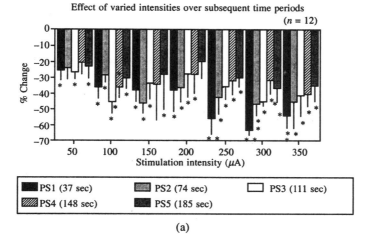

(a)

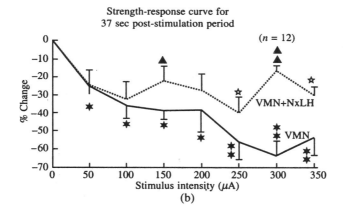

(b)

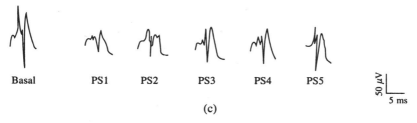

(c)

Fig. 5 (a) Effect of VMN stimulation (50-350 μA) on dEMG amplitude expressed as % change from basal. dEMG amplitude reduction is a function of intensity of tooth pulp stimulation vis-à-vis pain and recovery from it occurs correspondingly. (b) Compared with VMN stimulation pre (—) and post (. . . .) Nx administration at LHA. (c) Change in dEMG over subsequent time periods (37 sec, PS1 to 185 sec, PS5) after TP stimulation at one intensity (300 μA).

thioglucose, GTG) and electrolytic VMN lesions, the thresholds of flinch, jerk, jump and vocalisation were less as compared to their control counterparts indicating hyperalgesia in behaving rats. In our rats electrolytic or chemical (kainic acid) lesions of VMN produced a highly significant hyperalgesia as indicated by a decrease in tail flick latency, the thresholds of pain (tail flick, vocalization during and after stimulus) and an increase in tonic pain behavioural response to formalin injection (Fig. 4). In further support of it the stimulation of VMN has been reported from our laboratory as well as others to inhibit tooth pulp evoked responses recorded from m. digastricus (Fig. 5), reticular nuclei and to inhibit the response of spinal neurons to noxious inputs in anaesthetised animals [18].

The results indicate a significant inhibitory modulation by VMN in response to both phasic and tonic noxious stimuli when activated irrespective of the state (behaving/anesthetised) and type of noxious stimulus (phasic/tonic) unlike LHA. Moreover, the effects of either method utilised namely lesion or stimulation are not contradictory.

VMN lesion produced hyperalgesia in behaving rats as indicated by parameters related to phasic noxious stimuli (TFL, thresholds of TF, SV, VA, tail flinch, jerk, jump, vocalization) and tonic noxious stimulus related behaviour (formalin pain), while stimulation produced significant analgesia in rat TP-JOR, which was related to the intensity of stimulation. The results strongly suggest the role of VMN in tonic and phasic pain that involve various levels of neuraxis namely; spinal, trigeminal, brain stem or limbic areas. Besides, they also satisfy the fourth criterion of Daffny et al. [1].

Neuronal Basis of Pain Modulation by VMN

To further strengthen the contention it was attempted to identify the neurons involved in pain modulation since VMN contains different types of neurons. The neurons of the VMN respond to changes in the blood/CSF osmolarity, glucose, opioids, several other ions and related compounds [21]. A glucoresponsive neuron (GRN) was defined as the one whose activity increased dose dependently when subjected to direct electrophoretic application of glucose (through micropipette); the increase in activity is attributed to the membrane depolarisation caused by K^+ permeability [22] whereas, a neuron has been defined as a glucose sensitive neuron (GSN) if its spontaneous activity was dose dependently depressed by similar application of glucose. This is due to the membrane hyperpolarization caused by Na^+-K^+ pump activation [23]. GSN is feeding control and GRN is a satiation control neuron. The neurons affected by glucose when are also sensitive to sodium ions, are defined as the osmoreceptor cells. VMN does not possess any osmosensitive neurons whereas one-third neurons of LHA are osmosensitive.

We studied the precise role of VMN-GRN neurons in pain modulation by a slow uninterrupted delivery of 2-deoxy-d-glucosel (2DG) in micro quantities at a constant rate (1 µl/min) for 7 days in VMN. The 2 DG is an antimetabolite analogue of glucose, which prevents glucose utilisation by the neurons. It competes with glucose for hexokinase substrate (as they are structurally similar) leading to an artificial scarcity of glucose in the neurons, thereby inhibiting the phosphohexose isomerase reaction and membrane transport. The 2 DG was locally infused into the VMN to circumvent the stress related effects observed on systemic administration, including marked glucoprivation, peripheral sympathoadrenal discharge, hyperglycemia etc. [24]. Microinfusion of 2DG in VMN led to an increase in thresholds of motor response, stimulus induced vocalization during and post stimulus responses suggesting an analgesic response to phasic noxious stimuli; although the tail flick latency increased, it did not attain statistical significance (Fig. 6 b, c). However, the behavioural response to formalin pain was more during the late phase only (Fig. 6 d).

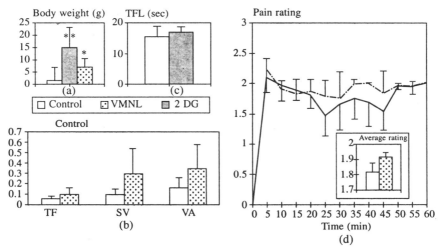

Fig. 6 Effect of 2DG (antimetabolite analogue of glucose) infusion (1 μl, constant, continuous for 7 days) in VMN of behaving rats on: (a) body weight, (b) threshold, (c) latency of phasic and (d) tonic pain. Open bars/continuous line depicts control group, dots show 2DG infused group and shaded is VMN lesion.

The role of GRN in pain modulation is strongly suggested by the hypoalgesia in TFL and thresholds in our rats following 2DG microinfusion in VMN. However, several researchers including us have reported electrical stimulation or activation of VMN, to produce analgesia (tooth pulp evoked response), while lesion (electrolytic/GTG lesion) to hyperalgesia (TFL, TF, SV, VA and tonic pain). Both these procedures involve a manipulation of a heterogenous population of neurons, thereby activating different sets of interneurons. Therefore, the data of lesion/stimulation has a limited value in extrapolating the results in terms of specific neuronal involvement. It is further supported by reports of iontophoretic glucose application to 43 neurons in VMN when only 24 neurons were excited and 19 were unaffected [25]. Obviously, the functional outcome is determined by the set of neurons activated since it is unlikely that any afferent information involves the neurons of the nucleus globally. In our experimental paradigm, 2 DG was specifically targeted to act on glucoresponsive neuronal population of VMH. The effect of intracarotid administration of 2DG on hypothalamic neuron activity was also reported to decrease the activity of VMN neurons only while there was no effect on those of anterior, middle or posterior nuclei of hypothalamus [26]. Conversely, iontophoretic application of 2DG produced no distinct response [27] while glucose increased the glucoreceptor neuronal activity [28]. This discrepancy in the effects of 2 DG is probably due to either insufficient quantity or time to exhibit the change. Nevertheless, 2DG competes with glucose, decreases the activity of VMN glucoreceptor neurons [28], thereby probably leading the neurons functionally inactive. The inactivity becomes apparent only when a stimulus/challenge is received and not otherwise. Possibly, this may leave the rest of the neurons unapposed, which may lead to a behaviour akin to VMN stimulation, i.e. analgesia rather than the expected hyperalgesia. It is, therefore, the interaction of several groups of neurons in a nucleus that ultimately determines the behaviour. Effects of knocking of all the neurons by lesion or stimulation per se on the behaviour should be interpreted carefully. The contention gets further support from the pattern of modulatory influence of LHA on nociceptive behaviour being dictated by the type of noxious stimulus and state of the animal.

The pattern of pain modulation by VMN and LHA are area specific although, the neuronal types are similar in LHA and VMN. However, the proportion of various neuronal types is different for example the GSN are predominant in LHA. They respond to glucose and morphine besides the noxious stimulus [10]. Out of the 52 glucosensitive neurons tested with noxious stimulation, 69% responded by a decrease in activity and 1% by an increase. The glucose-nonsensitive neurons participate in autonomic and behavioural regulation of food intake by monitoring the metabolic status of the body [23, 25, 27-30]. Glucose-nonsensitive neurons, do not respond to electrophoretically applied chemicals related to food intake control and their precise role in nociception is probably brought about by non-opioid substance. The convergence of multiple inputs on a single neuron in the LHA is necessary to integrate precise and vital control of food intake [29, 30]. The integrating network consists of the LHA microcircuit, with the GSN as an important element, receiving extrinsic sensory, intrinsic visceral and metabolic [28, 31] signals; second, the macrocircuit, involving extrahypothalamic structures such as the amygdala [32], globus pallidus, substantia nigra [33], prefrontal cortex and motor cortex [30]; third the effectors, i.e. neural substrates subserving feeding behaviour. Pain related sensory stimuli possibly inhibit the activity of GSN to set the integrating mechanisms in action; the final outcome is disturbance of feeding behaviour. Therefore, the GSN in the LHA are hypothesised to provide a logical integrating point for nociceptive inputs to participate in feeding control. The precise status of it is not hypothesised for VMN. VMN and LHA have a reciprocal influence on food intake but not so on nociceptive behaviour. Therefore, it is difficult to hypothesise the involvement of neuronal type as an integrating point for the two behaviours. Nevertheless, food intake and nociceptive behaviours influence each other and it can be extrapolated to VMN too since the behaviour of these neurons is similar although their proportion is less in VMN. However, the subtle differences in their controls over pain can be attributed to these differences in their numbers. Nonetheless, when phasic pain was repeatedly inflicted at unpredictable intervals and of unpredictably different types, there was a significant decrease in food intake on that day and when prolonged/tonic pain was given there was a significant decrease in the number of lever presses which was abolished by morphine pre-treatment suggesting the role of opioids in modulating the motivation for getting food (Fig. 7) [34-36].

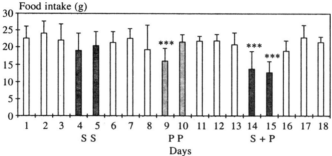

Fig. 7   Correlation of food intake (24 h) with sucrose ingestion (S) and/or painful stimuli (P) on food intake of that day. A nonsignificant influence of sucrose ingestion per se while a highly significant influence of sucrose in addition to painful stimuli on food intake.

These studies further satisfy the criterion 1 and 4 specifically by providing evidences for the specific neuronal group of VMN involved in modulating pain behaviour.

Pain Modulation by VMN

Role of Opioids

Histochemically, opiate and enkephalin receptors have been identified in cell bodies within the hypothalamus wherein the VMN has a robust, wide distribution of multiple opiate receptors. Recently, increase in beta-endorphin-like immunoreactivity was observed in the rat VMN and PAG during tonic pain induced by formalin injection in the forepaw. Immunohistochemistry reveals a high content of endogenous morphine-like oligopeptide, endorphin and enkephalin in its structures, which support its involvement and participation in pain perception and analgesia. Opioids have been implicated in both tonic and phasic pain. Subsequent intraventricular injection of normal rabbit beta-endorphin antiserum in rats produced a significant hyperalgesia in these rats, thus elucidating an opioidergic role of VMN in tonic pain [37-39]. Not only this, the single neuronal activity is also influenced by opioids; incidentally by the neurons which may or may not respond to glucose. Glucose administered to 43 neurons in the VMN excited only 24 neurons, morphine excited 17 neurons inhibited 2 while it did not affect 5. Out of 19 neurons unaffected by glucose in the VMN, 5 were excited by morphine and 14 were unaffected by it. Glucose and morphine administration produced similar results on LHA and VMN in terms of the latency, magnitude and dose effects except for the duration of the morphine effect which was double that of the glucose [40].

Exogenous administration of enkephalin had similar effects like morphine. In the LHA 2 were excited, 10 were inhibited and 2 were unaffected by enkephalin whereas in the VMN out of 11 neurons responding to glucose and morphine 10 also responded to enkephalin. Morphine antagonist (naloxone levellorphan) block the morphine and enkephalin action in LHA and VMN neurons but not those of glucose on the same neurons. It is possible that the effects of morphine and enkephalin on neurons associated with feeding are direct and not secondary [40], which is contrary to Yanaura et al. [41] who had shown that morphine has no effect on food intake and if at all, it decreases food intake secondary to the taste [42]. Therefore, we have reservations in suggesting from our study that the varying noxious stimuli at variable intervals to the rats reduced food intake directly or indirectly through opioid released as a part of the effort to reduce pain. Nonetheless, the decrease in food intake was potentiated when sucrose was ingested ad libitum by these rats [35], which is shown to activate opioid secretion in VMN [43]. These behavioural responses further support the observations.

Since both VMN and LHA are involved in pain modulation, which is similar in direction (atleast for some types of noxious stimuli) but not in magnitude and their morphological and functional closeness to each other; it was pertinent to explore their interaction specifically in pain modulation. Moreover, both these areas contain neurons, which have rich inter connections besides responding to glucose, opioids (enkephalins), naloxone and produce analgesia/hyperalgesia on stimulation/lesion albeit above mentioned differences. It was, therefore, proposed to study opiodergic interaction of LHA and VMN in pain modulation, besides their response to naloxone independently.

Effect of Naloxone Administration at VMN

Effect of naloxone administration per se or an equal volume of isotonic saline at VMN was studied on TP-JOR in anesthetised rats. A significant increase ($51.16 \pm 7.36\%$, $p < 0.01$) in the amplitude of dEMG as compared to basal was obtained when naloxone was administered, whereas there was no change in dEMG when isotonic saline was administered (Fig. 8).

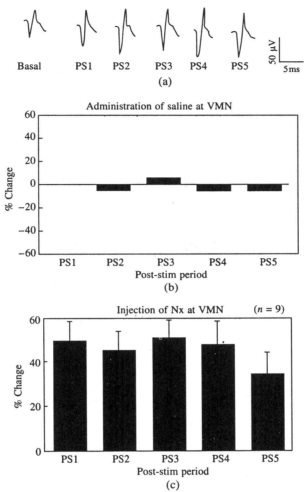

Fig. 8   Effect of naloxone administration at VMN on the tooth pulp stimulation produced
dEMG change in amplitude. (a, c) Effect (increase) on dEMG amplitude during
the period of observation (185 sec), (b) effect of saline administration at VMN
on TP-JOR.

Modulation of Pain by VMN and LHA

The VMN and LHA connect reciprocally through dorsomedial hypothalamus
and terminate commonly at perifornical regions, or through amygdala or
midbrain level where the medial forebrain bundle and the dorsal longitudinal
fasciculus (DLF) intermingle or through the reciprocal connection with PAG
[30]. The opioidergic interaction was studied by stimulating either LHA or
VMN and administering naloxone at the other site (VMN or LHA, respectively)
in the anesthetised rat utilising tooth pulp stimulation-jaw opening reflex
model.

Effect of VMN Stimulation Pre- and Post-naloxone Administration at LHA
Stimulation of VMN in anesthetised rats ($n = 18$) decreased the dEMG
amplitude (antinociception) when compared to the basal values. The effect
was proportional to the intensity of the stimulation and the maximal effect
was noted at 300 µA (Fig. 9).

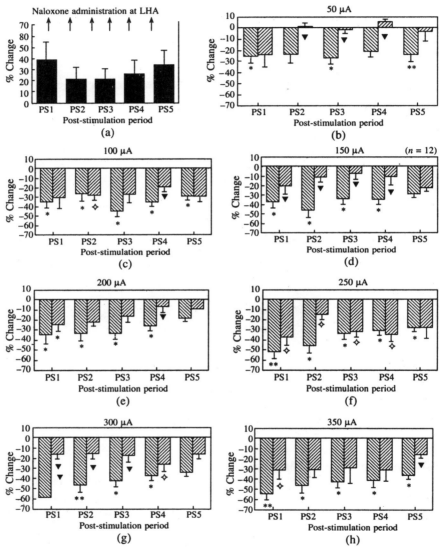

Fig. 9   Effect of varying stimulation intensity over subsequent time blocks (PS1-5)
within the period of observation on the amplitude of dEMG by TP stimulation.
(b-h) The data is compared post ▨ with pre Nx ▨ administration at LHA.
(a) effect of Nx per se on TP dEMG amplitude. *: Basal vs VMN ($p < 0.05$);
◇: Basal vs VMN + NxLHA ($p < 0.05$); ▼: VMN vs VMN + Nx LHA
($p < 0.05$).

Table 1   Effects of VMN or LHA stimulation and/or naloxone administration on TP-JOR of rat

S. No.	VMN	LHA	TP shock-anterior digastricus EMG amplitude
1	—	Electrical stimulus	Mild decrease
2	Saline administration	Electrical stimulus	Mild decrease
3	Naloxone administration	—	Strong hyperalgesia
4	Naloxone administration	Electrical stimulus	Attenuation of analgesia
5	Electrical stimulus	—	Moderate decrease
6	Electrical stimulus	Saline administration	Moderate decrease
7	—	Naloxone administration	Hyperalgesia (statistically NS)
8	Electrical stimulus	Naloxone administration	Attenuation of analgesia

Administration of naloxone per se at LHA (n = 12 rats) increased the amplitude of dEMG in comparison to the basal dEMG (although the change was not statistically significant), while that of isotonic saline at LHA failed to show any effect. However, when Nx was administered at LHA prior to VMN stimulation, the stimulation-produced-analgesia was attenuated (Fig. 9). The results suggest that VMN modulates pain possibly through LHA, which is opioid mediated.

Effect of LHA Stimulation Pre- and Post-naloxone Administration at VMN
The stimulation of LHA produced a decrement in dEMG amplitude (antinociception) as compared to basal, which was proportional to the intensity of stimulation. The effect was most evident immediately (37 sec) following the stimulus. However, when LHA stimulation was preceeded by Nx administration at VMN a reduction in this antinociception was observed although it (antinociception) still remained significant. Pre and post Nx difference in antinociception was more significant at lower current strengths than higher ones. However, when saline was administered into VMN there was no observable difference in its pre and post saline-LHA stimulation effects (Figs. 10 and 11).

In summary, it was observed that VMN stimulation-produced analgesia was greater than that produced by LHA stimulation, which was particularly evident at lower current strengths. VMN stimulation in comparison to that of LHA had the following features: (i) the antinociception was directly related to the intensity of stimulus, the pattern of which was similar to that of LHA albeit for the greater intensity of antinociception; (ii) the maximum

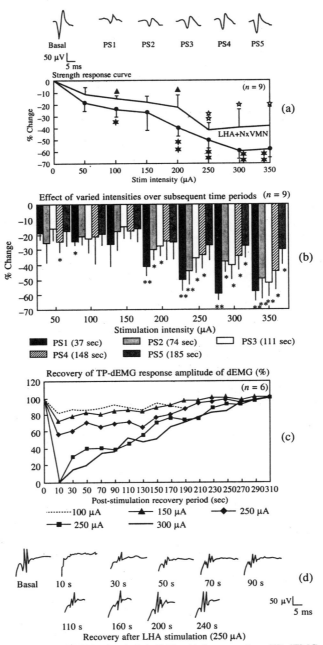

Fig. 10 (a) The effect of LHA stimulation (300 μA) (—•—•—) on TP-dEMG amplitude at various time intervals of 37 sec (PS1-5) and administration of Nx at VMN (—) while the lower panel shows effect of varying intensity of stimulation of LHA on the same (only at PS1) after administration of Nx at VMN. The data is compared: (i) basal with LHA stimulation (*), (ii) basal with LHA stimulation and Nx at VMN (✧) and (iii) between (i) and (ii) (▲). (b, c, d) Effect of varying intensity of LHA stimulation on the recovery of TP-dEMG amplitude until the period of observation.

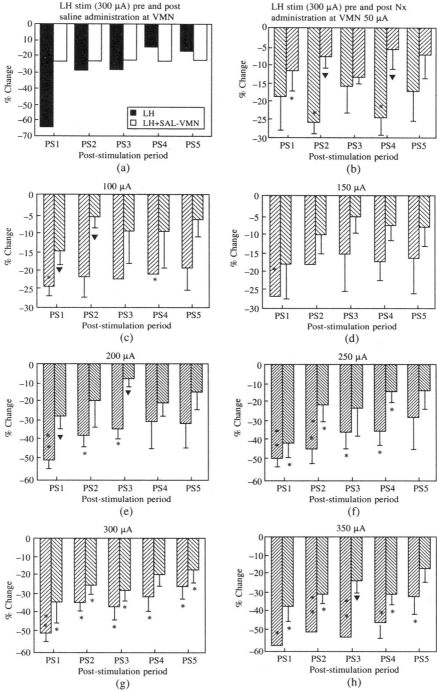

Fig. 11 Effect of varying intensity of stimulation at LHA over subsequent time blocks of 37 sec until the period of observation (185 sec) on TP stimulation induced change in dEMG amplitude. (b-h) The data is compared in pre ▨ and post ▨ Nx and (a) saline administration at VMN. *: comparison of basal versus LHA, ●: basal versus LHA + Nx VMN and ▲: LHA versus Nx VMN.

antinociception on VMN stimulation was obtained at an intensity of 300 µA whereafter no further increase in the effect was observed, which was similar to that of LHA; (iii) the increment in the effect with increasing intensity of stimulation was more in case of VMN. This influence is stronger than that acting via VMN when LHA is stimulated. This is probably because of the lower threshold of activation of the neurons at VMN, leading to a different/ more potent neurotransmitter release and/or a greater number of neurons engaged in pain modulation and (iv) as discussed earlier, comparison between the effects of Nx administration per se at the two areas revealed a significantly more hyperalgesia from VMN, which lasted for a longer duration. This could be taken as a reflection of a higher number of opioidergic neurons (large cells with multiple dendrites, exhibiting excitatory-inhibitory response) [30] in VMN than LHA accounting for more potent effects from of VMN stimulation. The other contributory factors in the characteristics of pain modulation by VMN are possibly smaller size of VMN, larger proportion of GSN and their activation thresholds.

Moreover, the results of LHA lesion/stimulation revealed that the effect on pain response is stimulus specific. It is therefore possible that within the nucleus/area even a differential activation of the various groups of neurons can determine a gamut of behavioural responses. For example, the activation of LHA 'nociceptive-on' and the 'nociceptive-off' cells by the noxious afferent input [1] of tail pinch leads to a short lasting increase in the activity of the 'on' cells but causes a decrease in the activity of the 'off' cells. It is assumed that the 'on' cells are connected directly with the spinal cord while the 'off' cells are connected to the spinal cord indirectly via interneurons located in LHA only or any other site. Incidentally, a direct ascending connection from the spinal cord to LHA has been demonstrated, which forms a direct reciprocal connection of LHA 'on' cells with spinal cord. The action of these cells may probably be similar to those at PAG [3, 44] where the 'off' cells activate the analgesic mechanism at the level of NRM and the 'on' cells supress it. Therefore, if naloxone blocks the activation of the 'off' cells in a similar way as in PAG, the predominance of activity of the 'on' cells at LHA may result in suppression of the antinociceptive effect at the spinal level via positive feedback through the LHA-spinal cord loop. Besides, through DLF and MFB monosynaptic connection to mid brain reticular formation, the information from VMN is transmitted to dorsal vagal nucleus and trigeminal nucleus, thereby modulating TP-JOR. It also sends descending input to trigeminal nuclei (oralis and caudalis) via NRM.

These evidences satisfy fifth criterion of Daffny et al. [1] namely local opioid application in this site should produce behavioural analgesia. It also covers criterion 2 in part, viz. remote focal electrical stimulation in a different albeit nearby "pain modulation" site should modulate the noxious evoked responses arriving at the investigated site which is further supported by studies involving some other sites such as PAG and NRM. The data of only former is presented here. It has been shown that either stimulation of PAG or microiontophoretic administration of morphine leads to inhibition of neuronal activity of VMN [45]. Suppression of cell firing in VMN was also observed on systemic [46, 47] and local opioid peptides [48, 49]. Thus, a highly predominant opioidergic mediation of phasic pain for VMN can be suggested which acts through LHA. Therefore, the effect of tooth-pulp stimulation was studied on the neurons of the PAG, which is the key area in the modulation of pain and the effect of LHA stimulation was studied on the single neuronal activity in the monkey [50].

Depending upon the type and grade of peripheral noxious stimuli applied, most of the neurons responded either by an increase or decrease in firing rate to at least mechanical and thermal noxious stimuli to all the four limbs. However, the receptive fields were non-specific without any limb-specific variation instead, the responses varied with the grades of noxious thermal or tooth-pulp stimuli, or on stimulation of LHA. As such, their responses were pooled together under different grades of stimuli. When the water was applied at temperatures varying from 45 to 60°C, the neurons responded by an either increase or decrease in the firing rate which was directly related to the intensity of stimulation, although former of the two was the predominant response (i.e. 11 = out of 12 or 91.7% of neurons). Effect of noxious pinch was studied on a total of 10 neurons on which 48 responses were recorded. An increase in firing rate was observed in 30 responses from 7 neurons (58.33%). A maximum increase of 3.14 ± 2.74 Hz was obtained from right limb pinching and a minimum of 1.80 ± 1.20 Hz from pinching left limb. Similarly, a majority of the neurons responded to LHA stimulation by an increase in the rate of firing which bore a good correlation with the strength of stimulation.

On the contrary, majority (62.50%) of the PAG neurons decreased their firing rate on tooth-pulp stimulation at all the test stimulus strengths (except 1 mA and 4 mA). However, no definite correlation was observed when the magnitude of response was compared with the grades of stimulation although, a maximum decrease in firing rate was observed at the highest intensity of stimulation (5 mA). The results indicate an influence of LHA on PAG nociceptive specific neurons.

Attributes of VMN Pain Modulation, Functional Significance: Evidence for opioidergic and glucoresponsive neuronal involvement

Both VMN and LH area reciprocate in control of eating behaviour. It is clear from the above discussion and outcome of the studies that VMN participates in modulation of the noxious stimuli and the role of VMN is not simply a reciprocal of LHA since both lead to hyperalgesia when stimulated. The specific pattern of modulation of each is discussed in the previous section. However, it is not sufficient to identify the pain modulatory area, since its identity is incomplete till a specific physiological significance is attached to it. In a VMN lesion animal the primary behavioural disturbances amongst others are hyperphagia, finickiness (preference for sucrose and high lipid food) and loss of diurnal variation in eating. Pari passu with this the specific attributes to the pain modulation by VMN were hypothesised to be in the related parameters, namely alteration in nociceptive behaviour, diurnal rhythm and the changes in both these after ingestion of palatable food. These objectives were studied in behaving intact, VMN lesion and 2DG (micro infused in VMN) models of rat.

The available literature strongly suggests a direct reciprocal relationship between the food intake vis-à-vis the hedonic properties of food, the endogenous opioids [51-54] and pain [51, 55-57]. Opioid agonist reduce pain, promote food intake [58] and alter food preference; (increase the preference for carbohydrates) [59, 60] while the effect of palatable foods on nociception is biphasic that is analgesia followed by hyperalgesia in the same rat. We reported that it is determined by the duration of sucrose availability, characteristics of noxious stimulus and gender of the subject [61-65]. Nonetheless, palatability of the food is the predominant factor in determining food intake and nociceptive status.

Emperical and sociocultural observations on post ingestional alterations in pain have led to a series of reports on the effect of some food components on pain perception. It is now well documented that the food intake in humans as well as in rat models alter sensitivity to pain. Components of food such as fat, lactose, proteins and sucrose have been studied although; we are still ignorant about their mechanism of action. The palatable substances like sucrose can enhance the analgesic properties of endogenous and exogenous opioids [51] and naloxone pre-treatment in rats abolishes the response indicating thereby involvement of opioidergic mechanism. In newborn infants also several painful procedures are being performed without anaesthesia [66]. Sucrose flavoured pacifier when used as an analgesic during the painful procedures in the newborn infants reduced crying and its effects namely; alterations in heart rate, palmar sweating, blood pressure, blood renin activity and plasma cortisol levels. Their hormonal profiles are indicative of a significant carbohydrate, protein, fat depletion; hyperglycemia; increased ketone bodies; increased lactate and pyruvate levels, which were naltrexone reversible [66]. Effectiveness of sucrose as an analgesic increased when it was combined with an analgesic cream [67] whereas in prepubertal and adults the analgesic response to sucrose ingestion is less and is limited to the recovery from the noxious stimuli. However, in our adult volunteers (male) sucrose induced analgesia lasted for approximately 20 min and we utilized both subjective and objective criterion for assessment of pain.

We studied systematically the influence of palatability on the behavioural responses to varied types of noxious stimuli. The effects were studied for various durations such as a few minutes to few months through several hours.

Effect of Ingestion of Palatable Food on Pain for Varied Durations

Effect of Ingestion of Palatable Substance (5-10 ml) for a Few Minutes on Pain Behaviour Until 60 min

The effect of ingestion of few ml (5-10 ml) sucrose for a few min (5 min) was studied on phasic and tonic pain. After sucrose feeding the pattern of tonic pain behaviour response including the initial severe pain remained the same as controls. Nonetheless, they spent more time in category 1 (least pain) and less time in categories 3 and 2 indicating an analgesic state (Fig. 12).

Whereas, in the phasic pain tests there was an increase in the latency to flick tail and threshold of tail flick indicating analgesia though no difference was observed in the threshold of simple vocalization and vocalization after discharge. However, in bilateral VMN lesion (electrolytic) rats, the analgesic effect of sucrose ingestion on phasic and tonic pain was not observed. Our results of the experiment suggest that an acute ingestion of a few mls of sucrose produces an immediate analgesia during both the phasic and tonic pain responses, which is mediated by VMN. A similar response viz; analgesia was reported by Blass et al. [69]. They infused sucrose directly into the mouths of 10 day old infant rats. It had an immediate effect of significantly elevating the paw lick latency to thermal noxious stimulus to all the paws. However, we are reporting for the first time such an effect in adult rats as well as to various phasic and tonic noxious stimuli. The threshold of tail flick, vocalisation during stimulus increased and the nociceptive behavioural rating decreased respectively indicating analgesia [61].

Acute effects of simple sugars or highly palatable substances is attributed by the direct evidence in favour of activation of the endogenous opioids vis-a-vis release of β-endorphins from hypothalamus. Short term sucrose feeding brings about a release of β-endorphins from the hypothalamus and increases the number of these receptors, which bring a brief period of analgesia [43].

Ingestion of sucrose stimulates the peripheral glucosensitive and glucoreceptor vagal units in the tongue. The stimulation is relayed on to the nucleus tractus solitarius (NTS) and area postrema. Here the initial integration of this information with information on vascular or ventricular (fourth ventricle) chemicals probably occurs. This integrated information can move in two directions: rostrally for higher integration and caudally by way of the dorso medial vagal nucleus, as a reflex from the NTS to produce responses in the appropriate viscera (or to control activity of hepatic enzymes or pancreatic hormones) and the information in the rostral direction goes, either directly or through the parabrachial nucleus to the hypothalamus. Glucose-responsive cells in these higher regions, the VMN and LHA sense systemic and the ventricular chemical information as discussed in the preceding sections. VMN neuronal correlates of eating and nociceptive behaviour have also been discussed in the preceeding sections. Therefore, further support to the previous results is provided by the VMN compromised rats, which do not

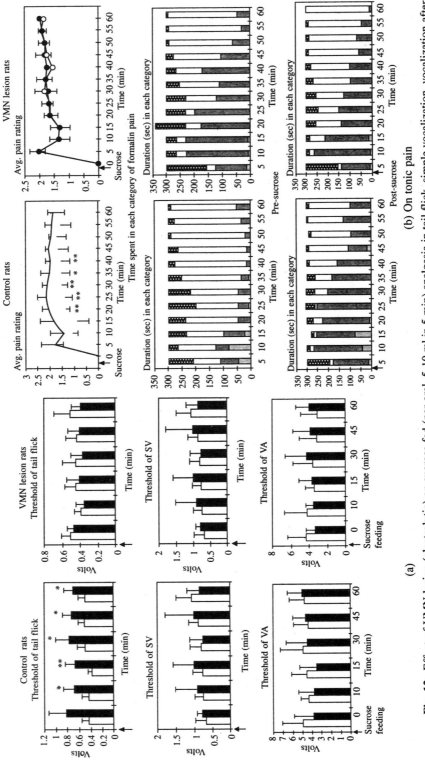

Fig. 12 Effect of VMN lesion (electrolytic) on sucrose fed (per oral, 5-10 ml in 5 min) analgesia in tail flick, simple vocalization, vocalization after discharge and the pain rating (average each category) during the period of observation (60 min). Arrow indicates presentation of sucrose.

respond to ingested palatable substances thereby suggesting the unique role of VMN in pain modulation. The probable flow of information is depicted in Fig. 13. This communication between the abovementioned association areas and the hypothalamus, plus further integration of information from other modalities, leads to feeding-related decision that go along paths parallel to those over which the afferent signals originally ascended in order to control visceral organs, and along other paths to the motor system by way of the motor cortex. Feeding-related regions of the central nervous system include the prefrontal cortex, the amygdala, and the parts of the reticular formation, which mediate signals from various sources and contribute, along with the hypothalamus, to integration of hunger and satiation signals.

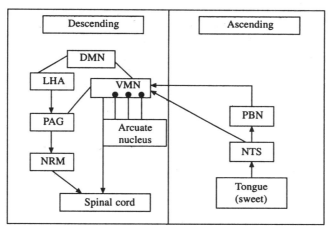

Fig. 13 Possible neural pathway for ingested sucrose to release beta endorphin (• • •) in VMN and the probable pathways for influencing TFL or SV.

Effect of Ingestion of Palatable Substance Until 5 h on Pain Behaviour
There is an initial analgesia for 45 min in TFL, 60 min in threshold of tail flick only (not in threshold of SV and VA) and tonic pain followed by eualgesia in all the tests and then to a significant hyperalgesia at 5 h in TFL, 6h in SV, VA and 3 h in tonic pain (Fig. 14). Surprisingly, threshold of tail flick remained eualgesic after an initial analgesia while the response to thermal noxious stimulus to paws was only hyperalgesic.

Only initial analgesia is reported to be opioidergic since Nx pretreatment abolished the responses to thermal noxious stimuli, while the late hyperalgesia is hypothesised to be ensuing from an effective decrease in opioids. There is no evidence regarding sparing effect on threshold of tail flick and hyperalgesia on hot plate or temporal variation in various responses. Nonetheless, it is pertinent to specify the conditions of stimulus and the nutritional status of the subject since both these factors modulate pain significantly.

Effect of Ingestion of Palatable Substance for 48 h on Pain Behaviour

The results of sucrose ingestion in addition to food and water ad libitum for varying durations, viz. 6-48 h on different pain responses reveal hyperalgesia. Vocalization during stimulus and after discharge are influenced by 6 h of sucrose ingestion, followed by tail flick latency and tonic pain rating after 12 h, whereas the threshold of tail flick remained unaffected (Fig. 15). Lesion (electrolytic) of VMN per se produces hyperalgesia, which was neither potentiated nor attenuated by sucrose ingestion, implicating a vital role of VMN in any pain modulation related to food intake.

In summary a moderately prolonged ingestion of sucrose for 6 h ad libitum (in addition to food and water) heightened the nociceptive responses to phasic noxious stimuli (both electrical and thermal) at the end of 6 h, while it attenuated the response to tonic noxious stimulus, thereby suggesting a

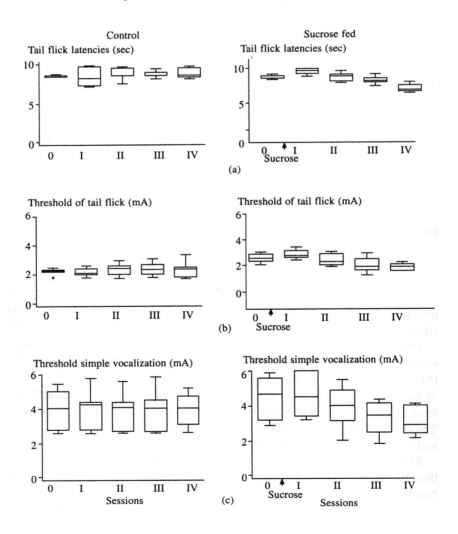

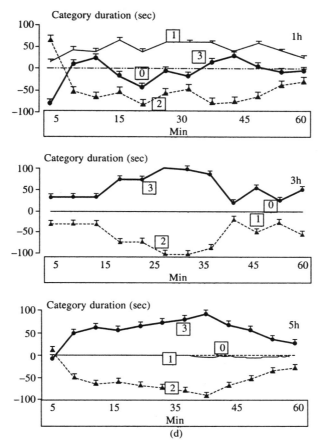

Fig. 14 Effect of sucrose ingestion ad libitum per orally for 5 h on pain responses in the same rat. (a, b) Latency and threshold of motor responses of tail from spinal cord, (c) motor response from brain stem, (d) change from control in pain rating during each category (0-3) of the formalin pain model.

hyperalgesic response to phasic and analgesic response to tonic noxious stimulus, which was absent in VMN lesion rats.

Our studies support the previous reports of analgesia after acute intake of sweet tasting fluids and hyperalgesia after chronic (more than 3-5 h) intake [51, 53, 54, 68]. We have determined the role of VMN in sucrose fed modulation of pain utilizing a wider spectrum of noxious stimuli while most scientists have reported generally on the basis of only the thermal noxious stimulus. These results again highlight a wide spectrum of responses ranging from nadir to increase or decrease depending on the stimulus variety.

Modulation by VMN as dictated by palatability is stimulus specific implying thereby that the susceptibility of responses to various noxious stimuli varies. Not only the thresholds for tail flick, simple vocalization and vocalization after discharge decrease, the response to tonic noxious stimulus also increases suggesting hyperalgesia [35, 62]. The threshold of vocalisation during and after stimulus are influenced by 6h of sucrose ingestion, followed by tail flick latency and tonic pain rating after 12 h while the threshold of tail flick remained unaffected even at the end of 48 h [35, 62]. Sucrose ingestion increases analgesic potency of morphine in male as well as female rats [53]. Long term sucrose feeding diminishes the capacity of the liver to metabolise

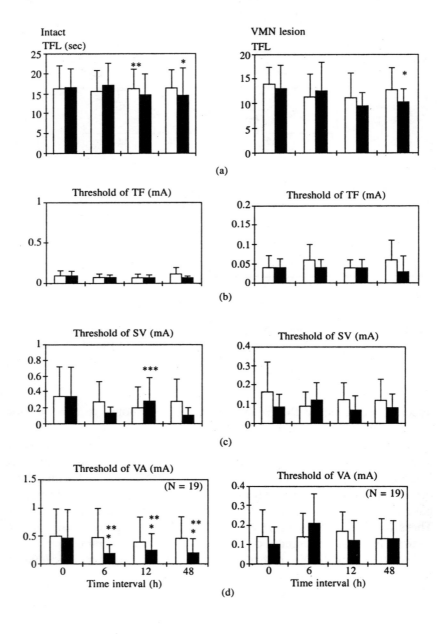

morphine leading to higher levels of plasma morphine and morphine analgesia. Long term sucrose feeding either/or initiates a mechanism that inhibits the tonic release of endogenous opioids or brings about a decrease in endogenous opioid functions or a mismatch between the rate of synthesis and a nearly continuous demand for its secretion. Any change in physiology resulting from sucrose exposure may be reversible. Nonetheless, an absolute or a relative decrease of endogenous opioids is hypothesised to lead to heightened sensitivity to pain. The results establish a close relationship between palatable food, opioids and nociceptive behaviour. It is suggested that ingestion of sucrose alters the activity at both mu and kappa receptors. The effect is naloxone reversible and discontinuing this sustained sucrose feeding aggravates morphine withdrawal [54].

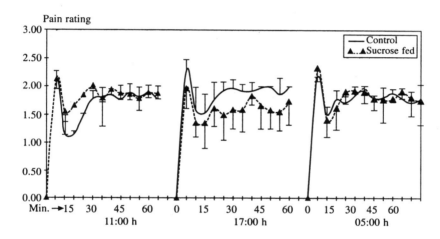

VMN lesion: Effect of sucrose feeding

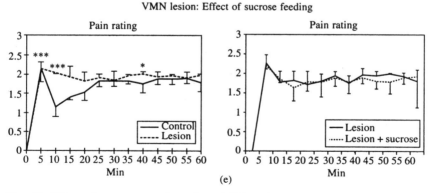

(e)

Fig. 15 Effect of acute sucrose ingestion ad libitum for 48 h (filled bars) on (a) latency, (b) threshold of tail flick, (c) simple vocalization, (d) vocalization after discharge and (e) tonic pain rating in intact and VMN lesion rats.

*Effect of Ingestion of Palatable Substance from Weaning to
Adulthood on Pain Behaviour*

Sucrose feeding for a few min to hours alters the pain behaviour of an
individual, however it is not known whether a prolonged, continued access
to sucrose in addition to normal diet during growth and development also
influences the pain responses in adults. We studied the responses to noxious
stimuli in rats having access to sucrose solution besides food and water after
weaning to adulthood. Most children during their period of growth may
receive such a favourable attention. To our surprise chronic availability vis-
à-vis ingestion of sucrose during childhood led to a highly significant decrease
in the threshold of TF, SV and VA and an increase in tonic pain rating
indicating a strong hyperalgesia.

The question now arises about the reversibility of the sucrose fed pain
modulation, which has not been addressed so far. Nonetheless, it appears
that prolonged sucrose ingestion leads to a situation akin to VMN lesion
since the hyperalgesia is comparable in both. This further supports our
previous conclusion that sucrose ingestion leads to functional inactivation
of VMN.

Influence of Gender

Palatability of the sweet ingesta, rather than its sweet content alone, may be
the critical factor in producing antinociception. Food induced pain modulation
results from an increase in central opioid activity that is dependent on the
reward value of food [43]. Since, other rewarding stimuli (electrical stimulation
of certain parts of the brain, sexual activtiy) also reduced the perception of
pain. Furthermore, the pain response is also a function of gender. It appears
that women are more sensitive to pain as compared to males. Hormones such
as estrogen and progesterone alter pain sensitivity by increasing the threshold
to painful stimulus [70].

There is an increased pain tolerance to experimental pain after ingestion
of palatable carbonated soft drinks containing glucose in healthy female
volunteers than males [71]. We studied gender specific pain response in
adult healthy volunteers systematically and objectively. We recorded the
nociceptive reflex (RIII) response. The thresholds of RIII response was
3.5 mA before sucrose ingestion in both the male and female volunteers but
after sucrose ingestion of sucrose the reflex response could not be elicited
until 11 mA in females for 5 min while in males until 15 min indicating the
shorter duration of analgesia in females than males.

There are reports of gender difference in the effect of prolonged sucrose
ingestion. Female rats at different stages of their estrous cycle were given
sucrose for 5 hours and then injected morphine. It was seen that diestrous
rats had prolonged pre morphine tail flick latencies compared to rats in
proestrous. No estrous cycle difference were seen after chronic consumption.
Also chronic consumption of sucrose attenuates hormonally induced differences

in nociception. Palatable sweet induction attenuated hormonally-induced-estrous cycle dependent differences in pain sensitivity in women.

The relationship between noxious stimuli, opioids and gonadal hormone (leutinising hormone) is reported in normal healthy volunteers, chronic headache, syndrome X patients etc. [72, 73].

We utilised a wide variety of paradigms and experimental pain models to investigate the role of VMN in pain modulation. It modulates pain through its gluco-responsive neurons which are sensitive to opioids too. However, the possibility of other neurons in integrating various other information cannot be ruled out. Nonetheless, VMN can be labelled as a pain modulation site according to the criterion set in the literature. We suggest that the functional specificity should be added to the existing list of criterion, which is being reported for VMN. The attributes of VMN modulation are described in terms of magnitude and direction of responsiveness, diurnal rhythm and reproductive functions specifically in response to palatable food.

Acknowledgement

The author sincerely appreciates the financial support from the Indian Council of Medical Research; Department of Science and Technology and All India Institute of Medical Sciences to support this research.

References

1. Dafny, N., Dong, W.Q., Prieto-Gomez, C., Reyes-Vazquez, C., Stanford, J. and Qiao, J.T. Lateral hypothalamus: site involved in pain modulation. *Neuroscience.* 1996; **70(2)**: 449–60.
2. Mayanagi, Y., Sano, K., Suzuki, I., Kanazawa, I., Aoyagi, I. and Miyachi, Y. Stimulation and coagulation of the posteromedial hypothalamus for intractable pain, with reference to beta-endorphins. *Appl Neurophysiol.* 1982; **45(1-2)**: 136–42.
3. Basbaum, A.I., Fields, H.L. Endogenous pain control systems: brainstem spinal pathways and endorphin circuitry. *Annu Rev Neurosci.* 1984; **7**: 309–338.
4. Carr, K.D., Uysal, S. Evidence of a supraspinal opioid analgesic mechanism engaged by lateral hypothalamic electrical stimulation. *Brain Res.* 1985; **335(1)**: 55–62.
5. Carstens, E., Fraunhoffer, M., Suberg, S.N. Inhibition of spinal dorsal horn neuronal responses to noxious skin heating by lateral hypothalamic stimulation in the cat. *J Neurophysiol.* 1983; **50(1)**: 192–204.
6. Gebhart, G.F., Sandkuhler, J., Thalhammer, J.G.., Zimmermann, M. Inhibition of spinal cord of nociceptive information by electrical stimulation and morphine microinjection at identical sites in midbrain of the cat. *J. Neurophysiol.* 1984; **51**: 75–89.
7. Lopez, R., Cox, V.C. Analgesia for tonic pain by self-administered lateral hypothalamic stimulation. *Neuroreport.* 1992; **3(4)**: 311–4.
8. Sinha. R., Sharma, R., Mathur, R., Nayar, U. Hypothalamo-limbic involvement in modulation of tooth-pulp stimulation evoked nociceptive response in rats. *Ind J.Physiol Pharmacol* 1999; **43(3)**: 323–331.

9. Nayar, U., Sharma, R., Sinha, R., Narasaiah, M. and Mathur, R. Endogenous pain control mechanisms. In : G.P. Dureja and T.S. Jayalakshmi (eds.), Current trends in pain research and therapy: Advances in pain research and therapy. 1996; 9–16.

10. Sikdar, S.K., Oomura, Y., Selective inhibition of glucose sensitive neurons in rat lateral hypothalamus by noxious stimuli and morphine. *J. Neurophysiol* 1985; **53** (1):17–31.

11. Jain, S., Functional recovery following neural tissue transplant in amygdalar-hypothalamic lesioned rats. Ph.D thesis submitted to AIIMS, New Delhi; 1997.

12. Wang, Q.A., Mao, L.M., Han, J.S. Analgesia from electrical stimulation of the hypothalamic arcuate nucleus in pentobarbital anaesthetised rats. 1990; **526 (2)**: 221–227.

13. Basbaum, A.I., Marley, N.J., O'Keefe, J., Clanton, C.H. Reversal of morphine and stimulus-produced analgesia by subtotal spinal cord lesions. *Pain*. 1977; **3(1)**: 43–56.

14. Truesdell, L.S., Bodnar, R.J., Reduction in cold water swim analgesia following hypothalamic paraventricular nucleus lesions. *Physiol. Behav.* 1987; **29**: 727–731.

15. Swanson, L.W., Immunohistochemical evidence for a neurophysin containing autonomic pathway arising in the paraventricular nucleus of the hypothalamus. *Brain Res.* 1977; **128**: 356–363.

16. Terman, G.W., Shavit, Y., Lewis, J.W., Cannon, J.T., Liebeskind, J.C. Intrinsic mechanisms of pain inhibition: activation by stress. *Science*. 1984; **226**(4680) : 1270–1277.

17. Frye, C.A., Cuevas, C,A,, Kanarek, R,B., Diet and estrous cycle influence pain sensitivity in rats. Pharmacol Biochem Behav. 1993; **45(1)**: 255–60.

18. Rhodes, D.L., Periventricular system lesions and stimulation-produced analgesia. *Pain* 1979; **7(1)**: 51–63.

19. Tseng, L.F., Mechanisms of Endorphin-Induced Antinociception. In: Tseng LF (ed.), The Pharmacology of Opioid Peptides. Harwood Academic Publishers, USA, 1995.

20. Turner, S.G., Sechzer, J.A., Liebelt, R.A., Sensitivity to electric shock after ventromedial hypothalamic lesions. *Exp Neurol.* 1967; **19(2)**: 236–44.

21. Ono, T., Nishino, H., Fukuda, M., Sasaki, K., Muramoto, K., Oomura, Y., Glucoresponsive neurons in rat ventromedial hypothalamic tissue slices in vitro. *Brain. Res.* 1982; **232**: 494–499.

22. Minami, T., Oomura, Y., Sugimori, M., Ionic basis for the electroresponsiveness of guinea-pig ventromedial hypothalamic neurones in vitro. *J Physiol.* 1986; **380**: 145–156.

23. Oomura, Y., Oomura, H., Sugimori, M., Nakamura, T., Yamada, Y., Glucose inhibition of the glucose sensitive neuron in the rat lateral hypothalamus. *Nature* (Lond.) 1974; **247**: 284–286.

24. Brown, J., Effects of 2-deoxyglucose on carbohydrate metabolism: review of the literature and studies in the rat. *Metabolism* 1962; **11**: 1098–1112.

25. Oomura, Y., Shimizu, N., Miyahara, S., Hattori, K., Chemosensitive neurons in the hypothalamus. Do they relate to feeding behavior? In: Hoebel BG, Novin D. Brunswick, ME (eds.) The neural basis of feeding and reward: Haer Institute for Electrophysiological Research 1982; 551–556.

26. Desiraju, T., Banerjee, M.G., Anand, B.K., Activity of single neurons in the hypothalamic feeding centers: effects of 2-deoxy-D glucose. *Physiol. Behav.* 1968; **3**: 757–760.

27. Oomura, Y., Ono, T., Ooyama, J., Wayner, M.J. Glucose and Osmosensitive neurons of the rat hypothalmus. *Nature (London)* 1969; **222**: 282–284.

28. Oomura, Y., Significance of Glucose, Insulin, and Fatty Acid on the Hypothalamic Feeding and Satiety Neurons. In: Novin, D., Wyrwicka, W., Bray, G. (eds). Hunger Basic Mechanisms and Clinical Implications. Raven Press, New York, 1976.

29. Ono, T., Oomura, Y., Nishino, H., Sasaki, K., Fukuda, M., Muramoto, K., Neural mechanisms of feeding behaviors. In : Katsuki Y, Norgren R, Sato M (eds). Brain Mechanisms of Sensation. Wiley, New York 1981; 271–286.

30. Oomura, Y., Input-output organization in the hypothalamus relating to food intake behavior. In: Morgane, P.J., Panksepp J (eds.) Handbook of the hypothalamus, Dekker, New York 1980; **2**: 557–620.

31. Oomura, Y., Glucose as a regulator of neuronal activity. In advances in metabolic disorders. *Adv Metab Disord* 1983; **10**: 31–65.

32. Oomura, Y., Ono, T., Ooyama, H. Inhibitory action of the amygdala on the lateral hypothalamic area in rats. *Nature (London)*. 1970; **228**: 1108–1110.

33. Oomura, Y., Nakamura, T., Manchanda, S.K., Excitatory and inhibitory effects of globus pallidus and substantia nigra on the lateral hypothalamic activity in the rat. *Pharmacol Biochem Behav.* 1975; Suppl **1.3**: 23–36.

34. Jain, S., Mathur, R., Sharma, R., Nayar, U. Effect of tonic pain on schedule specific feeding behaviour. *Indian Journal of Experimental Biology.* 2000; **38**: 834–836.

35. Mukherjee, K., Hypothalamic correlations between nociception and ingestive behaviour in rats. Ph.D. thesis submitted to AIIMS, 1998.

36. Mukherjee, K., Mathur, R., Nayar, U., Nociceptive responses to chronic stress of restrain and noxious stimuli in sucrose fed rats. *Stress and Health* 2001; **17**: 297–305.

37. Porro, C.A., Tassinari, G., Facchinetti, F., Panerai, A.E., Carli, G. Central beta-endorphin system involvement in the reaction to acute tonic pain. *Exp Brain Res.* 1991; **83(3)**: 549–54.

38. Facchinetti, F., Tassinari, G., Porro, C.A., Galetti, A., Genazzani, A.R., Central changes of beta-endorphin-like immunoreactivity during rat tonic pain differ from those of purified beta-endorphin. *Pain.* 1992; **49(1)**:113–116.

39. Oka, T., Oka, K., Hosoi, M., Aou, S., Hori, T., The opposing effects of interleukin -1 beta microinjected into the preoptic hypothalamus and the ventromedial hypothalamus on nociceptive behavior in rats. *Brain Res.* 1995; **700(1-2)**: 271–278.

40. Ono, T., Oomura, Y., Nishino, H., Sasaki, K., Muramoto, K., Yano, I., Morphine and enkephalin effects on hypothalamic glucoresponsive neurons. *Brain Res.* 1980; **185**: 208–12.

41. Yanaura, S., Tagashira, E., Suzuki, T. Physical dependence on morphine, phenobarbital and diazepam in rats by drug-admixed food ingestion. *Jap. J. Pharmacol.* 1975; **25**: 453–463.

42. Risner, M.E., Khavari, K.A. Morphine dependence in rats produced after five days of ingestion. *Psychopharmacologia* (Berl.) 1973; **28**: 51–62.

43. Dum, J., Gramsch, C., Herz, A. Activation of hypothalamic beta-endorphin pools by reward induced by highly palatable food. *Pharmacol Biochem. Behav.* 1983; **18**: 443–447.

44. Bodnar, R.J., Romer, M.J., Ekramer, E. Organic variables and pain inhibition: Role of gender and aging. *Brain Res. Bull.* 1988; **21**: 947–945.

45. Pittman, Q.J., Blume, H.W., Kearney, R.E., Renaud, C.P. Influence of midbrain stimulation on excitability of neurons in the medial hypothalamus of rats. *Brain Res.* 1979; **174**: 39–53.

46. Dafny, N., The hypothalamus exhibits electrophysiologic evidence for morphine tolerance and dependence. *Exp Neurol.* 1982; **77(1)**: 66–77.

47. Eidelberg, E., Bond, M.L. Effects of morphine and antagonists on hypothalamic cell activity. *Arch Int Pharmacodyn Ther.* 1972; **196(1)**: 16–24.

48. Gomez, B.P., Vasquez, C.R., Dafney, N. Microiontophoretic application of morphine and naloxone to neurons in hypothalamus of rat. *Neuropharmacol.* 1984; **23(9)**: 1081–1089.

49. Lakoski, J.M., Gebhart, G.F. Depression of neuronal activity in the hypothalamic ventromedial nucleus of the rat following microinjection of morphine in the amygdala or the periaqueductal gray. *Neuroscience* 1984; **12(1)**: 255–266.

50. Sharma, R., Sinha, R., Mathur, R., Nayar, U., Neuronal responses of periaqueductal gray to peripheral noxious stimulation. *Ind. J. Physiol. Pharmacol.* 1999; **43 (4)**: 449–457.

51. Kanarek, R.B., White, E.S., Biegen, M.T., Marks, K.R. Dietary influence on morphine-induced analgesia in rats. Pharmacol. *Biochem. Behav.* 1991; **38**: 681–684.

52. Marks, K.R., Karnarek, R.B., Delanty, S.N. Sweet-tasting solution modify the analgesic properties of morphine in rats. *FASEB* 1988; **2**: A1567.

53. Roane, D.S., Martin, R.J., Continuous sucrose feeding decrease pain threshold and increase morphine potency. *Pharma. Biochem. Behav.* 1990; **35**: 225–229.

54. Schoenbaum, G.M., Martin, R., Roane, D. Discontinuation of sustained sucrose-feeding aggravates morphine withdrawal. *Brain Res. Bull* 1990; **24**: 565–568.

55. Blass, E.M., Fitzgerald, E., Keoe, P., Interactions between sucrose, pain and isolation distress. *Pharmacol. Biochem. Behav.* 1987; **26(3)**: 483–489.

56. D'Anci, K.E., Kanarek, R.B., Marks-Kaufman, R., Duration of sucrose availability differentially alters morphine-induced analgesia in rats. *Pharmacol. Biochem. Behav.* 1996; **54**: 693–697.

57. Holder, M.D., Responsivity to pain in rats changed by the ingestion of flavoured water. *Behav. Neurl. Biol.* 1988; **49**: 45–53.

58. Morley, J.E., Levine, A.S., Yim, G.K., Lowey, M.T., Opioid modulation of appetite. *Neurosci Behav Rev* 1983; **7**: 281–305.

59. Marks, K.R., Increased fat consumption induced by morphine administration in rats. *Pharmacol. Biochem. Behav.* 1982; **16**: 949–955.

60. Belluzzi, J.D., Stein, L.. Endorphin mediation of feeding. In: Hoebel BG, Novin D (eds.) The neural basis of feeding and reward. Brunswick ME : Haer Institute 1982, 479–84.

61. Dutta, R., Mukherjee, K., Mathur, R., Effect of VMH lesion on sucrose-fed analgesia in formalin pain. *Jpn J Physiol.* 2001; **51(1)**: 63–69.

62. Mukherjee, K., Mathur, R., Nayar, U., Effect of VMH lesion on sucrose fed nociceptive responses. *Jpn J. Physiol.* 2000; **50 (4)**: 395–404.

63. Mukherjee, K., Mathur, R., Nayar, U., Ventromedial hypothalamic mediation of sucrose feeding induced pain modulation. *Pharmacol. Biochem. Behav.* 2001; **68 (1)**: 43–48.

64. Mukherjee, K., Mathur, R., Nayar, U., Hyperalgesic response in rats fed sucrose from weaning to adulthood: Role of VMH. *Pharmacol. Biochem. Behav.* 2002; **73(3)**: 601–610.

65. Bhattacharjee, M., Role of palatability on the nociceptive status of adult volunteers. M.D. thesis submitted to AIIMS, 2002.

66. Blass, E.M., Lisa, B., Hoffmeyer, M.A., Sucrose as an analgesic for newborn infants. *Paediatrics* 1991; **87**: 215–218.

67. Mohan, C.G., Risucci, D.A., Casimir, M., Gulrajani-LaCorte, M., Comparison of analgesics in ameliorating the pain of circumcision. *J Perinatol.* 1998; **18(1)**: 13–19.

68. Kanarek, B.R., Jeanne, P., D'Anci, K.E., Marks, K.R., Dietary modulation of Mu and Kappa opioid receptor-mediated analgesia. *Pharmacol. Biochem. Behav.* 1997; **58** (1): 43–49.

69. Blass, E.M., Shide, D.J., Weller, A., Stress reducing effects of ingesting milk, sugar and fats. *Ann NY Acad. Sci.* 1989; **575**: 292–305.

70. Frye, Ca, Bock, B.C., Kanarek, R.B., Hormonal milieu effects tail flick latency in female rats and may be attenuated by access to sucrose. *Physiol. and Behav* 1992; **52**: 699–706.

71. Mercer, E., Holder, M.D. Antinociceptive effects of palatable sweet ingesta on human responsivity to pressure pain. *Physiol. Behaviour.* 1997; **61(2)**: 311–318.

72. Stoffel E.F., Ulibarri, C.M., Folk, J.E., Rice, K.C., Craft, R.M. Gonadal hormone modulation of mu, kappa, and delta opioid antinociception in male and female rats. *Pain* 2005; **6(4)**: 261–74.

73. Holtman, J.R., Wala, E.P. Characterization of morphine-induced by hyperalgesia in male and female rats. *Pain* 2005; **114(1-2)**: 62–70.

74. Alreja, M., Mutalik, P., Nayar, U., Manchanda, S.K., The formalin test: a tonic pain model in the primate, *Pain*, 1977; **20**: 97–105.

6. Physiologically Significant Role in Emotional Learning, Memory and Autonomic Activity of Acidic Fibroblast Growth Factor

Yutaka Oomura

Department of Integrated Physiology, Faculty of Medicine, Kyushu University,
Fukuoka 812-0054, Japan

Abstract. Acidic fibroblast growth factor (aFGF) in the cerebrospinal fluid
(CSF) markedly increases during food intake. The ependymal cells located
in the III cerebral ventricle release aFGF in responding to an increase in the
glucose in the CSF during feeding. Released aFGF diffused into the brain
parenchyma and was taken by neurons in the hypothalamus and hippocampus
etc. Food intake was suppressed by aFGF reached to the lateral hypothalamic
area. The minimum suppressive dose of aFGF applied into the III cerebral
ventricle was picomole order and anti-FGF antibody facilitated food intake.
Emotional and spatial learning and memory were significantly more reliable
after taking aFGF in the hippocampus. At the cellular level to study the
learning and memory process long-term potentiation on CA1 neurons in
hippocamal slice preparations was also dose dependently facilitated by aFGF.
Marked dose dependent increases in plasma ACTH and corticosterone were
detected from 20 min to 2 h after intracerebroventricular or intravenous
administration of aFGF. Plasma epinephrine and norepinephrine also increased
for upto 120 min. Concomitant increases occurred in the activity in the
efferent sympathetic nerves as well as the body temperature. These findings
suggest that aFGF activates the hypothalamic-pituitary-adrenal axis and
sympathetic outflow. The phagocytosis in peritoneal macrophages was
enhanced by aFGF in a dose dependent manner. These results indicate that
aFGF is not only the most potent substance yet found for the suppression of
feeding, but it is also extremely effective substance as a memory facilitation,
sympathetic efferent as well as biodefence activations.

Acidic Fibroblast Growth Factor (aFGF) Increased in Cerebrospinal (CSF) During Food Intake

The aFGF is potent mitogens and is present throughout the nervous system. A
postprandial increase in aFGF was detected in rat CSF, and a dose dependent
increase was also observed after intraperitoneal (IP) injections of 7-300 mg/kg
of glucose (Fig. 1 upper and inset) [1]. The concentration of aFGF in CSF
which was 11.0 ± 3.0 pg/ml (0.73 ± 0.2 pmol) in prefeeding state, increased

to 10 ng/ml (0.7 nmol) 2 h after feeding. In rats, intra third cerebral ventricle (III ICV) microinfusion of aFGF (50-200 ng/rat), 1 h before dark period, dose responsively suppressed food intake whereas central infusion of inactivated aFGF was ineffective. The minimum effective dose of aFGF was 3.3 pmol, without influence on water intake. The III ICV infusion of 400-8000 ng/rat of the first 15 amino acide of aFGF (aFGF$_{1-15}$), 1 h before dark period, dose dependently decreased food intake for 3 and 8 h, respectively. Whole nighttime food intake (for 8 h), for example, decreased significantly (paired Student's *t*-test, $p < 0.01$) by almost 2 and 3 g from the control intake with the infusion of 400 and 800 ng, respectively. The aFGF$_{1-15}$ is 1/6 as potent as the complete aFGF [2]. The [16AL] aFGF$_{1-29}$ had about 4 times potency compared with that of aFGF$_{1-15}$. All of these fractions of aFGF had no mitogenic activity.

Modulation by Antibodies of Anti-aFGF on Food Intake

The night-time and total daily food intake were significantly (paired Student's *t*-test, $p < 0.05$) increased by bilateral intralateral hypothalamic area (LHA, feeding center) administration of anti-aFGF antibody (total 240 ng/rat) when applied at 1900 [2]. Daytime food intake was not changed. The increase in food intake, for example, was 1.2 g for the first 3 h at nighttime and 2 g for the whole nighttime (for 8 h) in both cases. Infusion of 240 ng/rat preimmune immunoglobulin (IgG) did not affect on food intake.

The antibody of the aFGF$_{1-15}$ fraction (240 ng/rat) effectively increased food intake. The increase in food intake was 1.6 g for the first 3 h at nighttime. This result was probably due to the effective blockade of binding on the receptor sites by the anti-aFGF$_{1-15}$ antibody. The net result would appear as a decrease in the effectiveness of the total aFGF population.

Effects of aFGF on Neurons in the LHA and Ventromedial Hypothalamic Nucleus (VMH)

Effect of aFGF on Glucose-Sensitive Neurons in the LHA

The neuronal activity of glucose-sensitive neurons (GSNs) in the LHA was reversively suppressed with long latency and duration by electrophoretic applications of aFGF using multibarrel glass capillary technique (Fig. 1, lower) [1]. The latency of the suppression of aFGF was 7.0 ± 2.3 min and the duration was 10.6 ± 4.1 min. The difference in effects of aFGF on GSNs and nonGSNs was statistically significant (χ^2-test, $p < 0.01$). To explain the extremely long latency and duration of the aFGF effect on GSNs, we examined the effects of a direct activator of protein kinase C, 1-oleoyl-2-acetylglycerol (OAG) on 42 LHA neurons. The effects of OAG on 16 neurons out of the 42 were nearly identical to the effects of aFGF, including the long latency and duration [2]. The effect of aFGF on GSNs may be through its activation of protein kinase C. Neurons in the VMH, satiety center, were not affected by aFGF.

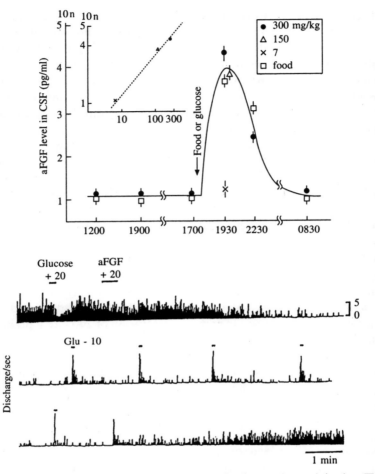

Fig. 1. Top: aFGF change in CSF before and after feeding or glucose injection. □, food intake. ●, △, ×, glucose, IP injection. Mean ± SD, $n = 7$. Inset: Dose dependent effect of glucose injection; symbols, same as above; mean values only. Bottom: Effects of electrophoretic application of aFGF on LHA glucose-sensitive neuron. Record, from top to bottom. Upper bars: Application time of indicated substances at current specified (nA). Glucose, inhibitory effect. aFGF inhibition after latency of about 6 min, and this lasts for 16 min. Glu, excitation by glutamate, nonspecific excitant, during aFGF inhibition (reproduced with permission from [1]).

Localization of FGF Receptor

The localization of FGF receptor-1 in rat brain by immunohistochemistry using a polyclonal antibody against an acidic peptide sequence of chicken FGF receptor-1 was investigated [6]. Positive neurons were distributed widely in various brain regions, but were particularly abundant in such regions as the LHA, substantia nigra, locus coeruleus and raphe unclei. The FGF receptor-1 could not be found in the VMH neurons.

Production of aFGF in the Brain

Histochemical staining of the brain with anti-aFGF antibody usually revealed aFGF in ependymal cells in the III cerebral ventricle walls [3]. However, 2 h after a meal or a 300 mg/kg glucose IP injection, the ependymal cells were clear and aFGF appeared in neurons in the LHA, dorsomedial septum, hippocampus, amygdale, and other central regions, but not in the VMH [2, 3]. When cDNA of the 30-100 base from the middle part of aFGF were synthesized and hybridized, only ependymal cells were stained [2, 3]. This revealed mRNA in the ependymal cells only, so aFGF is produced in those cells.

New Type of Glucose Sensor

To clarify this migration of aFGF, the glucose (0.2 mg/10 μl, 3.3 mM, at 300 μl of CSF volume) was applied directly III ICV and the level of aFGF was determined by *Hydra* bioassay [1]. After meal, glucose in CSF doubles from 2 to 4 mM. Before the glucose injection, aFGF level in CSF was 0.7 pmol, within 15 min this increased to 2.6 nmol; it peaked at 7.5 nmol at 45-60 min; decreased to 0.7 nmol at 2 h, and returned to 4.6 pmol at 3 h. The same amount of mannitol or Krebs Ringer solution injection had no effect. The minimum effective dose of 3.3 pmol to suppress feeding is thus well within the physiological limits. This action of glucose on ependymal cells to release aFGF is complementary to the action of glucose on pancreatic β cells to release insulin. Also the same as β cells, aFGF is released by III ICV applications of L-leucine or arginine. Production and release of aFGF is thus an endocrine phenomenon in the brain that is parallel to a visceral phenomenon.

Plastic Effect of aFGF on the Hippocampus

The neuronal uptake of aFGF in the hippocampus 2 h after meal or glucose IP injection led us to investigate the plastic effects of endogenous and exogenous aFGF [4].

Emotional Learning and Memory: Passive Avoidance Task

Four group of mice were injected IP with 300 mg/kg glucose 1, 2, 3 or 5 h before giving electric shock when they entered a dark box (acquisition). After 24 h the same trials were repeatd (retention, affective memory). Fig. 2 (upper) shows that behavior of the 1, 3 and 5 h groups were not significantly different from that of the controls. Mice injected with Krebs Ringer solution were the controls. The latency of the 2 h group to enter the dark box, 68.5 ± 14.2 s (mean $\pm$ SEM, $n = 19$) was significantly longer than that of the controls, 15.2 ± 2.3 s (Student's t-test, $p < 0.002$, $n = 20$) and that of the 1, 2 and 5 h groups [4]. In similar trials, anti-aFGF antibody (total 2.2 μg/mouse, bilateral) was administrated III ICV and glucose was injected 30 min later. Based on the first trials as controls, all comparisons were made after 2 h. In these trails, the latency, 26.6 ± 7.3 s ($n = 19$), tended to be longer than the acquisition time,

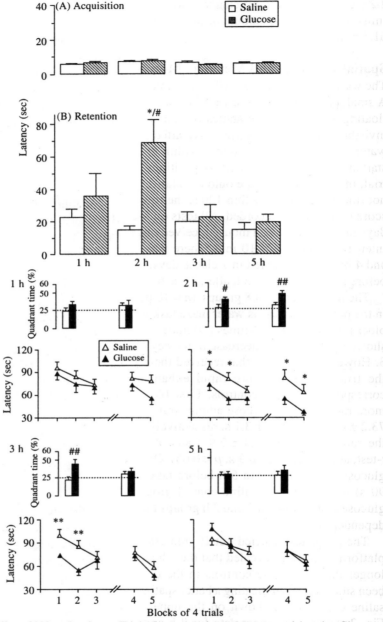

Fig. 2. Effect of 300 mg/kg glucose IP injection on learning and memory task by mice. Glucose or control saline administered at various times before the task. Upper: Passive avoidance task. Retention trial, carried out 24 h after acquisition trial. Ordinates: Latency (mean ± SEM) for acquisition trial, (A) and retention trial (B) $n = 20$ for each group. *$p < 0.002$ (vs 2 h saline group, t-test); #$p < 0.04, 0.02, 0.002$ (vs 1 h, 3 h and 5 h glucose groups, respectively; one-way ANOVA followed by Fisher's PLSD). Lower: Water maze task $n = 8$ for each group. Latency to escape onto the platform, shown for each block (mean ± SEM). Mean time spent in platform quadrant in the 100 s after the last trial of block 2 and 4 (probe test; shown as a percentage) is shown in the insets for glucose group (filled bar) and saline group (open bar). *$p < 0.05$, **$p < 0.01$ (vs saline group of the same block, t-test); #$p < 0.05$, ##$p < 0.01$ (vs saline group, t-test) (reproduced with permission from [4]).

8.2 ± 0.7 s, but was significantly shorter than that of the glucose alone group. Infusion of the same amount of preimmune IgG did not affect the retention, 61.3 ± 13.2 s ($n = 19$).

Spatial Learning and Memory: Morris Water Maze Task

The water maze pool was a 100 cm diameter, 20 cm deep plastic water tank. A small platform was fixed 1 cm below surface of the water made opaque by floating styrene foam granules on the surface such that the platform was invisible to the mouse. A trial was started by placing a mouse by and into the water at one of four locations. Within each block of 4 trials, each mouse started at each of the 4 starting positions, was changed randomly. In each trial, the latency to escape onto the platform was recorded. If the mouse did not find the platform within 120 s, the trial was terminated and a maximum score of 120 s was recorded. All tests on one mouse were done on alternate days in one week. Each mouse received one block of 4 trials in one day with inter-trial intervals of 10 min. There was one day interval between block, and 4 blocks were tested in 7 elapse days. Food was deprived from 7 to 10 h before the trials until to 3 h after, in each testing day.

The mean latency of 8 groups ($n = 10$ per group) to climb on the platform in the pool in the Morris water maze task was measured [4]. Each point (one block) is the mean of 4 times (10 mice × 4 times each). Generally the mice showed a progressive decrease in latency as they underwent blocks 1, 2 and 3. However, only mice that received their glucose injection 2 or 3 h before the trial showed a more rapid enhancement of performance than the corresponding saline controls. First block performance was significantly more rapid after IP glucose administration 2 and 3 h before each first trial, 73.2 ± 6.8 s and 73.4 ± 3.1 s, respectively, than after saline administration at the same intervals, 96.4 ± 7.9 s and 99.8 ± 5.2 s, respectively (Student's t-test, at 2 h, $p < 0.01$, at 3 h, $p < 0.05$). On the other hand, mice that received glucose injections 1 and 5 h before task, had latencies similar (more than 90 s) to those of the saline control group. These results indicate that the glucose application on 2 and 3 h groups facilitated spatial memory with time dependent inducton.

The probe test, carried out 10 min after the last trail in block 2 with the platform removed, revealed that the 2 h and 3 h glucose injected mice spent longer than the saline controls in the quadrant in which the platform had been situated, thus indicating a better spatial awareness than the corresponding saline controls. As shown on the upper side of the appropriate insets in Fig. 2 (lower), the exact data for 2 h and 3 h groups were 38.0 ± 2.4 s vs 26.1 ± 4.5 s and 43.7 ± 5.3 s vs 22.0 ± 4.0 s, respectively (Student's t-test, $p < 0.05$ and < 0.01 for the 2 h and 3 h groups).

Afer a no-test interval of three days for extinction, the platform was moved and the mice trained to learn the new location (blocks 4 and 5, Fig. 2, lower). All mice showed a rapid decrease in latency between block 4 and 5.

However, a statistically significant difference between the glucose and saline groups was observed, only in the groups injected 2 h before the trials (repeated-measures ANOVA).

Either anti-aFGF antibody (total 2.2 µg/mouse, bilateral, $n = 18$) or the preimmune IgG ($n = 8$) was applied to mice 30 min before glucose injection. The latency of the antibody (plus glucose) group to climb on the platform, 98.5 ± 3.0 s, was significantly longer than that of the control IgG (plus glucose) group, 81.4 ± 6.4 s, in the first block (Student's t-test, $p < 0.05$).

The probe test also showed a better spatial awareness by the IgG plus glucose group than by the IgG plus saline group (*post hoc* Fisher's PLSD, $p < 0.001$). However, preinjection of the anti-aFGF antibody completely abolished the glucose induced effects.

These indicate that facilitation of spatial memory by glucose was due to aFGF in the central nervous system.

Electrophysiological Basis on the Plastic Effect of aFGF

Effects of aFGF (0.5-25 ng/ml) on synaptic transmission were investigated in rat hippocampal slice preparations[5]. Stimulaton was applied to the Schaffer collateral/commissural afferents and evoked synaptic potentials were recorded at the apical dendrites in CA1 pyramidal cell layer. When brief tetanic stimulation (7 pulses at 100 Hz) was applied just after the perfusion of aFGF for 30 min, evoked synaptic potentials increased in magnitude after the tetanus and facilitated the generation of long-term potentiation (LTP) as shown in Fig. 3. These effects of aFGF were dose dependent. The facilitation of LTP was not evident when aFGF was applied immediately or 10 min after the tetanus. Similar facilitations were obtained by $aFGF_{1-15}$ (100-400 ng/ml). The results suggest that aFGF modulates synaptic efficacy through FGF receptor-1[6] and can facilitate learning and memory through mechanisms related to the generation of LTP. The hippocampal CA1 neurons take up aFGF released from the ependymal cells during food intake. Therefore, feeding is important, because it not only maintains body energy homeostasis, but also leads to preparation of readiness for memory facilitation.

Effect of aFGF on the Hypothalamic-Pituitary-Adrenal Axis

During food intake, released aFGF in the brain parenchyma reaches the parvocellular paraventricular nucleus (pPVN) and facilitates the neuronal activity, thus activates the hypothalamic-pituitary-adrenal axis (HPA-A) [7].

Modulation of Plasma Corticosterone and ACTH by aFGF

Marked increases in plasma corticosterone were evoked in a dose dependent manner in response to III ICV administrated aFGF (at 1 and 10 ng, Fig. 4a). The corticosterone levels reached a maximal level at 60 min and remained elevated for upto a further 120 min after the administration. The integrated corticosterone responses (for the 180 min after the administration) also showed

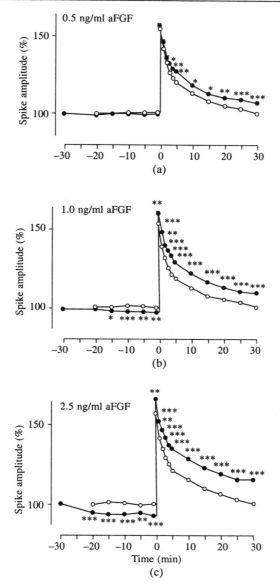

Fig. 3. Effect of aFGF on long-term potentiation on CA1 neurons in hippocampal slices induced by 7 pulses at 100 Hz tetanus. Ordinate: Evoked synaptic potential amplitude expressed % change of mean basal evoked synaptic amplitude before tetanic stimulation defined as 100%. After the control potentiation (open circles) induced by the first tetanus was observed for 30 min in Krebs Ringer solution, aFGF was perfused for 30 min. The second tetanic stimulation was applied 30 min after beginning of aFGF perfusion (A, B and C). Effect of 0.5 ($n = 5$), 1.0 ($n = 9$) and 2.5 ($n = 9$) ng/ml aFGF on potentiation (filled circles) induced by the second tetanic stimulation, respectively, *$p < 0.05$, **$p < 0.01$, ***$p < 0.001$ (reproduced with permission from [5]).

a dose dependent increase (Fig. 4a, inset). When 10 ng aFGF was administered via the III ICV route, the ACTH concentration was already increased significantly at 5 min after the injection; it continued to increase and peaked at 15 min after the injection (Fig. 4b). Thereafter, it gradually decreased, but remained elevated until 150 min after the injection, it had returned to the basal level at 180 min. At this time, the plasma corticosterone was still at an

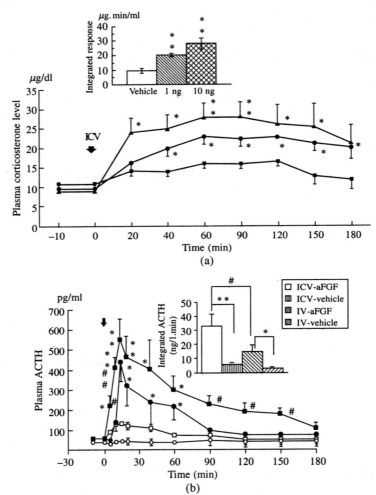

Fig. 4. Effect of aFGF administration on plasma corticosterone and ACTH. (a) III ICV administration of aFGF on plasma corticosterone. ■, vehicle, $n = 6$; ●, aFGF 1 ng/rat, $n = 7$; ■, aFGF 10 ng/rat, $n = 5$. Inset: Corticosterone responses integrated over 180 min after administration of aFGF. Mean ± SE., *$P < 0.05$, **$p < 0.01$ (10 ng/rat) vs vehicle applied (at arrow). (b) III ICV or IV administration of aFGF on plasma ACTH. ■, ICV aFGF, $n = 6$;. □, ICV vehicle, $n = 5$; ●, IV aFGF; ○, IV vehicle, $n = 5$. #$p < 0.05$ vs IV aFGF (reproduced with permission from [8]).

elevated plateau level after its peak at 60 min (Fig. 4a). Fig. 4b shows that the responses of ACTH to aFGF administrated via this route were significantly greater than those evoked via the intravenous (IV) route, the integrated responses in the former experiments being greater than those in the latter by almost twofold at 1 ng and 1.4 fold at 10 ng ($P < 0.05$ in each case). The pretreatment with anti-CRH antibody ICV significantly attenuated the increase in corticosterone evoked by ICV administration of aFGF, but had almost no effect on the response to its IV administration. These pieces of evidences suggest that endogenous aFGF (given ICV) directly stimulates CRH secretion from pPVN neurons and that this CRH then activates the HPA-A.

The aFGF concentration in the CSF may be within the physiological range after an ICV administration of 10 ng (0.7×10^{-12} mol) aFGF. In fact, if we assume that the total volume of the rat CSF is 300 µl, the concentration of aFGF in the CSF would be 2 pmol/ml. This would seem to lie within the normal range, because the aFGF concentration in rat CSF increases from 0.7 pmol/ml to 0.7 nmol/ml at 15 min, 7.5 nmol at 45 min and 4.6 mpol/ml at 3 h after 4 mM glucose application into the cerebral ventricle [9] and after food intake [1]. The figure of 4 mM glucose corresponds to the glucose level in the CSF after food intake or IP injection of 300 mg/kg glucose [1].

Plasma Catecholamine and aFGF
Administration of 1 to 10 ng/rat aFGF III ICV induced dose dependent increases in the plasma levels of both epinephrine (Epi) and norepinephrine (NE) [10]. A significant increase to 250 pg/ml by 1ng and 600 pg/ml by 10 ng aFGF in Epi from the basal 150 pg/ml was first detected at 60 min, and the response seemed to be peaking at 150 min (600 pg/ml, by 1 ng; 1700 pg by 10 ng). At 180 min after aFGF administration (when sampling ended), it was showing no sign of returning to the basal level. Similar changes we observed in plasma NE levels. Injection of heat-treated aFGF (10 ng) induced no such increases in plasma catecholamines. The similar increases in Epi and NE were also occurred by IV injection of aFGF, though in the absolute terms, aFGF via this route showed almost one-tenth size compared with that via the ICV route.

Activation of Sympathetic Efferent Outflow Caused by aFGF
In response to applications of 10 ng aFGF III ICV the sympathetic efferent discharges in the adrenal nerve showed a clear increase (in term of the multi-unit discharge rate) starting at 15 min and reaching significance at or before 30 min (Fig. 5a). The mean discharge rate showed a dose dependent increase, and the increases induced by 1 or 10 ng/rat aFGF were both significantly greater than that induced by vehicle (Fig. 5a, inset). When IV administrated 10 ng/rat aFGF again markedly facilitated the discharge (Fig. 5b). By comparison with the basal level, the mean discharge rate at 90 min after the 10 ng/rat administration was increased by 86% (ICV) or 67% (IV) (Fig. 5a b,

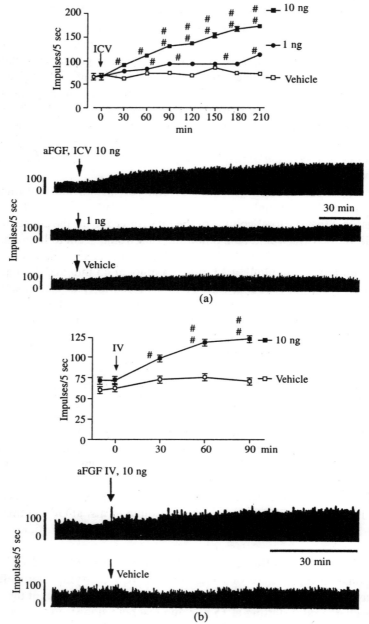

Fig. 5. Effect of III ICV or IV administration of aFGF on the efferent firing rate in a sympathetic branch of the left adrenal nerve. (a) Efferent discharge rate in response to ICV vehicle (bottom) or aFGF at 1 (middle) or 10 ng/rat (top). Inset: Mean discharge rates (±SE) for ICV vehicle ($n = 3$) and for 1 ($n = 10$) and 10 ng ICV aFGF at 10 ng (top). (b) Efferent discharge rate in response to IV vehicle (bottom) or IV aFGF at 10 ng (top). Inset: Mean discharge rates (±SE) for IV vehicle ($n = 3$) and IV 10 ng aFGF ($n = 10$). # $p < 0.05$, ## $p < 0.01$ vs vehicle control at the same time point (reproduced with permission from [10]).

inset). Quite similar activations were observed in sympathetic efferent discharge to the liver, spleen, brown adipose tissue (BAT) by aFGF administration via the two routes.

Relationship Between Neuroimmune Function and aFGF

Central Immune Activity Induced by aFGF
A further area of interest is the link between aFGF and the immune system. Splenic sympathetic natural killer cells cytotoxicity is reduced by activation of the splenic sympathetic outflow. Furthermore, it has become clear that catecholamines, as well as glucocorticoids, should be viewed as physiological inhibitors of inflammatory responses and as immunosuppressive mediators [11]. These data suggest that aFGF would be expected to affect the neuro-immune system.

Phagocytosis in Mouse Peritoneal Macrophages and aFGF
Macrophages play an important role in innate and acquired immunity. They are distributed as resident cells throughout tissues of the normal animal and express altered endocytosis and biosynthesis properties after inflammatory recruitment and immune activation. The phagocytic and digestive capacities of macrophages are initial representative responses to activate the immune system. FGF receptors (FGFR-1, 2) has been observed in monocytes which also contain FGF. The effects of aFGF and its fragments on macrophage phagocytosis including attachment and ingestion were analyzed using flow cytometry in this study [12].

aFGF enhanced the phagocytosis of latex particle in a dose dependent manner. The threshold concentration of aFGF is lower than 10^{-9} M. The enhancement of phagocytosis at 5×10^{-8} M was $202 \pm 18\%$ (mean $\pm$ SD, $n = 4$) for percentage of phagocytic cells, defined as the % of macrophages that ingested one or more particles (PP) and $249 \pm 35\%$ ($n = 4$) for the phagocytic index, defined as the average number of particles ingested per macrophage (PI), as compared to the unstimulated control phagocytosis.

Effect of aFGF Fragments on Macrophages
$aFGF_{1-15}$ had little effect at a concentration of 10^{-7} M. However, $aFGF_{1-20}$ clearly enhanced phagocytic activity. Longer fragment, $aFGF_{1-29}$ demonstrated a significant enhancement 1.4 times more compared with $aFGF_{1-20}$. By eliminating residues 1-8, the enhancement by $aFGF_{9-29}$ was slightly reduced (1.2 times more than $aFGF_{1-20}$). Among the fragments used, $aFGF_{1-29}$ was most effective in inducing the phagocytic enhancement. Fig. 6 shows $aFGF_{1-29}$ enhanced phagocytosis of latex particles in a dose dependent manner upto 10^{-6} M. The threshold concentration of $aFGF_{1-29}$ may be close to 10^{-9} M. The percentage enhancement of phagocytosis at 5×10^{-8} M was $35.5 \pm 5.5\%$ (mean $\pm$ SD, $n = 6$) for PP and $53.7 \pm 6.5\%$ ($n = 6$) for PI, compared

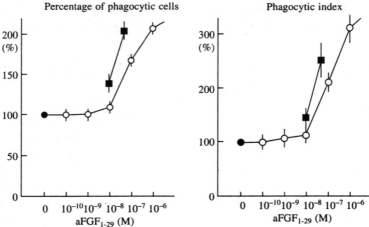

Fig. 6. Concentration-response curve showing the enhancement of phagocytosis in peritoneal macrophage by aFGF$_{1-29}$ and full length of aFGF. O: Data of aFGF$_{1-29}$, mean ± SD, $n = 6$ for all concentrations (10^{-8} M, $n = 5$). ■: Data of full length aFGF at concentrations 10^{-8} and 5×10^{-8} M ($n = 4$). The left PP and right PI graphs represented as % of control phagocytosis (100%) in the absence of aFGF (reproduced with permission from [12]).

with unstimulated conrol phagocytosis. These evidences indicate that aFGF is an immunoregulator factor as a stimulator for the immune system, although splenic natural killer cell cytotoxicity is reduced by activation of the splenic sympathetic outflow, and the antigen and antibody reaction is reduced by corticosterone released by the HPA-A activation.

Conclusion

Figure 7 (upper) shows the conclusive variegated physiological significance of aFGF and its fragments. By food intake, aFGF is released from the ependymal cells in the III cerebral ventricle which responds to an increase in glucose concentration from 2 to 4 mM in the CSF during food intake. Released aFGF diffuses into the brain parenchyma and first reaches the LHA and suppresses food intake through inhibiting the activity of GSNs which induce feeding. This inhibition is antagonized by application of anti-aFGF antibody. Secondly, aFGF reaches the hippocampus and facilitates synaptic plasticity and improves emotional and spatial learning and memory performance. Thirdly, aFGF reaches the pPVN neurons and facilitates CRH release and also activates not only HPA-A but also efferent sympathetic outflow.

Corticosterone released can also modulate the LTP in CA1 neurons [13] and promote the learning and cognitive processes [14]. In fact, the clinical data suggest that CRH deficiencies can be detected in the brain in patients with neurodegenerative dementia [15]. The parallel activation of the sympathetic outflow to the adrenal and BAT may show that aFGF has a multifunctional role in the control of neural and/or endocrinological activity.

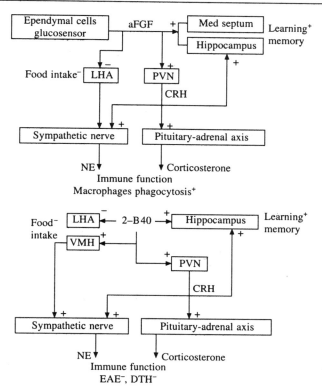

Fig. 7. Deduced physiological action of endogenous satiety substances. Upper: aFGF released by food intake. Ependymal cells located in III cerebroventricle release aFGF responding to an increase in glucose in CSF during food intake. aFGF reaches the glucose-sensitive neurons in the lateral hypothalamic area (LHA, feeding center) and inhibits the neuronal activity. aFGF reaches the hippocampus and facilitates emotional and spatial learning and memory. aFGF reaches the neurons in the parvocellular paraventricular nucleus (pPVN) and activates these neurons causing CRH release. These neurons and CRH activate efferent sympathetic outflow and pituitary-adrenal axis. Splenic sympathetic activation and released corticosterone modulate immune function. aFGF stimulates of phagocytosis of macrophages. Lower: 2-B4O increased in blood during food deprivation. The physiological concentration of 2-B4O enters in the brain. 2B4O reaches the glucose-sensitive neurons in the LHA and inhibits the neuronal activity. 2-B4O facilitates the neuronal activity in the ventromedial hypothalamic nucleus (VMH, satiety center). Thus 2-B4O is one of satiety substances; facilitates spatial learning and memory; reaches the pPVN and activates these neurons, causing CRH release. These neurons and released CRH as well as VMH facilitation, activate the efferent sympathetic outflow and pituitary-adrenal axis. Splenic sympathetic activation and released corticosterone suppress the immune function. 2-B4O also suppresses experimental allergic encephalomyelitis, model for human multiple lateral sclerosis, a typical autoimmune disease. 2-B4O also suppresses DTH, delayed-type hypersensitivity, a T-cell immune response. Thus 2-B4O is a potent suppressant of autoimmune function (reproduced with permission from [16]).

The IV administration of glucose as well as aFGF also induces a long-lasting hyperthermia of < 1°C, corresponding to the postprandial hyperthermia, in awake and freely moving rats (our unpublished observation). These results suggest that the long-lasting fever induced by exogenous aFGF given via the IV or ICV route is caused, at least in part, by activation of sympathetic nerves innervating the adrenal and BAT via the release of CRH in the brain.

Corticosterone and splenic sympathetic activation attenuates the immune function, in other words, the autoimmune reaction is reduced. That is a benefit to the living machinery. The aFGF, however, enhances the phagocytosis of the macrophages thus biodefence activity.

Figure 7 (lower) outlines the physiological significance of another endogenous satiety substance, 2-buten-4-olide (2-B4O) [16]. 2-B4O begins to increase at 24 h and peak at 48 h after food deprivation. The physiological concentration of 2-B4O enters the brain parenchyma, and first reaches the LHA and VMH, where it controls food intake. 2-B4O suppresses the neuronal activity of GSNs and facilitates that of glucoreceptor neurons in the VMH. Thus, 2-B4O acts as a satiety substance. Secondly, 2-B4O reaches the pPVN, facilitates CRH release, and activates not only the HPA-A, but also the efferent sympathetic outflows. These effects produce hyperglycemia, together with increase in the plasma Epi, NE and corticosterone levels. Thirdly, 2-B4O facilitates emotional and spatial learning and memory performance in the hippocampus through the aFGF release that occurs in response to the hyperglycemia induced by 2-B4O [17]. In addition, 2-B4O acts as an immunomodulator, suppressing the activity of the immune system. 2-B4O potentially suppresses the clinical severity of experimental allergic encephalomyelitis, a model for human multiple sclerosis and for autoimmune disease.

aFGF and 2-B4O, both endogenous satiety substances, play quite similar physiological role, albeit in the presence or absence of alimentation, respectively. These evidences indicate that food intake and deprivation, both maintain not only the body energy homeostasis but also prime the brain for important functions.

References

1. Hanai, K., Oomura, Y., Kai, Y., Nishikawa, K., Morita, H., Plata-Salamon C.R. Central action of acidic fibroblast growth factor in feeding regulation. *Am J. Physiol.*, 1989; **256**: R217–223.
2. Oomura, Y., Sasaki, K., Hanai, K. Chemical and neuronal regulation of flood intake. In: Oomura Y., Tarui, S., Baba, S. Inoue, S. (Eds). Progress in obesity research 1990; London: John Libbey, 1991: 3–12.
3. Tooyama, I., Hara, Y., Yoshihara, O., Oomura, Y., Sasaki, K., Muto, T., Suzuki, K., Hanai, K., Kimura, H. Production of antisera to acidic fibroblast growth factor and their application to immunohistochemical study in the rat brain. *Neuroscience*, 1991; **40**: 769–779.

4. Li, A.J., Oommura, Y., Sasaki, K., Suzuki, K., Tooyama, I., Hanai, K., Kimura, H., Hori, T. A single pre-training glucose injection induces memory facilitation in rodents performing various tasks: contribution of acidic fibroblast growth factor. *Neuroscience* 1998; **85**: 785–794.

5. Sasaki, K., Oomura, Y., Figrov, A., Yagi, H. Acidic fibroblast growth factor facilitates generation of long-term potentiation in rat hippocampal slices. *Brain Res. Bull.*, 1994; **33**: 505–511.

6. Matsuro, A., Tooyama, I., Isobe, S., Oomura, Y., Akiguchi, I., Hanai, K., Kimura, J., Kimura, H. Immunohistochemical localization in the rat brain of an epitope corresponding to the fibroblast growth factor receptor-1. *Neuroscience*, 1994; **60**: 49–66.

7. Sasaki, K., Oomura, Y., Urashima, T., Shiokawa, A., Tsukada, A., Kawarada, A., Yanaihara, N. Effect of acidic fibroblast growth factor on neuronal activity of the parvocellular part in rat paraventricular nucleus. *Neurobiology*, 1995; **3**: 329–338.

8. Matsumoto, I., Oomura, Y., Niijima, A., Sasaki, K., Aikawa, T. Acidic fibroblast growth factor activates hypothalamo-pituitary-adreocortical axis in rats. *Am J. Physiol.*, 1998; **274**: R503-509.

9. Oomura, Y., Sasaki, K., Suzuki, T., Muto, T., Li., A.-J, Ogita, Z., Hanai, K., Tooyama, I., Kimura, H., Yanaihara, N. New brain glucosensor and its physiological significance, *Am J Clin Nutr*, 1992; **55**: 278S-282S.

10. Matsumoto, I., Niijima, A., Oomura, Y., Sasaki, K., Tsuchiya, K., Aikawa, T. Acidic fibroblast growth factor activates adrenomedullary secretion and sympathetic outflow in rats. *Am J Physiol*, 1998; **275**: R1003–1012.

11. Van der Poll, T., Lowry, S.F. Epinephrine inhibits endotoxin-induced IL-1β production: roles of tumor necrosis factor-α and IL-10. *Am J. Physiol*, 1997; **273**: R1885–R1890.

12, Ichinose, M., Sawada, M., Sasaki, K., Oomura, Y. Enhancement of phagocytosis in mouse peritoneal macrophages by fragments of acidic fibroblast growth factor (aFGF). *Int J Immunopharmacol*, 1998; **20**: 193–204.

13. Rey, M., Carlier, E., Talmi, M., Soumireu-Mourat, B. Corticosterone effects on long-term potentiation in mouse hippocampal slices. *Neuroendocrinology*, 1994; **60**: 36–41.

14. Behan, D.P., Heinrichs, S.C., Troncoso, J.C., Liu, X.J., Kawas, C.H., Ling, N., De Souza, E.B. Displacement of corticotrophin releasing factor from its binding protein as a possible treatment for Alzheimer's disease. *Nature*, 1995; **378**: 264–287.

15. De Souza, E.B., Whitehouse, P.J., Kuhar, M.J., Price, D.L., Vale, W.W. Reciprocal changes in corticotrophin-releasing factor (CRF)-like immunoreactivity and CRF receptors in cerebral cortex of Alzheimer's disease. *Nature*, 1986; **319**: 593–595.

16. Oomura, Y., Aou, S., Matsumoto, I., Sakata, T. Physiological significance of 2-buten-4-olide (2-B4O), an endogenous satiety substance increased in the fasted state. *Exp Biol Med*, 2003; **228**: 1146–1155.

17. Li, X-L., Aou, S., Li, A.-J., Hori, T., Tooyama, I., Oomura, Y. 2-Buten-4-olide, an endogenous feeding suppressant, improves spatial performance through brain acidic fibroblast growth factor in mice. *Brain Res Bull*, 2001; **56**: 531–536.

Pain Updated: Mechanisms and Effects
Edited by R. Mathur

7. Amygdalar Influences on Pain

Suman Jain[1], M. Narasaiah[2], U. Nayar[3] and R. Mathur[1]

[1]Department of Physiology, All India Institute of Medical Sciences,
New Delhi-110029, India

[2]Department of Anatomy, School of Medicine, The University of California,
San Francisco (UCSF), CA94143, USA

[3]Department of Medicine and Medical Sciences, Arabian Gulf University,
P.O. Box 22979, Bahrain

Introduction

Pain is a universal phenomenon and yet remains a universal mystery. There is no one who has not known pain, as there is no one who understands it all. Art and science, medicine and law, all have sought to expound the philosophy of pain, but have served only to add new dimensions to the enigma. Pain is defined as "an unpleasant sensory and emotional experience associated with actual or potential tissue damage or described in terms of such damage" [1]. Pain is a subjective and multifaceted experience. It has various dimensions such as sensory, emotional and cognitive [2]. Each component of pain is mediated by different areas of the central nervous system.

The afferent pathways that convey information on noxious stimuli to the central nervous system arise from neurons of the substantia gelatinosa. Shortly after their origin they cross to the opposite side where they ascend centrally via spinothalamic tract. On reaching the brain stem, information from the spinothalamic tract is also passed to the reticular formation. These latter tracts are thought to carry afferent nerves which mediate pain provoked autonomic responses such as pupillary dilatation, swelling and the vasomotor collapse which accompanies severe pain. The spinothalamic tract ends in the thalamus. It is here that pain is thought to be processed emotionally. The greatest part of the spinothalamic tract fades out in the region of the posterior inferior ventral nucleus (NVPL), the smaller part in the intralaminar nuclei. From the specific thalamic nuclei, i.e. NVPL, it projects to the specific sensory areas in the postcentral gyrus of the cerebral cortex, where the quality of pain is consciously appreciated. From the thalamus a significant contribution of projections is also relayed to different areas of the limbic system, i.e. amygdala, hippocampus, septum, etc., which influences the emotional and motivational component of the pain [3].

The Amygdala

The amygdaloid complex is situated in the dorsomedial portion of the temporal lobe, anterior and superior to the tip of the inferior horn of the lateral ventricle. It is divided into two main nuclear masses, a corticomedial nuclear group and a basolateral nuclear group. The corticomedial amygdaloid complex has central, medial and cortical amygdaloid nuclei, the nucleus of the lateral olfactory stria and a transitionally ill differentiated anterior amygdaloid area. The basolateral amygdaloid complex is large and well differentiated and has lateral, basal and accessory basal amygdaloid nuclei.

The amygdaloid complex receives afferents from diencephalon, specific and non-specific thalamic nuclei, brain stem reticular formation, neocortex and olfactory areas. Fibers arising in the rostral half of the hypothalamus pass via the stria terminalis and ventral to basal ganglia to all the amygdaloid nuclei [4-5]. The neocortical projections are from the inferior temporal gyrus to the basolateral and central nuclei of the amygdala [6-7]. The orbitofrontal and a limited number of afferent fibers from parietal, occipital and temporal areas pass to the lateral amygdaloid nucleus via the posterior limb of the anterior commissure [8].

The stria terminalis is the most prominent efferent pathway from the amygdaloid nuclear complex. Most of the fibers in this bundle originate from the corticomedial nuclear group of the amygdaloid complex [9-10]. It terminates in the nuclei of the stria terminalis which is located lateral to the fornix and dorsal to the anterior commissure [9, 11]. However, some of the fibers also terminate in the anterior hypothalamus, ventromedial nucleus of the hypothalamus, medial preoptic area and medial forebrain bundle [9, 11-12]. Another important efferent pathway is the ventral amygdalofugal projection. It emerges from the dorsomedial part of the amygdala and pass to the substantia innominata and enter into the lateral preoptic and hypothalamic areas, the septal region and the nucleus of the diagonal band [4, 13].

The main entry point as suggested by Pitkanen et al. [14] and Pare et al. [15] for the sensory information to the amygdaloid complex is through the lateral nucleus. The projections from auditory cortex and auditory thalamus terminate in the lateral division of the lateral nucleus [16-17]. The medial division of the lateral nucleus receives input from higher order polysensory association regions. The lateral nucleus gives heavy projections to basal and accessory basal nuclei [15, 18], which in turn mainly project to central and medial nuclei of the amygdala. The basal nucleus also projects to a number of cortical areas including sensory processing areas as well as prefrontal and temporal neocortical areas and perirhinal and entorhinal cortices [19-21]. The lateral nucleus also projects to the periamygdaloid complex [22]. The central and medial nuclei gives rise to projections to hypothalamic and brain stem areas involved in the control of behavioural, autonomic and endocrine responses associated with emotional and motivated states [20]. The central nucleus of amygdala has also recently been shown to receive nociceptive signals from the parabrachial area, i.e. the spino-ponto-amygdaloid nociceptive pathway [23]. This pathway is involved in the affective-emotional (fear, memory of aggression), behavioural (vocalization, freezing, flight, defense and offense) and autonomic (papillary dilatation, cardiorespiratory and adreno-cortical responses and micturition) reactions to the noxious and/or visceral events [23-25].

Role of Amygdala in Pain Modulation

The amygdala is a subcortical complex of nuclei, which plays a role in the mediation of emotionality [26] and fear related processes [27]. Bilateral CeA lesions have been shown to significantly increase the thresholds for simple vocalizations and vocalization after-discharge [28], without affecting the tail flick latency (TFL) in the noxious thermal test and the average pain rating in the formalin test. Charpentier [29] and Calvino et al. [30] also reported an increased threshold for vocalizations after bilateral amygdalectomy indicating a reduction in the emotional nociceptive reactivity. Al-Rodhan et al. [31] observed no change in the TFL following microinjections of the carbachol into the CeA. However, Klamt and Prado [32] observed an increase in the tail flick latency following microinjections of the carbachol into the CeA. Manning and Mayer reported no change in the TFL [33] and the pain rating in the formalin test [34] following bilateral CeA lesions. Administration of neurotensin, an endogenous peptide, into the central nucleus of amygdala has been shown to increase the nociceptive threshold in jump or paw lick latency in the hot plate test. Bilateral stimulation of basolateral nuclei of amygdala produced analgesia in the noxious thermal tail flick test [35]. Stimulation of CeA also has been shown to produce analgesia in the jaw-opening reflex of cats [36], while no effect was observed on the non-nociceptive reflex such as jaw closing reflex. In anaesthetized guinea pigs amygdalar stimulation has been shown to produce two different types of responses. Stimulation of lateral amygdala produced analgesia as demonstrated by reduction in vocalization, motor and respiratory movements while stimulation of the medial nucleus of amygdala resulted in an increase in vocalization intensity, motor and respiratory responses indicating hyperalgesia [37]. The analgesia following amygdalar stimulation is suggested to be mediated by opioid receptor mechanisms. The amygdaloid complex is known to have opiate receptors and enkephalins [38-39] and electrical stimulation of amygdala is known to release endogenous opioids [40]. In 1968, Melzack and Casey [2] suggested that the amygdala might be involved in the emotional and affective component of pain. The amygdala has extensive connections with the areas involved in the processing of the sensory information [17], which transmit emotionally neutral sensory signals. The amygdala also receives inputs from the hippocampal formation, which is involved in higher cognitive functions [41]. Thereby, thoughts and memories receive emotional coloration by way of information transmission to the amygdala.

Opioidergic Pain Modulation

Endogenous and exogenous opioids have been implicated in many behavioral studies of pain, stimulation produced analgesia and stress-produced analgesia [42-43]. Opiates have been shown to exert direct effects on the sensitivity of pain fibers [43]. In the experiments carried out in our laboratory [35] naloxone (3 mg/kg) produced varying effects in the tail flick and vocalization tests. Subcutaneous injection of naloxone (3 mg/kg) alone did not produce a significant change in thresholds for tail flick, but naloxone combined with amygdalar stimulation produced analgesia as revealed by an increase in the threshold for TF. Woolf et al. [44] reported that the electrical stimulation of tail itself activate opioid mediated inhibition in the spinal circuitry. It has been shown that low doses of systemic naloxone (1-50 µg/kg) facilitated the spinal reflexes to electrical stimuli which is sufficient to activate either A fibers alone or A and C together [45]. Intravenous injection of low titres of β-endorphin has been shown to decrease while high titres of β-endorphin increase the thresholds for tail flick. The analgesic effects of endorphin were blocked by naloxone [46]. In the vocalization tests, naloxone alone produced a hyperalgesic response in our study. However, naloxone with amygdalar stimulation increased the thresholds for vocalization showing analgesic effects. Kayser and Gullibaud [47] have also shown that injection of low doses of morphine and naloxone (3-10 µg/kg) produced a significant increase in thresholds for vocalization in arthritic rats as compared to normal rats. On the contrary, a high dose of naloxone (1 mg/kg) decreased the threshold for vocalization. The amygdaloid complex is known to have high concentrations of opiate receptors and enkephalins and high dose of naloxone was suggested to be acting at post-synaptic level in the amygdala, thereby producing hyperalgesic response [38-39, 48]. The analgesic effect of naloxone and amygdalar stimulation may be mediated via opiate receptors in the amygdala. Electrical stimulation of amygdala is known to release endogenous opioids [40].

Cholinergic Pain Modulation

The role of cholinergic system has been implicated in nociceptive mechanisms [49]. The endogenous cholinergic mechanisms are known to modulate mechanical and thermal nociceptive transmission in the spinal cord. In rats, systemic administration of choline, atropine, mecamylamine or apomorphine produced analgesia in the formalin test [50]. Muscarinic receptor antagonists (scopolamine, atropine and pirenzepine) produced a dose dependent decrease in the thresholds of tail flick involving both mechanical and thermal stimuli. It has been suggested that cholinergic component is directly involved in the emotional-affective aspect of pain. In rats, subcutaneous injection of oxotremorine (muscarinic receptor agonist) at subconvulsive doses (30-67 µg/kg) increased the thresholds in a dose dependent manner for vocalization after-discharge. Atropine antagonized the antinociceptive effects of oxotremorine on vocalization during and after-discharge [51]. Systemic administration of methylscopolamine has been shown by Grau et al. [52] to attenuate the shock-induced vocalization. In the experiments done in our laboratory, bilateral systemic administration of cholinergic receptor antagonist, atropine (5 mg/kg) produced hyperalgesia in tail flick test but had no effect on the pain rating in the formalin test. However, bilateral amygdalar stimulation after systemic administration of atropine produced analgesia in both the tail flick and formalin test [35]. These results suggest that cholinergic receptors of amygdala may be involved in the endogenous pain modulation. Green and Kitchen [53] have suggested that an interaction exists between endogenous opioids and cholinergic receptors involved in pain modulation. In our study very low doses of atropine (10 µg) produced analgesia in the tail flick test [35]. This have been suggested to be mediated by selective inhibition of presynaptic muscarinic receptors, while the hyperalgesic effects with high dose of atropine may be due to blocking of postsynaptic muscarinic receptors [54].

GABAergic Pain Modulation
GABAergic mechanisms modulate the nociceptive behavior at both spinal and supraspinal levels. Peripheral administration of GABAergic agents have been shown to produce an increase in morphine induced analgesia while the central injection of GABAergic drugs produced inhibition of antinociceptive effects. In rats, 6,7-dimethoxy-4-ethyl-carboline-3-caroxylic acid methyl ester (DMCM), a benzodiazepine agonist produced dose dependent analgesia in the formalin test [55]. The analgesia was accompanied by emotional reactions such as defecation and urination. The opioid anatagonist, naltrexone did not alter these behaviors but reversed the conditioned analgesia. In monkeys, intraperitoneal injection of baclofen produces a dose-dependent analgesia in formalin induced chemoinflammatory pain which is suggested to be mediated via presynaptic inhibition of primary afferents involving GABA-B receptors [56]. The GABA agonist, muscimol (5 µg) when injected intrathecally produced a significant elevation of vocalization thresholds for tail flick latency to radiant heat [57]. At low doses (1 µg) it produced a significant elevation of vocalization thresholds, but tail flick latency to radiant heat was not altered [57]. Mena et al. [35] observed that systemic administration of baclofen (2 mg/kg), a GABA-B agonist produces analgesia in the formalin test. Induction of inflammatory pain in the hind limb of rats has also been shown to increase GABAergic cells and GABA neurotransmitter levels in the dorsal horn laminae (I-III) of spinal cord [58]. In cats, it has been shown that stimulation of primary nociceptors by noxious thermal stimuli release GABA and inhibits the spinal neuronal activity [59]. In our study bilateral amygdalar stimulation along with baclofen produced significant analgesia in the formalin pain test and tail flick test [35]. These analgesic effects of baclofen and amygdalar stimulation may be mediated by GABA-B or benzodiazepine or NMDA

receptors of the amygdala.. Amygdalar nuclei, especially basolateral nucleus has been shown to have a large number of benzodiazepine receptors [60]. Recently, it has been demonstrated that the microinjection of diazepam into the basolateral amygdala decreased hypoalgesia in the formalin test [61]. The benzodiazepine inverse agonist, DMCM has been shown to occupy the GABA-A receptor complex as a result of which the inhibitory effects of GABA are reduced. Amygdalar stimulation has been shown to modulate the GABA and NMDA receptors in the amygdala and produces long lasting changes in the neurons [62]. Analgesia produced by baclofen and amygdalar stimulation, in our study, may be due to interaction of GABA and enkephalins at the spinal level. Immunohistochemical evidence shows that a relationship between GABA and enkephalins exists for the transmission of pain impulses. Thus disinhibition of opioid neurons in the nociceptive circuitry of the spinal cord may be an important mechanism in antinociception [63].

Electrophysiology of Amygdala

The lateral capsular subdivision (CeLC) of the CeA is considered to be the "nociceptive" subdivision [64]. In this subdivision 78% of the neurons get excited by noxious stimuli, whereas, neurons in other CeA subdivisions get inhibited by noxious stimuli or remain unresponsive. The CeLC receives a strong and specific nociceptive input from a pontine parabrachial area. It also receives projections from several thalamic areas like parafascicular, paraventricular nuclei, medial geniculate nucleus that provide additional sources of nociceptive input. It also receives substantial afferent projections from the rostral infralimbic cortex and also from entorhinal and posterior agranular insular cortex. These projections may modulate aversive emotional aspects of pain.

In the CeLC approximately 80% of the total nociceptive neurons respond exclusively or preferentially to the noxious mechanical or thermal stimuli and only 20% are influenced by other innocuous, somesthetic or heterosensory stimuli [65]. These nociceptive neurons of CeLC are basically of two types, viz. those that get activated by the peripheral noxious stimuli and those that get inhibited. Both of these types of neurons have been shown to have large peripheral receptive fields, indicating that these neurons do not have a role in sensory discriminative aspect of pain. Although most of these neurons respond to all the parts of the body in a similar fashion, but there are some that respond preferentially to the restricted areas of the body. It is reported [65] that these neurons also have the ability to encode different intensities of the stimuli within the noxious range. However, these two types of neurons are not homogenously distributed in and around CeA. The neurons inhibited by noxious stimuli are preferentially located in the central nucleus, whereas, those which get excited are located in the peripheral edges or in the rostral portion of the lateral capsular subdivision of the central nucleus. Hence, Bernard et al. [23] suggested that amygdala have a dual role in the pain modulation. In the experiments carried out in our laboratory majority of amygdalar units recorded from medial, lateral and basolateral nuclei responded to different peripheral noxious stimuli [66]. A large number of amygdalar neurons (67%) showed an increase while a small number (33%) showed a decrease in firing rate in response to peripheral noxious stimuli. The neurons from the lateral and medial amygdaloid nuclei showed after discharge to strong noxious electrical stimuli. Bernard et al. [23] also showed majority of neurons responding to noxious electrical stimuli and found an increase in peak latency when transcutaneous electrical stimuli were applied to the tail. These peak responses were correlated with the conduction velocities of Aδ and C fibers. In the study by Mena [66], a large majority of neurons also responded to thermal stimuli ranging from 45-60 °C. Although the after discharges were shown by only medial amygdaloid neurons. The application of noxious mechanical pinch to different parts of the body (forelimbs, hindlimbs and tail) also produced an increase in amygdalar neuronal activity in our study with medial amygdalar neurons showing after-discharges in response to contralateral hind limb pinch. Bernard et al. [23] have also shown an increase in amygdalar firing rate when thermal stimulus [50 °C] was applied to forelimbs and in response to mechanical pinch applied to forelimbs, hindlimbs and face of the animal. They reported weak after-discharges from the ventral portion of the globus pallidus when noxious mechanical pinch was applied to contralateral forepaw. These studies suggest that CeA have neurons which are nociceptive specific and have wide dynamic range. It is hypothesized that elicitation of after-discharge from the amygdalar neurons may be mediated through NMDA receptors, GABAergic or monoaminergic neurons. Amygdalar regions have been shown to have a high density of benzodiazepine receptors and monoaminergic neurons [67].

Neural Tissue Transplant

Neural tissue transplantation today is recognized to be a valuable technique for studying normal development and regeneration in the central nervous system. Till date successful transplantation of practically every region or specialized group of neurons, or encapsulated group of neurons/cells from the foetal brain or biotechnologically engineered or cultured neurons into adult/young host, are vigorously being pursued in both animals and humans.

Luschekina and Podachin [68] first showed that embryonic amygdala when transplanted into the cortex survived poorly whereas in the subcortical structures it survived the best. They also showed the differentiation of nerve and glial cells, growth of capillaries and formation of neuropil between the graft and host. Luschekina et al. [69] also reported that amygdalar tissue transplantation is most successful when done five days after amygdalectomy. In the study by Jain et al. [28], amygdalar tissue transplantation at the CeA lesioned site significantly decreased the thresholds for vocalization when compared with the lesioned only group. However, when compared with the basal group it showed an increase, indicating partial recovery of the vocalization response following amygdalar tissue transplantation. Amygdalar tissue transplantation did not have any effect on the tail flick latency and pain rating in the tail flick test and formalin test, respectively. These studies suggest that even amygdalar tissue transplants are capable of inducing recovery of the nociceptive behavior (emotional and affective component).

Conditioned Antinociceptive Responses

More recently, amygdala has been demonstrated to be critical for the expression of conditioned antinociceptive responses or conditioned hypoalgesia. It refers to the antinociceptive response that is elicited by an earlier neutral stimulus that has come to predict the onset of an aversive stimulus. In other words, if neutral stimuli like tone (conditioned stimulus, CS) that cannot itself elicit any behavioral response if is paired with an aversive stimuli like footshock (unconditioned stimulus, UCS), starts eliciting the behavioral responses which were earlier elicited by footshock. If conditioned stimulus is now associated with pain testing there is activation of the endogenous analgesic system resulting in the hypoalgesia. Normally, all innate or learned danger signals besides activating defensive behavioral system activate endogenous analgesic system irrespective of the type of environmental aversive stimuli and the defensive behaviour being recruited. The amydaloid complex which shares extensive reciprocal connection with the ventral periaqueductal gray is thought to be involved in the conditioned hypoalgesia. Helmstetter and Bellgowan [70] observed no change in the baseline tail flick latency in response to noxious heat stimulus following bilateral large amygdaloid lesions. However, the conditioned hypoalgesia of the tail flick was attenuated following the lesions. Watkins et al. [71] also observed no effect of the amydalar lesions on the unconditioned tail flick latency but there was a blockage of conditioned hypoalgesia of TFL. He therefore suggested that amygdala might be more critically involved in the expression of conditioned reactions to the aversive events than in the mediation of the unconditioned reactions. Helmstetter [72] reported similar results with formalin test. He observed no change in the baseline pain rating after CeA or BL lesions, but complete blockage of conditioned hypoalgesia of pain rating. Harris and Westbrock [73] reported a reduction in the conditioned hypoalgesia of the hot plate test following microinjections of benzodiazepine unilaterally into the basolateral amygdala of the rats. Good and Westbrock [74] also observed a reduction in the conditioned hypoalgesic responses to the hot plate test after microinjections of the morphine into the basolateral nucleus. They suggested that amygdala is a critical site in the circuitry by which learned danger signals activate antinociceptive mechanisms in the brainstem thereby provoking hypoalgesic responses. Helmstetter and Bellgowan [61] also suggested that the amygdala might not be involved in the organization or expression of the animals' normal response to the noxious stimulation, but in the conditioned antinociceptive responses. It was suggested by Fanselow et al. [75] that defensive and hypoalgesic responses co-occur because antinociceptive mechanisms are controlled by activity in defensive system. It was also proposed that all innate or learned danger signals involve amygdala based fear system, which in turn activates distinct neural circuits in the periaqueductal gray (PAG) through direct projections [76]. These PAG circuits then coordinate a variety of defensive responses such as freezing [77] and hypoalgesia [78]. Thus, amygdala seems to represent a critical component of a "defensive behavior system" that controls the expression of anxiety and fear related responses [79]. Conditioned hypoalgesia thus is an integrated component of this defensive behavior pattern.

Conclusion

Amygdala, although seems to be playing an important role in the modulation of pain, it appears that it is not involved in the organization or expression of the animals' normal response to the noxious stimulation. As the amygdala is an important site of neural plasticity during Pavlovian conditioning it is possible that the nociceptive inputs to this structure are directly related to the animals ability to learn about and remember noxious environmental events.

References

1. Mersky, H. Pain terms: A list with definitions and notes on usage. Recommended by the IASP subcommittee on taxonomy. *Pain*, 1979; **6**: 249–252.
2. Melzack, R. and Casey, K.L. Sensory, motivational and central control determinants of pain: A new conceptual model. In: The skin senses, edited by D. Kenshalo, Springfield, 1968; 423–443.
3. Wall, P.D. and Melzack R. Introduction: Basic aspects. In: Textbook of pain. 4th edition, Chuchill Livingstone.
4. Cowan, W.M., Raisman, G. and Powell TPS. The connexions of the amygdala. *J. Neurol. Neurosurg. Psychiat.*, 1965; **28**:137–151.
5. Szentagothai, J., Flerko, B., Mess, B. and Halasz, B. Hypothalamic control of the anterior pituitary. An experimental-morphological study. Akademiai Kiado, Budapest 1968.
6. Whitlock, D.G. and Nauta, W.J.H. Subcortical projections from the temporal neocortex in *Macaca mulatta*. *J. Comp. Neurol.*, 1956; **106**: 183–212.
7. Lammers, H.J. and Lohman, A.H., Experimental anatomisch onderzoek naar de verbindingen van piriform cortex en amygdala kernen bij de kat. *Nederld Tijdschr Geneesk*, 1957; **101**: 1–2.
8. Alphen, H.A.W. Van. The anterior commisure of the rabbit. *Acta Anat.* 1969; **74** (suppl): 9–11.
9. DeOlmos, J.S. The amygdaloid projection field in the rat as studied with the cupric-silver method. In: Eleftheriou, B.E. (eds). The neurobiology of the amygdala. Plenum Press, New York, 1972.
10. Lammers, H.J. The neural connections of the amygdaloid complex in mammals. In: Eleftheriou, B.E. (eds). The neurobiology of the amygdala. Plenum Press, New York, 1972; 123–144.

11. Heimer, L. and Nauta, W.J.H. The hypothalamic distribution of the stria terminalis in the rat. *Brain Res.*, 1969; **13**: 284–297.

12. Heimer, L., Ebner, F.F. and Nauta, W.J.H. A note on the termination of commissural fibers in the neocortex. *Brain Res.* 1967; **5(2)**:171–7.

13. Leonard, C.M. and Scott, J.W. Origin and distribution of amygdalofugal pathways in the rat. An experimental neuroanatomical study. *J. Comp. Neurol.* 1971; **144**: 313–330.

14. Pitkanen, A., Stenfanacci, L., Farb, C.R., Go G.G., LeDoux, J.E. and Amaral, D.G. Intrinsic connections of the rat amygdaloid complex: projections originating in the lateral nucleus. *J. Comp. Neurol.* 1995; **356**: 288–310.

15. Pare, D., Smith, Y. and Pare, J.F. Intra-amygdaloid projections of the basolateral and basomedial nuclei in the rat *Phaseolus vulgaris*—Leucoagglutinin anterograde staining at the light and electron microscopic level. *Neurosci.*, 1995; **69(2)**: 567–583.

16. LeDoux, J.E., Farb, C.R. and Ruggerio, D.A. Topographic organization of neurons in the acoustic thalamus that project to the amygdala. *J. Neurosci.* 1990; **10**: 1043–1054.

17. LeDoux, J.E. Emotion and the amygdala. In: Aggleton, J.P. (ed). The amygdala: neurobiological aspects of emotion, memory and mental dysfunction. Wiley-Liss, New York 1994; 339–352.

18. Krettek, J.E. and Price, J.L. Amygdaloid projections to subcortical structures within the basal forebrain and brainstem in the rat and cat. *J. Comp. Neurol.* 1978; **178**: 225–254.

19. Sripanidkulchai, K., Sripanidkulchai, B. and Wyss, J.M. The cortical projection of the basolateral amygdaloid nucleus in the rat: a retrograde fluorescent study. *J. Comp. Neurol.* 1984; **229**: 419–431.

20. Price, J.L., Russchen, F.T. and Amaral, D.G. The limbic region. II. The amygdaloid complex. In: Bjorklund et al. (eds). Handbook of chemical neuroanatomy, vol. 5. Integrated systems of the CNS. Part I. Amsterdam, Elsevier, 1987; 279–388.

21. Amaral, D.G., Price, J.L., Pitkanen, A. and Carmichael, S.T. Anatomical organization of the amygdaloid complex. In: Aggleton, J.P. (ed). The amygdala: neurobiological aspects of emotion, memory and mental dysfunction. Wiley-Liss, New York, 1994; 1–66.

22. Luskin, M.B. and Price, J.L. The topographic organization of associational fibers of the olfactory system in the rat including centrifugal fibers to the olfactory bulb. *J. Comp. Neurol.*, 1983; **216**: 264–291.

23. Bernard, J.F., Huang, J.F. and Besson, J.M. The nucleus centralis of the amygdala and the globus pallidus ventralis: electrophysiological evidence for its involvement in pain process. *J. Neurophysiol*, 1992; **68**: 551–569.

24. Bernard, J.F. and Besson, J.M. The spino (trigemino) pontoamygdaloid pathway: electrophysiological evidence for its involvement in pain process. *J. Neurophysiol*, 1990; **63**: 473–490.

25. Bernard, J.F., Huang, J.F. and Besson, J.M. The parabrachial area: electrophysiological evidence for an involvement in visceral nociceptive processes. *J. Neurophysiol.* 1994; **71**: 1646–1660.

26. LeDoux, J.E. Emotion. In: Plum, F. (ed). Handbook of Physiology: Nervous system V. Washington, DC, American Physiological Society, 1987; 419–459.

27. Davis, M. The role of the amygdala in conditioned fear. In: Aggleton, J.P. (ed). The amygdala: Neurobiological aspects of emotion, memory and mental dysfunction. Wiley-Liss, New York 1992; 256–306.

28. Jain, S., Mathur, R., Sharma, R. and Nayar, U. Amygdalar tissue transplants

improve recovery of the nociceptive behaviour. *Restorat Neurol Neurosci*, 2000; **16**(2): 143–7 .

29. Charpentier, J. Modifications de la reaction a la douleur provoqvees par diverse lesions cerebrales, et leurs effects sur la sensibilite a la morphine. *Psychopharmacol*, 1967; **11**: 95–121.

30. Calvino, B., Levesque, G. and Besson, J.M. Possible involvement of the amygdaloid complex in morphine analgesia as studied by electrolytic lesions in rats. *Brain Res*, 1982; **233**: 221–226.

31. Al-Rodhan, Chipkin, R., Yaksh, T.L. The antinociceptive effects of SCH-32615, a neutral endopeptidase inhibitor microinjected into periaqueductal gray, ventral medulla and amygdala. *Brain Res*, 1990; **520**: 123–130.

32. Klamt, J.G. and Prado, W.A. Antinociception and behavioural changes induced by carbachol microinjected into identified sites of the rat brain. *Brain Res*, 1991; **549**: 9–18.

33. Manning, B.H. and Mayer, D.J. The central nucleus of the amygdala contributes to the production of the morphine antinociception in the rat tail flick test. *J. Neurosci.*, 1995a; **15**: 8199–8213.

34. Manning, B.H. and Mayer, D.J. The central nucleus of the amygdala contributes to the production of the morphine antinociception in the formalin test. *Pain*, 1995b; **63**: 141–152.

35. Mena, N.B., Mathur, R. and Nayar, U. Amygdalar involvement in pain. *Ind. J. Physiol. Pharmacol.*, 1996; **39**: 339–346.

36. Kowada, K., Kawarada, K. and Matsumoto, N. Conditioning stimulation of the central amygdaloid nucleus inhibits the jaw-opening reflex in the cat. *Jpn. J. Physiol.*, 1992; **42**: 443–458.

37. Lico, M.C., Hoffman, A. and Covian, M.R. Influence of some limbic structures upon somatic and autonomic manifestation of pain. *Physiol. Behav.*, 1974; **12**: 805–811.

38. Kuhar, M.J., Pert, C.B. and Synder, S.H. Regional distribution of opiate receptor binding in monkey and human brain. *Nature*, 1973; **245**: 447–450.

39. Hokfelt, T., Elde, R., Johansson, O., Terenius, L. and Stein, L. The distribution of enkephalin immunoreactive cell bodies in the rat central nervous system. *Neurosci. Lett*, 1977; **5**: 25–31.

40. Frenk, H., Engel, J., Jr., Ackermann, R.F., Shavit, Y. and Liebeskind, J.C. Endogenous opioids may mediate post-ictal behavioral depression in amygdaloid-kindled rats. *Brain Res.*, 1979; **167**(2):435–40.

41. Squire, L.R. Memory: Neural organization and behaviour. In: Plum, F. (ed). Handbook of Physiology, Section I: The nervous system. Vol. V, Higher function of the brain. *Bethesda*: American Physiological Society, 1987; 295–371.

42. Akil, H., Watson, S.J., Young, E., Lewis, M.E., Khachaturian, H. and Walker, J.M. Endogenous opioids: Biology and function. *Ann. Rev. Neurosci*, 1984; **7**: 223–225.

43. Smith, A.P. and Lee, N.M. Pharmacology of dynorphin. *Ann. Rev. Pharmacol. Toxicol.*, 1988; **28**: 123–140.

44. Woolf, C.J., Mitchell, D. and Barrett, G.D. Antinocicpetive effect of peripheral segmental electrical stimulation in the rat. *Pain*, 1980; **8**: 237–252.

45. Hartell, N.A. and Headley, P.M. The effect of naloxone on spinal reflexes to electrical and mechanical stimuli in the anaesthetized spinalized rat. *J. Physiol.*, 1991; **442**: 513–526.

46. Litinova, S.V., Kalyuzhnyi, L.V., Shulgovskii, V.V., Aristova, V.V. and Salieva, R.M. Action of β-endorphin antiserum of different antibody titres on thermal or tail shock pain in rats. *Biomed. Sci.*, 1990; **1**: 471–474.

47. Kayser, V. and Gullibaud, G. Local and remote modifications of nociceptive sensitivity during carrageenin induced inflammation in the rat. *Pain*, 1990; **28**: 99–107.

48. Basbaum, A.I. and Fields, H.L. Endogenous pain control systems: Brainstem spinal pathways and endorphin circuitry. *Ann. Rev. Neurosci.*, 1984; **7**: 309–338.

49. Pert, A. Cholinergic and catechalaminergic modulation of nociceptive reactions-interactions in opiates. In: Pain and Headache, Vol. 9, Basel: Karger 1987; 1–63.

50. Dennis, S.G. and Melzack, R. Effects of cholinergic and dopaminergic agents on pain and morphine analgesia measured by three pain tests. *Exp. Neurol.*, 1983; **81**: 167–176.

51. Paalzow, G., Paalzow, P. Antinociceptive action of oxotremorine and regional turnover of rat brain noradrenaline, dopamine and 5-HT. *Eur. J. Pharmacol.*, 1975; **31**: 261–272.

52. Grau, J.W., Illich, P.A., Chen, P.S. and Meagher, M.W. Role of cholinergic systems in pain modulation. I. Impact of scopolamine on environmentally induced hypoalgesia and pain reactivity. *Behav, Neurosci*, 1991; **105**: 62–81.

53. Green, P.G. and Kitchen, I. Antinociception, opioids and the cholinergic system. *Prog. Neurobiol.*,1986; **26**: 119–146.

54. Ghelardini, C., Malmberg-Aiello, P., Giotti, A., Malcangio, M. and Bartolini, A. Investigation into atropine induced antinociception. *Br. J. Pharmacol.*, 1990; **101**: 49–54.

55. Fanselow, M.S., Kim, J.J. Benzodiazepine inverse agonist DMCM as an unconditional stimulus for fear induced analgesia: Implications for the role of GABA-A receptors in fear related behaviour. *Behav Neurosci.*, 1992; **106**: 336–344.

56. Sharma, R., Mathur, R., Nayar, U. and Gaba, B. Mediated analgesia in tonic pain in monkeys. *Ind. J. Physiol. Pharmacol.*, 1993; **37**: 189–193.

57. Roberts, L.A., Beyer, C. and Komisaruk, B.R. Nociceptive responses to altered GABAergic activity at the spinal cord. *Life Sci.*, 1986; **39**: 1667–1674.

58. Castro-Lopes, J.M., Tavares, I., Tolle, T.R., Coito, A. and Coimbra, A. Increase in GABAergic cells and GABA levels in the spinal cord in unilateral inflammation of the hindlimb in the rat. *Eur. J. Neurosci.*, 1992, **4**: 296–301.

59. Morris, R. Evidence for the possible involvement of gamma-aminobutyric acid in cutaneous and muscle-nerve evoked inhibitions of responses of cat spinal neurons to noxious thermal stimulation. *J. Physiol.*, 1985; **364**: 42p.

60. Niehoff, D. and Kuhar, M.J. Benzodiazepine receptors : localization in rat amygdala. *J. Neurosci*, 1983; **3**: 2091–2097.

61. Helmstetter, F.J. and Bellgowan, P.S. Stress induced hypoalgesia and defensive freezing are attenuated by application of diazepam to the amygdala. *Pharmacol. Biochem. Behav.*, 1993a; **44**: 433–438.

62. Gean, P.W., Gallangher, P.S. and Anderson, A.C. Spontaneous epileptiform activity and alteration of GABA and NMDA mediated neurotransmission in amygdala neurons kindled in vivo. *Brain Res.*, 1989; **494**: 171–181.

63. Liu, H., Llewellynsmith, I.J., Pilowsky, P. and Basbaum, A.I. Ultrastructural evidence for GABA mediated disinhibitory circuits in the spinal cord of the cat. *Neurosci. Lett*, 1992; **138**: 183–187.

64. Bourgeais, L., Gauriau, C. and Bernard, J.F. Projections from the nociceptive area of the central nucleus of the amygdala to the forebrain: a PHA-L study in the rat. *Eur. J. Neurosci.*, 2001; **14(2)**: 229–255.

65. Bernard, J.F., Bester, H. and Besson, J.M. Involvement of the spino-parabrachio-amygdaloid and -hypothalamic pathways in the autonomic and affective emotional aspects of pain. *Prog. Brain. Res.*, 1996; **107**: 243–55.

66. Mena, N.B. The role of limbic system in pain modulation: A behavioural and electrophysiological study in rats. Ph.D. thesis submitted to All India Institute of Medical Sciences, New Delhi, India. Personal Communication.

67. Fallon, J.H. and Ciofi, P. Distribution of monoamines within the amygdala. In: Aggleton, J.P. (ed), The Amygdala: Neurobiological aspects of emotion, memory and mental dysfunction, Wiley-Liss, 1992, pp. 97–144.

68. Luschekina, E.A. and Podachin, V.P. Survival of embryonic amygdala grafted into various parts of the adult rat brain. *Neurophysiol.*, 1987; **19**: 443–450.

69. Luschekina, E.A., Kurbatova, M.B., Khonicheva, N.M. and Podachin, V.P. Transplantation of embryonic amygdalar tissue into the brain of amygdalectomized rats. *Zh Vyssh Nervn Deyat Pavlova*, 1988; **38**: 769–772.

70. Helmstetter, F.J. and Bellgowan, P.S. Lesions of the amygdala block conditioned hypoalgesia on the tail flick test. *Brain Res.*, 1993b; **612**: 253–257.

71. Watkins, R.I., Weirtdak, P.E. and Maier, F.S. The amygdala is necessary for the expression of conditioned but not unconditioned analgesia. *Behav. Neurosci.*, 1993; **107**: 402–405.

72. Helmstetter, F.J. The amygdala is essential for the expression of conditioned hypoalgesia. *Behav. Neurosci.*, 1992; **106**: 518–528.

73. Harris, J.A. and Westbrock, R.F. Effects of benzodiazepine microinjection into the amygdala of periaqueductal gray on the expression of conditioned fear and hypoalgesia in rats. *Behav. Neurosci.*, 1995; **109**: 295–304.

74. Good, J.A. and Westbrock, R.F. Effects of a microinjection of morphine into the amygdala on the acquisition and expression of conditioned fear and hypoalgesia in rats. *Behav. Neurosci.*, 1995; **109**: 631–641.

75. Fanselow, M.S., Kim, J.J., Young, S.L., Calcagnetti, D.J., DeCola, J.P., Helmstetter, F.J. and Landeira-Fernandez, J. Differential effects of selective opioid peptide antagonists on the acquisition of pavlovian fear conditioning. *Peptides*, 1991; **12(5)**: 1033–7.

76. Rizvi, T.A., Ennis, M., Behbehani, M.M. and Shipley, M.T. Connections between the central nucleus of the amygdala and midbrain periaqueductal gray: topography and reciprocity. *J. Comp. Neurol.*, 1991; **303**: 121–131.

77. Kim, M. and Davis, M. Electrolytic lesions of the amygdala block fear potentiated startle even with extensive training but do not prevent reacquisition. *Behav. Neurosci.*, 1993; **107**: 586–595.

78. Helmstetter, F.J. and Landeira-Fernandez, J. Conditioned hypoalgesia is attenuated by naltrexone applied to the PAG. *Brain Res.*, 1990; **537**: 88–92.

79. Killgore, W.D. and Yorgelun-Todd, D.A. Social anxiety predicts amygdala activation in adolescents viewing fearful faces. *Neuroreport*, 2005; **16**: 1671–1675.

Pain Updated: Mechanisms and Effects
Edited by R. Mathur

8. Nociceptors and the Spinal Reflexes

Shripad B. Deshpande

Department of Physiology, Institute of Medical Sciences,
Banaras Hindu University, Varanasi-221005, India

Abstract. The sensation of pain indicates the tissue injury and/or damage and brings the appropriate protective responses. Fast pain originates from the thinly myelinated Aδ-nociceptors and the slow pain is through the unmyelinated C-nociceptors. The thermal, chemical and mechanical stimuli activate the nociceptors via diverse sets of ion channels or ligands involving wide range of second messenger systems. The tissue injury or inflammation liberates chemicals which increase the sensitivity of nociceptors. These in turn make even an innocuous stimulus to be very painful. The Aδ- and C-fibres make synaptic contact with the dorsal horn neurons where glutamate is a transmitter. Thus, glutamate receptors modulate the pain transmission by involving other transmitters (opiates, substance-P, 5-hydroxytryptamine etc.). The N-methyl-D-aspartic acid (NMDA) receptors are concerned with the ultimate 'wind up' mechanism of pain and prevent the tolerance development to opiates. The non-NMDA receptors are implicated in the chronic pain conditions. The painful stimuli evoke flexor reflexes, which involve polysynaptic pathway. The polysynaptic reflexes also involve NMDA receptor mediated mechanism. The NMDA antagonists diminished the pain sensation and also decreased the occurrence of tolerance to opioid analgesics. However, the NMDA antagonists interfere with the memory, learning and higher functions. Thus, there is a need for newer class of analgesics. The *in vitro* spinal cord preparation and its modification are good models more suited to explore the nociceptive neural networking at the spinal level.
Pain is a complex experience that involves not only the transduction of noxious environmental stimuli, but also the cognitive and emotional processing by the brain. Pain is a sensation that alerts us to the real impending injury and triggers appropriate protective responses. The molecular mechanisms whereby primary sensory neurons detect pain producing stimuli is referred to as nociception.

Classification of Nociceptors

The term nociception arose from the conclusions of Sherrington [1] relating to the stimuli capable of compromising the integrity of the organism, or in other words, which produce tissue damage or injury. The nociceptors have characteristic thresholds that distinguish them from others. That means the noxious heat, intense pressure or irritant chemicals produce a sensation of pain but not the innocuous stimuli such as warmth or light touch or pressure

[2]. Hence, it is similar to any other sensation in the body such as vision, olfaction or touch, where stimuli of certain quality or intensity are detected by the cells with appropriately tuned receptive properties.

Most but not all Aβ fibres detect innocuous stimuli applied to skin, muscle and joints and thus do not contribute to pain [3, 4]. Indeed stimulation of large fibres can reduce pain as occurs when these fibres are activated by rubbing. By contrast small and medium diameter cell bodies give rise to most of the nociceptors. including the unmyelinated slowly conducting C-fibres and thinly myelinated Aδ-fibres, respectively [4]. It has long been assumed that Aδ- and C-nociceptors mediate 'first' and 'second' pain, respectively (Fig. 1). Thus, Aδ-nociceptors mediate rapid, acute, sharp pain and C-fibres mediate the delayed more diffuse dull pain [5].

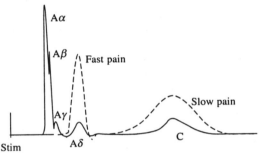

Fig 1. The representation of compound action potential indicating different nociceptors. The compound action potential has Aα, Aβ, Aγ, Aδ and C peaks depending upon their conduction velocity and the degree of myelination [47]. The Aδ (thinly myelinated with conduction velocity 5-15 m/sec) and C-fibres (unmyelinated with conduction velocity < 1 m/sec) conduct the fast and slow nociceptive impulses, respectively, indicated by dashed line.The stimulus artifact is indicated as stim. The time scale and amplitude are drawn to the proportion as mentioned in Erlanger and Gaser [47].

Nature of Stimuli for Nociceptors Activation

Both the classes of nociceptors respond to intense mechanical stimuli, but can be distinguished by their differential responsiveness to intense heat or their response to tissue injury. The C-fibre nociceptors are polymodal in nature, and respond to themal, mechanical and chemical stimuli [6]. On the other hand, the Aδ-nociceptors are mechanically insensitive and respond to noxious heat. Most of the C-fibre nociceptors also respond to noxious chemical stimuli such as acid or capsaicin. The natural stimuli for some of the nociceptors are difficult to define. These so called 'silent' or 'sleeping' nociceptors are responsive only when sensitized by tissue injury [3].

Diversity of Nociceptors

The nociceptors originate mainly from the skin, but also from other tissues [6]. The stimulation of corneal afferents by capsaicin or even by innocuous touch produce pain. In teeth almost any stimulus always produce pain. Visceral pain is unique in that there are no first (fast) or second (slow) components; instead pain is often poorly localized and dull. Distension or stretch is good enough to produce the pain without the tissue damage [7]. The pain of ischemia may have unique features that reflect innervation of vasculature by distinct subsets of acid sensitive primary sensory nociceptors. These features illustrate the vagueness of nociceptors and their diversity.

Molecular Mechanisms of Nociception

The nociceptors use different intracellular signalling mechanisms to detect the physical, thermal or chemical stimuli. Noxious heat mediates its action through the transient receptor (TRP) channels. Vanilloid receptors (VR-1 and VRL-l) belong to this family. The mechanical stimuli are detected by epithelial sodium channels (ENaC) or degenerin (DEG) channels [8]. The molecular transducers for detecting the noxious cold are yet to be identified [3].

The thresholds for the activation of cold sensitive fibres may not be as distinct as they are for the heat. First, the threshold for cold-evoked pain is not as precise as heat. Secondly, the noxious cold excites only 15% of the C-nociceptors as against 50% in response to heat in the same area of the hind paw of rodents [9]. Thus, it was proposed that noxious heat and cold are detected by distinct mechanisms. The mechanisms underlying the depolarization of nerve terminal by cold is not known, but appears to be mediated by inhibiting Na^+-K^+ ATPase or K^+ current [10] or by promoting Ca^{2+} and/or Na^+ influx [11, 12].

The nociceptors can be activated by mechanical stretch resulting from direct pressure, tissue deformation or changes in osmolarity. The detection of pressure or deformation is through the mechanically gated proteins involving brain sodium channel (BNC-l) or acid sensing ion channel-2 (ASIC-2) [8].

The nociceptors are activated by the diverse stimuli such as the chemicals released from tissue injury (protons, H^+ capsaicin, etc.), the thermal stimuli (increase/decrease in temperature) or the mechanical stimuli (pressure or stretch). Each of these involve different type of cell signalling pathways. The noxious chemicals such as capsaicin or H^+ are detected through VR-l receptors, Sometimes a single type of stimulus can interact with multiple detectors e.g. H^+ activate VR-l and ASIC-2, the latter belong to the family ENaC/DEG channel family. Other mechanisms might involve a mechano-chemical process, whereby, stretch evokes the release of a diffusible chemical messenger that then excites nearby primary sensory nerve terminal. Extracellular ATP excites primary sensory neurons via the ATP gated channels [13]. Even all these things may be brought about by a single nociceptor enabling the cell to integrate the information. Hence, the nociceptor must be equipped with large repertoire of transduction pathways.

Inflammatory Mediators in Nociception

The injury heightens the pain threshold by increasing the sensitivity of nociceptors to both the thermal and mechanical stimuli. This phenomenon results, in part, from the production and release of chemical mediators from the sensory terminal and/or from the non-neural cells [14]. The large group of molecules or chemicals are released during inflammation. They include protons, ATP, 5-hydroxytryptamine (5-HT) and lipids (Table 1) and alter the excitability by interacting with ion channels on the nociceptor surface, whereas, bradykinin and nerve growth factor (NGF) bind to the metabotrophic receptors and mediate their effects via second messenger signalling pathway [15].

Table 1 Substances present in the exudate of inflammation known as inflammatory soup [3] and the corresponding sites for their action

Chemicals	Channels or receptors
Nerve growth factor (NGF)	Tyrosine kinase A (TrkA)
Bradykinin (BK)	BK_2
5-Hydroxytryptamine (5-HT)	$5HT_3$
ATP	P_2X_3
Protons (H^+)	VR-1
Lipids	PGE_2/VR-1
Thermal (heat or cold)	VR-1/VRL-1
Mechanical (pressure/stretch)	ENaC/DEG

Allodynia

The receptive properties of the primary afferent nociceptors can be modulated by various factors. The persistent and pathological painful condition is known as allodynia. The nociceptors not only signal the acute pain but also contribute to the production of allodynia. This occurs in the setting of injury wherein pain is produced by innocuous stimuli [5, 16]. Allodynia can result from two different conditions: increased responsiveness of spinal cord pain transmission neurons (central sensitization), or by lowering the threshold for nociceptor activation (peripheral sensitization). With central sensitization, pain can be produced by activity in non-nociceptive primary sensory fibres. Peripheral sensitization is produced when nociceptors terminals become exposed to the products of tissue damage and inflammation, referred collectively as inflammatory soup (Table 1). Such products include extracellular protons, arachidonic acids and other lipid metabolites, 5-HT, bradykinin, nucleotides and nerve growth factors. All of them interact with the receptors or ion channels on the sensory nerve endings. The nociceptors release peptides and neurotransmitters (substance P, calcitonin gene related peptide, 5-HT and ATP), ₁rom their peripheral terminal when activated by noxious stimuli. These chemicals facilitate the production of inflammatory soup by promoting the release of factors from the local non-neuronal cells and vascular tissue. This phenomenon is known as neurogenic inflammation [5].

Glutamate in Nociceptive Transmission

All the primary nociceptors make synaptic connections with the neurons in the grey matter (dorsal horn) of the spinal cord. Some of these neurons transmit pain messages to higher centres including the reticular formation, thalamus and ultimately the cerebral cortex [6]. The neural circuitry within the dorsal horn is very complex. It is very much essential to understand the subclasses of primary sensory nociceptors and spinal circuits they engage.

Advances have been made in identifying the higher cortical areas that process the pain signals. But, far greater advances have been made in the understanding of the molecular mechanisms whereby primary sensory neurons detect pain producing stimuli and process them. Glutamate is the predominant excitatory transmitter at peripheral and central sites of nociception [17]. The central sites involve the processing at spinal cord or higher up where other transmitters such as substance-P, 5-HT are also involved [18]. Further, at the primary sensory nociceptors make synaptic connections with the neurons in the grey matter (dorsal horn) of the spinal cord. Subsets dorsal horn neurons in turn project axons and transmit pain messages to higher centers [4]. These subsets of neurons involve enkephalinergic and serotonergic neurons [18]. For the opioid receptors., the source of endogenous ligand is dear as the interneurons in the superficial dorsal horn synthesize opioid peptides that can target presynaptic opioid receptors and regulate the neurotransmitter release by decreasing Ca^{2+} conductance [5]. As noted above, it is likely that spinal cord derived PGE_2 targets the central terminal of the nociceptor. Functional presynaptic purinergic receptors have also been described and source of ATP can be identified [19]. By contrast presynaptic vanilloid receptors will never be exposed to noxious thermal temperatures or to the magnitude of pH changes that regulate VR-1 gating at the peripheral terminal of the nociceptor, and thus other ligands must be considered. Lipid mediators, such as anandamide, may be relevant. There is evidence for the presynaptic regulation of neurotransmitter release through an action of anandamide at both cannabonide (CB1) and vanilloid receptors in the dorsal horn [4]. Thus, the neural circuitry within the dorsal horn is incredibly complex. Understanding the subclasses of primary sensory nociceptors and the spinal circuits that are involved in the pain will be of great help for relieving the pain.

Nociception and Spinal Reflexes

The nociceptor stimulation evoke reflexes that protect the organisms from the impending danger. These include flexion reflexes (withdrawal reflexes), autonomic reflexes (regulating the heart and respiratory rates, dilatation of the pupil) and behavioral reflexes such as flight reactions, vocalization etc. [18]. The flexor or withdrawal reflexes involve polysynaptic pathways in the spinal cord. The polysynaptic reflexes can be recorded in spinal cord preparations *in vitro* and shown in Fig. 2 or elsewhere [20-24]. In this preparation, stimulation of dorsal root produce temporally dispersed reflex potentials in the corresponding segmental ventral root (Fig. 2). The first reflex potential has a latency of about 5 msec and is considered as monosynaptic reflex (MSR). Subsequent reflexes involve polysynaptic pathways (latency> greater than 15 msec) and known as polysynaptic reflexes (PSR). More than 2-3 PSRs were observed (Fig. 2). Our results show that PSRs were abolished in the presence of Mg^{2+} or NMDA receptor antagonist, 2-amino-5-phosphonovaleric acid (APV) in the medium [20, 24].

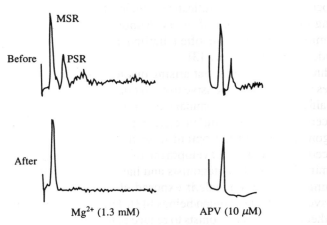

Fig. 2. Actual tracings of the reflex potentials recorded at L4 ventral root by stimulating the ipsilateral L_4 dorsal root in 6 day old neonatal rat spinal cord *in vitro*. The *first* reflex potential is a monosynaptic reflex (MSR) having a latency around 5 msec and the subsequent potentials have greater than 15 msec latency. They are polysynaptic reflexes (PSR). The PSRs were sensitive to Mg^{2+} and NMDA receptor antagonist, 2-amino-5-phosphonovaleric acid (APV) as evidenced by the reflexes in the bottom row. Vertical calibration=1 mV and horizontal calibration=10 msec.

The NMDA receptor complex has several sites, viz. NMDA, dizocilpine, Mg^{2+}, Zn^{2+}, polyamine and strychnine resistant $glycine_B$ [25]. The glycine binding site is distinct from the strychnine sensitive-glycine inhibitory receptors and is known as $glycine_B$ site [25]. The $glycine_B$ site is antagonized by 7-chlorokynurinic acid and D-serine is an agonist at this site [25]. The reports elsewhere show that 7-chlorokynurinic acid blocked the polysynaptic reflexes which could be reversed by D-serine [21, 22, 24]. Thus, the PSR is mediated through NMDA receptors involving $glycine_B$ site.

The *in vitro* spinal cord preparation is a good model to study the neuronal circuitry including the role of NMDA receptors and its modulation by other neurotransmitters [5-HT, GABA, acetylcholine) [26-30], neuropeptides (TRH, substance-P) [28, 31-34], or toxins (*Ptychodiscus brevis* toxin, organophosphorous compounds etc. [23. 24, 30, 35)]. Further, this preparation can be extended to spinal cord-hind limb preparation [36] or spinal cord-tail preparation [37] or spinal cord-nerve preparation [38] to investigate the nociceptor pathways.

NMDA Antogonists for the Treatment of Pain

One of the main challenges is to understand how both of the specific physiological properties of nociceptors and the circuits that they engage in the central nervous system determine the pain perception and the resultant behaviour. Molecular markers make it possible to identify and manipulate the activity of subsets of nociceptors. It is important to understand the function of the many neurotransmitters, receptors and transducers that are expressed by nociceptors and the significance of their transcriptional and post-translational setting in the regulation of injury. Although opioids and non-steroidal anti-inflammatory agents are often limited by their unacceptable side effects outside the pain pathway [3].

Chronic pain such as that arising due to the injury of peripheral or central nerves is often non-responsive to even opioids. Low dose of ketamine reduced the pain resulting chronic spinal cord injury [39, 40]. Amantidine significantly reduced the chronic pain in cancer patients [41]. Further, these NMDA antagonists reduced the opioid dose in the treatment of chronic pain and reduced the tolerance development by the narcotics [42]. Amantidine and ketamine are NMDA antagonists and have grave side effects on *memory* and learning of the individuals if exposed chronically. Ketamine even produce the psychotic state in human beings [43]. These considerations have prompted for other glutamate antagonists to reduce pain. Combined use of therapeutically safe glycine$_B$ antagonists with the opioids in the treatment of chronic pain is shown to be useful and synergistic with others. The glycine$_B$ antagonists even have been shown to block the development of chronic pain status and lower the development of tolerance to the opiates analgesics [44, 45]. The non-NMDA receptors include α-amino-3-hydroxy-5-methyl-4-isoxazole propionic acid (AMPA) and kainate site. The antagonists at these sites also exhibited analgesic effects [46]. These receptors are implicated for the chronic pain model and the NMDA receptors for the 'wind up' and to decrease the tolerance.

Conclusion

The nociception is a complex sensation, requiring diverse group of receptors and fibres, excited by the wide spectrum of stimuli. Further, the molecular mechanisms for the processing of nociception involve variety of ion channels and second messengers. Even a single nociceptor can involve multiple mechanisms. The *in vitro* preparations of spinal cord or spinal cord-tail or spinal cord-hind limb or spinal cord-nerve preparations will be useful to delineate the complex processing pathways and networking concerning the pain. These are so required to identify newer class of analgesics having no tolerance development and effective in reducing the pain.

References

1. Sherrington, C.S. The integrative action of the nervous system, New York: Scribner, 1906.
2. Burgress, P.R. and Perl, E.R. Myelinated afferent fibres responding specifically to noxious stimulation of the skin. *J. Physiol.*, 1967; **190**: 541–562.
3. Julius D. and Basbaum A.I. Molecular mechanisms of nociception. *Nature* 2001; **413**: 203 210.
4. Djouhri. L, Bleazard, L. and Lawson, S.N. Association of somatic action potential shape with sensory receptor properties in guinea pig dorsal root ganglion neurones. *J. Physiol.*, 1998; **513**: 857–872.
5. Basabaum, A.I. and Jessen, T.M. In: Kendel, E.R., Schwartz, J.H. and Jessell, T.M. (eds) Principles of Neuroscience. New York, McGraw-Hill, 2000; 472–491.
6. Raja, S.N., Meyer, R.A., Ringcarnp, M. and Campbell, I.N. In: Wall, P.D. and Melzack, R. (eds). Text book of pain. Edinburgh: Churchill Livingstone, 1999: 11–57.
7. Oebhart, O.F. Visceral polymodal receptors. *Frog. Brain. Res.*, 1996; **113**; 101–112.
8. Lingueglia, E., de Wille, J.R., Bassilina, F., Heurteux, C., Sakai, H., Waldmann, R. and Lazdunski, M. A modulatory subunits of acid sensing ion channels in brain and dorsal root ganglion cells. *J. Biol. Chem.*, 1997; **272**: 29778–29783.
9. Caterina, M.J., Leffler, A., Malmberg, A.R., Martin, W.J. Trafton J., Peterson-Zeitz, K.R., Koltzenburg, M., Basbaum, A.J. and Julius, D. Impaired nociception and pain sensation in mice lacking the capsaicin receptor. *Science*, 2000; **288**: 306–313.
10. Reid, G. and Fonta, M. Cold transduction by inhibition of a background potassium conductance in rat primary sensory neurones. *Neurosci. Lett*, 2001; **297**: 171–174.
11. Akswith, C., Benson, C., Welsh, M. and Snyder, P. DEG and ENaC ion channels involved in sensory transduction are modulated by cold temperature. *Proc Natl Acad Sci USA* 2001; **98**: 6459–6463.
12. Suto, K. and Gotoh, H., Calcium signalling in cold cells studied in cultured dorsal root ganglion neurones. *Neurosci*, 1999; **92**: 1131–1135.
13. Krishtal, O.A., Marchenko, S.M. and Obukhov, A.G. Cationic channels activated by extracellular ATP in rat sensory neurons. *Neurosci*, 1988; **27**: 995–1000.
14. Bevan, S., In: Wall, P.D., Melzack, R. (eds). Text book of pain. New York, Churchill Livingstone, 1999: 85–103.
15. Woolf, C.J. and Salter, M.W. Neuronal plasticity: increasing the gain in pain. *Science*, 2000; **288**: 1765–1767.
16. Basbaum, A.I. and Woolf, C.J. Pain. *Curr. Biol.*, 1999; **9**: R429–R431.
17. Weidner, C., Schmelz, M., Schmidt, R., Hansson, B., Handwerker, H.O. and Torebjork, H.E. Functional attributes discriminating mechano-insensitive and mechano-responsive C nociceptors in human skin. *J. Neuroscience*, 1999; **19**: 10184–10190.
18. Besson, J-M. and Chaouch, A. Peripheral and spinal mechanisms of nociception. *Physiol. Rev.*, 1987; **67**: 67–186.
19. Gu, J.G. and MacDermott, A.B. Activation of ATP P2X receptors elicits glutamate release from sensory neuron synapse. *Nature*, 1997; **389**: 749–753.
20. Deshpande, S.B. Significance of monosynaptic and polysynaptic reflexes in rat spinal cord *in vitro*. *Ind. J. Expt. Biol.*, 1993; **31**: 850–854.
21. Maruoka, Y., Ohno, Y., Tanaka, H., Yasuda, H., Ohtani, K.I., Sakamoto, H.,

Kawabe, A., Tamamura, C. and Nakamura, M. Selective depression of the spinal polysynaptic reflexes by the NMDA receptor antagonists in an isolated spinal cord *in vitro*. *Gen Pharmacol*, 1997; **29**: 645–649.

22. Maruoka, Y., Ohno, Y., Tanaka, H., Yasuda, H., Ohtani, K.I., Tamamura, C. and Nakamura, M. Effect of novel tricyclic quinoxalinedione and its analogs on N-methyl-D-aspartate (NMDA) receptor mediated synaptic transmission in the isolated neonatal rat spinal cord *in vitro*. *Jpn. J. Pharmacol*. 1998; **76**: 265–270.

23. Singh, J.N., Das Gupta, S., Gupta, A.K., Dube, S.N. and Deshpande, S.B. Relative potency of synthetic analogs of *Ptychodiscus brevis* toxin in depressing synaptic transmission evoked in neonatal rat spinal cord *in vitro*. *Toxicol. Lett.*, 2002; **128**: 177–184.

24. Singh, J.N. and Deshpande, S.B. Involvement of N-methyl-D-aspartate receptors for the *Ptychodiscus brevis* toxin-induced depression of monosynaptic and polysynaptic reflexes in neonatal rat spinal cord *in vitro*. *Neurosci*, 2002 (in press).

25. Dansyz, W. and Parsons, C.G. Glycine and N-methyl-D-aspartate receptors: Physiological significance and possible therapeutic applications. *Pharmacal. Rev.* 1998; **50**: 597–664.

26. Deshpande, S.B. and Warnick, J.E. Temperature dependence of reflex transmission in the neonatal rat spinal cord *in vitro:* Influence on strychnine and bicuculline sensitive inhibitions. *Neuropharmacology*, 1988; **27**: 1033–1037.

27. Deshpande, S.B. and Warnick, J.E. Receptor subtypes involved in mediating serotonin induced depression of the spinal monosynaptic reflex *in vitro*. In: Manchanda, S.K., Selvamurthy, W., Mohan Kumar, V. (eds). Advances in Physiological Sciences. New Delhi, Macmillan India Ltd, 1992; 631–635.

28. Deshpande, S.B. and Warnick, J.E. Thyrotropin-releasing hormone reverses the supersensitively depressed monosynaptic transmission by serotonin in 5,7 dihydroxytryptamine treated neonatal rats *in vitro*. *Brain Research* 1994; **655**: 263–266.

29. Warnick, J.E., Deshpande, S.B., Yang, Q.Z. and Das Gupta, S. Biphasic action of sarin on monosynaptic reflex in the neonatal rat spinal cord *in vitro*. *Arch Toxico*, l1993; **67**: 302–306.

30. Das Gupta, S., Deshpande, S.B. and Warnick, J.E. Segmental depression caused diisopropylphosphorofluoridate and sarin is reversed by thyrotropin-releasing hormone in the neonatal rat spinal cord. *Toxicol Appl. Pharmacal.*, 1988; **95**: 499–506.

31. Deshpande, S.B., Pilotte, N.S. and Warnick, J.E. Gender specific action of thyrotropin-releasing hormone in the mammalian spinal cord. *FASEB J*, 1987; **1**: 478–482.

32. Deshpande, S.B. and Warnick, J.E. Interaction of thyrotropin-releasing hormone and methylsergide on the monosynaptic reflex in isolated mammalian spinal cord. *Neurosci Lett*, 1990; **116**: 141–148.

33. Deshpande, S.B. and Warnick, J.E. Thyrotropin releasing hormone-induced potentiation of spinal monosynaptic reflex in rats *in vitro*. *Ind. J. Expt. Biol.*, 1993; **31**: 112–114.

34. Deshpande, S.B. and Warnick, J.E. Analogs of thyrotropin-releasing hormone in potentiating the spinal monosynaptic reflex *in vitro*. *Eur J. Pharmacol.*, 1994; **271**: 439–444.

35. Deshpande, S.B. and Das Gupta, S. Diisopropylphosphorofluoridate-induced depression of segmental monosynaptic transmission in neonatal rat spinal cord is also mediated by increased axonal activity. *Toxicol. Lett*, 1997; **90**: 177–182.

36. King, A.E., Thompson, S.W.N. and Woolf, C.J. Characterization of the cutaneous input to the ventral horn *in vitro* using the isolated spinal cord-hind limb preparation. *J. Neurosci. Meth.*, 1990; **35**: 36–46.

37. Otsuka, M. and Yanagisawa, M. and Effect of a tachykinin antagonist on a nociceptive reflex in the isolated spinal cord-tail preparation of the new born rat. *J. Physiol.*, 1988; **395**: 255–270.

38. Yoshioka, K., Sakuma, M. Otsuka, M. Cutaneous nerve-evoked cholinergic inhibition of monosynaptic reflex in the neonatal rat spinal cord: Involvement of M2 receptors and tachykininergic primary afferents. *Neuroscience.*, 1990; **38**: 195–203.

39. Eide, K., Stubhaug, A., Oye, I. and Breivik, H. Continuous subcutaneous administration of the N-methyl-D-aspartic acid (NMDA) receptor antagonist ketamine in the treatment of post-herpetic neuralgia. *Pain*, 1995; **61**: 221–228.

40. Eisenberg, E. and Pud, D. Can patients with chronic neuropathic pain be cured by acute administration of the NMDA receptor antagonist amantidine? *Pain*, 1998; **74**: 337–339.

41. Pud, D., Eisenberg, E., Spitzer, A., Adler, R., Fried, G. and Yarnitsky, D. NMDA receptor antagonist amantadine reduces surgical neuropathic pain in cancer patients: A double blind, randomized, placebo controlled trial. *Pain*, 1998; **75**: 349–354.

42. Dingledine, R., Borges, K., Bowie, D., Traynclis, S.F. The glutamate receptor ion channels. *Pharamacol. Rev.*, 1999; **51**: 7–61.

43. Krystal, J.H., Karper, L.P., Seibyl, J.P., Freeman, G.K., Delaney, R., Bremner, J.D., Heninger, G.R., Bowers, M.B. Jr, Charney, D.S. Subanaesthetic effects of the noncompetitive NMDA antagonist, ketamine, in humans. Psychotomimetic, perceptual, cognitive and neuroendocrine responses. *Arch. Gen. Psychiatry.*, 1994; **51**: 199–214.

44. Eide, P.K., Stubhaug, A. and Stenehjcm, A.E. Central dysesthesia pain after traumatic spinal cord injury is dependent on *n*-methyl-D-aspartate receptor activation. *Neurosurgery*, 1995; **37**: 1080–1087.

45. Eliott, K., Kest, B., Man, A., Kao, B. and Inturrisi, C.E., N-mcthyl-D-aspartate (NMDA) receptors, mu, kappa opioid tolerance and perspective in new analgesic drug development. *Neuropsycopharmacol.*, 1995; **13**: 347–356.

46. Simmons, R.M.A., Li, D.L., Hoo, K.H,, Deverill, M., Omstein, P.L. and Iyengar, S., Kainate, GluR5 receptor subtype mediates the nociceptive response to formalin in the rat. *Neuropharmacology*, 1998; **37**: 25–36.

47. Erlanger, J. and Gaser, H.S. Electrical signs and nervous activity. Philadelphia, University of Pennsylvania Press, 1938.

Pain Updated: Mechanisms and Effects
Edited by R. Mathur

9. Mechanisms Underlying Progression of Acute to Chronic Pain: Role of Autonomic Nervous System

Neena Bhattacharya[1] and Abhijit Bhattacharya[2]

Departments of [1]Physiology and [2]Anesthesiology,
University College of Medical Sciences, Delhi-110095, India

Introduction

Chronic pain is markedly different from acute pain, be it the cause, its function, characteristic features, underlying patho-physiology or management. It is considered to be *pathological* because of underlying chronic pathological process in either somatic, viscera or neural tissue besides a significant involvement of psycho-social and environmental factors. While acute pain has been identified as *physiological* which sub-serves a very useful function (most of the time), of warning and protecting the body tissues from harmful effects of chemical, mechanical or thermal trauma. The duration of pain that will qualify its inclusion into the category of chronic pain is controversial. A wide variety of duration varying from 3 to 6 months have been mentioned in different reports. However, the most logical criteria has been suggested by Bonica [1] which is now widely accepted. It states that "the pain which persists for a month beyond the usual course of an acute disease or reasonable time for an injury to heal, or that which recurs at intervals for months or years is chronic pain".

Chronic pain cannot be considered as a mere prolongation of acute pain, it is certainly as a result of changes induced in peripheral and/or central nervous system by untreated/persistent pain. Development and progression of acute to chronic pain may primarily involve the following areas:

(a) Peripheral nociceptors
(b) Spinal and higher neural mechanisms
(c) Psycho-socio environmental factors

In this article mechanisms at the former two levels are being elaborated.

Mechanisms Involving Peripheral Nociceptors

Nociception starts with the noxious stimulation of the nociceptors and liberation of algogenic substances like serotonin, histamine, bradykinin, prostaglandins

(PG) etc. (Fig. 1). These substances act directly on the cell membrane of the nociceptor and excite it resulting in the production of the excitatory neurotransmitters such as glutamate and substance P from primary afferents at the dorsal horn or the equivalent brain stem neurons and an impulse, which is conducted along different neural pathways to the central nervous system [2].

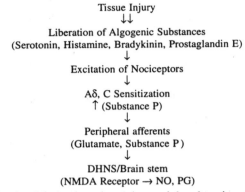

Fig. 1.   Mechanisms involving peripheral nociceptors.

The algogenic substances not only act on the nociceptor cell membrane but also cause increased capillary permeability resulting in edema and a further increase in chemical mediators causing progressive nociceptor stimulation. In addition, substance P is brought via retrograde route to the nociceptor terminals. The inflammatory mediators can cause continuous low frequency discharge in the nociceptor afferent. The chemical environment created around the nociceptor is complex nevertheless a simplified version of it is shown in Fig. 2 [4].

Up regulation of genes encoding sequence of afferent neuropeptides (Substance P, Neurokinin A) also results as a consequence of persistent afferent stimulation as shown in Freund's adjuvant-induced monoarthritis in the rat [5]. Tissue injury thus begins the inflammatory process. However, if it is immediately checked, the situation returns to normal. But, when it is not checked, it leads to the development of sensitization of receptors and accompanying allodynia and hyperalgesia. Neurophysiological studies conducted on arthritic animal pain model have significantly contributed towards the understanding of this mechanism. In these animals the nociceptors were easily excited by even a mild mechanical stimulus in contrast to their pre-arthritis condition, when they responded to only noxious stimuli. Thus persistent stimulation of nociceptors leads to the development of nociceptor sensitization. Sensitization of C polymodal nociceptors has been suggested in various types of nerve injuries, inflammatory diseases, and also reflex sympathetic dystrophy [6].

Effect of tissue damage on C-fiber terminals can further add to the sensitization of nociceptor by the C-fiber mediated axon-reflex causing vasodilatation and neurogenic edema [7]. Additionally when an axon is cut, it begins to regress, sprint towards the periphery and generate chronic afferent barrages, which can continue indefinitely if reconnection is not established [8]. Persistent stimulation and subsequent sensitization of nociceptors probably contribute towards chronic pain associated with growing cancer of viscera and tumors obstructing blood vessels.

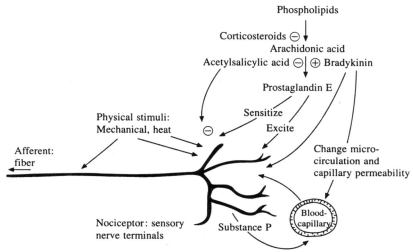

Fig. 2. Nociceptor and its environment. The nociceptor, represented histologically as the terminal arborization of an afferent fiber, is excited or has its excitability enhance by physical stimuli and/or endogenous algesic substances. These substances are also vasoactive: they affect microcirculation and muscular permeability, which in turn change the microenvironment of the nociceptor resulting in facilitation. Algesic substances exert facilitatory interactions, e.g. the facilitation (+) of prostaglandin synthesis by bradykinin. Peripherally acting analgesic drugs such as acetylsalicylic acid inhibit (−) the synthesis of prostaglandin and the excitability of the nociceptor (adapted from [4]).

Fortunately, most of the mechanisms at the peripheral receptor level such as those associated with inflammatory pain leading to persistent nociceptor stimulation have been studied in details. Therefore, this is the primary site where the noxious information can be interferred with to relieve pain. Synthetase inhibitors, or local anaesthetics are commonly utilized to relieve pain because of their peripheral site of action. In the development of chronic pain, there is a significant contribution of peripheral mechanism. Therefore, peripheral nociceptors are one of the convenient sites for the prevention of development of chronic pain. This is further evidenced by the peripheral site of action of most pain relief measures in chronic pain (Table 1).

Therapy targeted towards peripheral pathophysiology treats causalgia seen initially in peripheral nerve injuries. If effective therapy is not carried out early, the patho-physiological changes shift to central neuraxis and may even

Table 1 Relief in pain by measures acting locally

Sr. No.	Painful conditions/Sites	Pain relief measures
1	Arthritis	Drug: PG synthesis inhibitors (Aspirin, Indomethacin)
2	Coronary artery disease	Bypass surgery
3	Myofascial tendonitis (joints, tendons)	Drug: Local anesthetics in muscle
4	Pain due to chronic degenerative changes in the knee	Knee replacement

become irreversible. Some chronic pain conditions have a predominant peripheral component namely arthritis, myofascial syndrome, chronic tendonitis, neuritis, some neuropathic disorders, headaches, pancreatitis and peripheral vascular disease etc.

Persistent peripheral stimulation leads to the plasticity in central neuraxis which further supports chronicity of the pain. Hence, untreated acute pain, when allowed to persist, can cause detrimental effects.

Decreased Peripheral Input/Nerve Dissociation Theory

This theory was originally proposed by Noordenbos [9] to explain pain associated with peripheral nerve disorders. These disorders lead to a reduction in the large nerve fibers, which reduces the inhibition of synaptic transmission among dorsal horn neurons. The concept was later incorporated into the Melzack and Wall theory of pain. Nerve dissociation theory, however, has lost popularity as it has become evident that a selective reduction in large myelinated fibers does not necessarily result in pain. Moreover, microneurography has shown absence of any ongoing activity in nociceptive fibers [6].

There are attempts to explain chronic pain on the basis of ectopic impulse generation in partially or totally transected nerves undergoing regeneration. These nerves are capable of generating abnormal discharges. Most often the source of ectopic impulses are fine sprouts and demyelination plaques in peripheral nerves. Studies on regenerating nerve fibers have revealed spontaneous and mechano-sensitive discharges in these fibers, which could be the probable basis of chronic pain felt by patients with partially or completely transected nerves. Similarly, an increased firing in sensory units under conditions of chronic nerve compression, e.g. in herniated inter-vertebral disc may lead to chronic pain.

At the Spinal Cord and Brainstem Level

Persistent nociceptive stimulation not only results in peripheral nociceptor sensitization but also leads to increased excitability of spinal cord neurons. Afferent input into the spinal cord is processed by dorsal horn neurons in a specific manner wherein the responses of the neurons are not static or stereotyped but are in a state of continuous dynamism. They change according to the situation. At any given time spinal neuronal pools are under the influence of peripheral input, higher neural descending activity and their own intrinsic excitatory state coupled to neurotransmitter levels. Spinal neurons can be visualized as undergoing continuous change in excitability, leading to hypo- to hyperalgesic state. This concept has been described by Woolf [10]. A shift in neuronal excitability can be brought about by a number of external and/or internal factors including continuous peripheral nociceptive inputs.

Increased responsiveness of spinal neurons located in deep dorsal and ventral horns, along with expansion of their peripheral receptive fields under conditions of persistent peripheral sensory input have been demonstrated most conclusively by elegant neuro-physiological studies in both human and animal experimental models [11, 12]. Spinal sensitization has been mostly shown to occur in wide dynamic range (WDR) neurons, which receive input from both nociceptors and low threshold mechanoceptors. This also explains mechanism of secondary hyperalgesia and allodynia.

Increased levels of neurotransmitters like glutamate, substance P, neurokinin A, calcitonin gene related peptide linked to the development of prolonged depolarization and EPSP within 2-3 weeks in peripheral inflammation are well documented [3, 12, 13]. At the dorsal horn neurons (DHNS) glutamate mediated N-methyl-D-aspartate (NMDA) receptor activation leads to Ca^{2+} influx and initiation of an enzyme cascade. The latter finally evokes the release of nitric oxide (NO) and prostaglandins (PGs). NO and PGs in turn have been hypothesized to further increase the release of glutamate leading to an ongoing activity in the primary afferents thereby contributing towards peripheral and central sensitization [13, 14]. A mutual potentiation of NO, PG, glutamate and NMDA receptor and their involvement in the initiation as well as maintenance of facilitated nociception has been suggested in several reports [15, 16, 17]. Therefore, NO and PGs may be subserving an important role in the chronification of pain. To explain the central neural involvement in the genesis of chronic pain several theories have been propounded.

One of the earliest theories is 'central summation theory' according to which intense stimulation from the damaged nerve and tissue activates internuncial pools of neurons in the spinal cord creating reverberating activity in closed self exciting neuron loops. This prolonged activity spreads to spinal cord pain transmission neurons as well as those in the lateral and ventral horns. Spread of activity to the former group of neurons explains the sympathetic while that to the latter explains motor effects. Thus, pain is accompanied by sympathetic outflow and motor effects (muscle spasm). This hypothesis is the most accepted conceptualization of pathophysiological mechanism underlying chronic pain. It has been supported by experimental studies that have revealed increased neuronal discharge in laminae I, V and also deeper laminae of spinal cord [10, 18].

Central Pain Mechanisms

The hypothesis offered by Haugen [19] was based on the complexity and dynamic plasticity of central nervous system (CNS). It explains the fate of sensory information after entering into CNS. The information may be transmitted or ignored, accentuated or diminished and may ascend to consciousness or short-circuited in the vicious circle of activity within short chains of internuncial neurons. The later possibility is seen in chronic pain. Pre-existing back ground activity in the internuncial pool and brain stem reticular activating neurons play a very important role in providing the dynamic characteristic to CNS. The concept is quite useful in explaining persistence of activity after the utility of sensory input passes away.

Central biasing mechanism (CBM) can be visualized as a further extension of Haugen's hypothesis utilized by Melzack [20] to explain pain of phantom limb, causalgia and other peripheral nerve injuries. According to this hypothesis a portion of the brain stem reticular formation has been conceptualized as CBM which exerts a tonic inhibitory influence or 'a bias' on transmission at all synaptic levels of somato-sensory system (Fig. 3). This inhibitory function

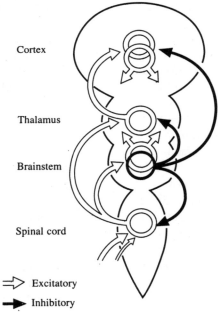

Fig. 3. Central biasing mechanism proposed by Melzack. Large and small fibers from a limb activate a neuron pool in the spinal cord, which excites neuron pools at successively higher levels. The central biasing mechanism, represented by inhibitory projection system that originates in the brain stem reticular formation modulates activity at all levels. When sensory fibers are destroyed after amputation or peripheral nerve lesion the inhibitory influence decreases and this decrease results in sustained activity at all levels that can be triggered by the remaining fibers (adapted from [1]).

of CBM depends on normal sensory input into it. Thus, when there is a loss of sensory input into the system, namely, after nerve lesion, amputation etc. would weaken this (CBM) inhibitory system and produce persistent pain.

Injury/lesion of certain parts of the nervous system can cause spontaneous burning or aching pain. It may occur during accidental injuries of spinal cord, surgical interruption of pain pathways or diseases like tabes dorsalis, syringomyelia and multiple sclerosis.

Role of Autonomic Nervous System in Chronic Pain

The sympathetic nervous system has been implicated in maintaining a number of pain states [19, 21]. It is, therefore, implied that the afferent sympathetic neurons could be targeted for the therapeutic purposes. Reflex sympathetic pain syndromes are now well recognized conditions exhibiting causalgia and sympathetic overactivity [22]. Pain associated with a number of conditions is relieved by sympatholytic therapy [23, 24, 25, 26]. Further, $\alpha1$-receptors are significantly involved in sympathetically maintained pain [27]. A state of anxiety/overactivity of sympathetic nervous system potentiates chronic abdominal pain in some patients due to the development of post-operative intestinal adhesions [19]. A relief in their pain by splanchnectomy further supports the involvement of sympathetic activation in this group of patients [28]. It is well known that constrictive spasm of blood vessels can lead to pain and the stimulation of sympathetic nerve fibers produce maximal vasoconstriction. Therefore, sympathetic nervous system has a vital role in a number of chronic pain conditions of vascular origin, namely, angina pectoris and intermittent claudication.

Several studies from our laboratory have revealed an involvement of autonomic nervous system in acupuncture analgesia. In anaesthetized cats, acupuncture like stimulation of sciatic nerve evoked pressor and depressor blood pressure responses. A trend towards potentiation of depressor and inhibition of pressor response was seen at the end of acupuncture stimulation [29]. It was explained on the basis of a shift in autonomic balance towards increased parasympathetic and/or decreased sympathetic activity. This was further supported by a study conducted on pain patients undergoing acupuncture therapy for pain relief. Blood flow measurement using venous occlusion plethysmography following acupuncture stimulation on the contralateral limb revealed varying degrees of increase in blood flow (Table 2).

In addition to this, a variable degree of fall in BP and pupillary constriction was seen in these patients following acupuncture analgesia. The data strongly suggests a shift towards parasympathetic activation and sympathetic inhibition with a concommitant pain relief resulting from acupuncture therapy [30].

Several experimental studies have demonstrated modulation of nociception by nor adrenergic system. Iontophoretic application of norepinephrine has been shown to inhibit the discharge of dorsal horn neurons evoked by noxious stimulation [31]. Electrical stimulation of brain stem noradrenergic nuclei

Table 2 Blood flow in contralateral limb following acupuncture stimulation

Sr. No.	Patient name	Age	Sex	Diagnosis	Rate of blood flow (ml/min)		
					Before	After	Increase %
1	JK	30	M	Gangrene toe	8.16	8.72	6.86
2	JAYA	28	F	Raynaud's	3.9	5.67	45.38
3	SK	42	F	Osteoarthritis	8.18	9.3	13.69
4	AJ	11	F	Bell's palsy	5.17	7.38	42.75
5	AL	25	M	Facial palsy	5.69	6.34	11.42
6	SB	24	M	Bronchial asthma	8.84	10.85	22.74
7	VW	60	F	Facial palsy	6.89	9.37	35.99
8	NB	40	F	Facial palsy	3.44	4.45	29.36
9	DC	30	M	Facial spasm	6.79	9.69	42.71
10	MC	56	M	Bronchial asthma	4.15	5.33	28.43

has been reported to produce analgesia [32, 33]. In line with these are several observations on clonidine (a central $\alpha 2$-adrenoceptor agonist) of analgesic effects [34, 35, 36, 37].

Experimental work has revealed mechanisms through which sympathetic activity contributes to abnormal pain sensation. Wall and Gutnick [38] have shown that the sprouts formed by regenerating axons develop a sensitivity to nor-epinephrine (NE) mediated by α-adrenergic receptors. After injury NE receptors on the terminals of severed primary afferent axons are expressed.

Effect of adrenergic and cholinergic blockers on tail flick latencies of wistar rats was examined. A decrease in tail flick latency [TFL) was noted with both adrenergic (propranalol) and cholinergic (atropine) blockade. However, the decrease in TFL (hyperalgesia) was much more significant with cholinergic blockers. Furthermore, it occurred even in spinal animals, although the decrease in TFL was lesser (Table 3) [30].

These results suggest an inhibitory role of both the adrenergic and cholinergic activation on nociception wherein, the latter influence was more pronounced. However, association of pain with sympathetic overactivity and its relief with decreased sympathetic and increased parasympathetic activity has been seen in several other situations [39].

In order to understand the mechanisms underlying genesis and progression of chronic pain one needs to identify factors that increase the excitability of nociceptors and those involved in the maintenance of it for prolonged

Table 3 **Effect of propranalol (4 mg/kg I/P) and atropine (1 mg/kg) on tail flick latency of intact and spinal rats**

Intact	Group	Before	After	P value
	Saline	3.32 ± 0.25	2.98 ± 0.18	NS
	Propranalol	3.35 ± 0.25	2.68 ± 0.21	$P < 0.02$
	Atropine	3.49 ± 0.22	2.48 ± 0.13	$P < 0.001$
	Saline	2.68 ± 0.32	2.51 ± 0.22	NS
		2.83 ± 0.19	2.53 ± 0.22	
Spinal				
	Propranalol	2.46 ± 0.30	2.53 ± 0.22	NS
	Atropine	2.17 ± 0.32	1.71 ± 0.06	$P < 0.02$

duration. Pathophysiology underlying genesis of chronic pain may be at the nociceptor level, while its increase in intensity and maintenance may be by dorsal horn neurons, higher neural centers or the autonomic interaction with the pain system. An understanding and recognition of the above mentioned sites is necessary in the institution of the most appropriate and effective therapy.

Acknowledgement

Authors gratefully acknowledges the help received from some of their colleagues from the department of Physiology and Anaesthesiology Critical Care, University College of Medical Sciences and GTB Hospital, Shahdara, Delhi while conducting these studies.

References

1. Bonica, J.J. General considerations of chronic pain. In : Bonica J.J., Lea and Febiger (Eds), Management of Pain. Philadelphia, London, 1990; 180–196.
2. Lawand, N.B., McNearney, T., Westlund, K.N. Amino acid release into the knee joint: key role in nociception and inflammation. *Pain*, 2000; **86**: 69–74.
3. Schaible, H.G., Schmidt, R.F. (Eds) Time course of mechanosensitivity changes in articular afferents during a developing experimental arthritis. *J. Neurophysiology*, 1988; **60**: 2180–2195.
4. Zimmermann, M. Basic concepts of pain and pain therapy. In : Sharma KN et al. *Current Trends in Pain Research and Therapy* 1988; **3**: 1–13.
5. Donaldson, L.F., Harmar, A.J., McQueen, D.S. and Seckl, J.R. Increased expression of preprotachykinin, calcitonin gene-related peptide, but not vasoactive intestinal peptide messenger RNA in dorsal root ganglia during the development of adjuvant monoarthritis in the rat. *Molecular Brain Research* 1992; **16**: 143–149.
6. Ochoa, J.L., Torebjork, E., Marchettini, P. and Sivak, M. Mechanisms of neuropathic pain: Cumulative observations, new experiments and further speculation. In : H.L. Fields, R. Dubner, F. Cervero and L.E. Jones (Eds). Advances in Pain Research and Therapy. Vol. 9 New York, Raven Press, 1985; 431–450.
7. Wall, P.D. Introduction. In: P.D. Wall and R. Melzack (Eds). Textbook of Pain, New York, Churchill Livingston, 1985; 1–16.

8. Whitehead, W. Chronic Pain : An overview. In: Thornas W. Miller (Ed). Chronic Pain, International University Press, Inc. Connecticut 1988; 5–48.

9. Noordenbos, W. Pain. Amsterdam, Elsevier 1959.

10. Woolf, C.J., Wall, P.D. Relative effectiveness of C. Primary afferent fibers of different origins in evoking a prolonged facilitation of the flexor reflex in the rat. *J. Neurosci.*, 1986; **6**: 1433–1442.

11. Grubb, B.D., Stiller, R.U., Schaible, H.G. Dynamic changes in the receptive field properties of spinal cord neurons with ankle input in rats with chronic unilateral inflammation in the ankle region. *Experimental Brain Research*, 1993; **92**: 441–452.

12. Neugebauer, V., Schaible, H.G. Evidence for a central component in the sensitization of spinal neurons with joint input during development of acute arthritis in cat's knee. *J. Neurophysiology*, 1990; **64**: 299–311.

13. Wu, J., Lin, Q., McAdoo, D.J., Willis, W.D. Nitric oxide contributes to central sensitization following intradermal injection of capsaicin. *Neuro. Report*, 1998; **9**: 589–592.

14. Kawamata, T. and Omote, K. Activation of spinal N-methyl-D-aspartate receptors stimulates a nitric oxide/cyclic guanosine 3,5-monophosphate/glutamate release cascade in nociceptive signaling. *Anesthesiology*, 1999; **91**: 1415–1424.

15. Dickenson, A.H. A cure for wind up: NMDA receptor antagonists as potential analgesics. *Trends Pharmacol. Sci.*, 1990; **11**: 307–309.

16. Minami, T., Onaka, M., Okuda, Ashitaka, E., Mori, H., Ito, S. and Hayaishi O. L-NAME, an inhibitor of nitric oxide synthase, blocks the established allodynia induced by intrathecal administration of prostaglandin E2. *Neurosci. Lett*, 1995; **201**: 239–242.

17. Muth-Selbach, U.S., Tegeder, I., Brune, K., Geisslinger, G. Acetaminophen inhibits spinal prostaglandin E_2 release after peripheral noxious stimulation. *Anesthesiology*, 1999; **91**: 231–239.

18. Blumberg, H. and Janig, W. Changes of reflexes in vasoconstrictor neurons supplying the cat hind limb following chronic nerve lesions : a model for studying mechanisms of reflex sympathetic dystrophy. *J. Auton. Nerv. Syst.*, 1983; 7: 399–411.

19. Haugen, F.P. The autonomic nervous system and pain. *Anesthesiology*, 1968; **29**: 785–792.

20. Melzack, R. Phantom limb pain: Implications for treatment of pathologic pain. *Anesthesiology*, 1971; **35**: 409–419.

21. Koltzenburg, M. and McMahon, S.B. The enigmatic role of the sympathetic nervous system in chronic pain. *Trends Pharmacol. Sci.*, 1991; **12**: 399–401.

22. Merskey, H. Classification of chronic pain, description of chronic pain syndromes and definition of pain terms. IASP Press, *Seattle*, 1994; 40–43.

23. Bell, S.N., Cole, R. and Roberts-Thomson I.C. Coeliac plexus block for control of pain in chronic pancreatitis. *Br. Med. J.*, 1980; **281**: 1604.

24. Waldman, S.D. Celiac plexus block. In : Weiner RS (Ed). Innovations in Pain Management. Orlando, PMD Press, 1990; 10–15.

25. Waldman, S.D. Management of acute pain. *Postgrad. Med.*, 1992; **87**: 15–17.

26. Raj, P. Stellate ganglion block. In : Waldman and Winnie (Ed.). Interventional Pain Management. Philadelphia, WB Saunders, 1996; 269.

27. Torebjork, E. In: Stanton Hicks, M., Janig, W. and Boas, R.A. (Eds). Reflex Sympathetic Dystrophy. Kluwer Academic Publisher, 1990; 71–80.

28. White, J.C. and Smithwich, R.H. (Eds). The Autonomic Nervous System. Anatomy, Physiology and Surgical Application. Second edition, New York, Macmillan, 1941.

29. Bhattacharya, N., Radhakrishnan, V., Sharma, K.N. and Bhattacharya, A. Modification of somato-autonomic responses by electro acupuncture stimulation. In : Sharma, K.N. and Nayar, U. (Eds). Basic Mechanisms and Clinical Applications, Indian Society for Pain Research and Therapy, 1985; 215–221.

30. Bhattacharya, N., Vaney, N. and Sharma, K.N. Effect of adrenergic and cholinergic antagonists on pain sensitivity in intact and spinal rats. In : Sharma, K.N. et al. (Eds). Pain Sensitivity and Management of Pain Syndromes. *Indian Society for Pain Research and Therapy*, 1989; **5**: 27–38.

31. Belcher, G., Ryall, R.W. and Schaffner, R. The differential effects of 5-hydroxytryptamine, noradrenaline and raphe stimulation on nociceptive and non-nociceptive dorsal horn interneurones in the cat. *Brain Res*, 1978; **151**: 307–321.

32. Akaike, A., Shibata, M.S. and Takagi, H. Analgesia induced by microinjection of morphine into and electrical stimulation of the nucleus reticularis and paragigantocellularis of rat medulla oblongata. *Neuropharmacology*, 1978; **17**: 775–778.

33. Segal, M. and Sandberg, D. Analgesia produced by electrical stimulation of catecholamine nuclei in the rat brain. *Brain Res.*, 1977; **123**: 369–372.

34. Kulkarni, S.K. Heat and other physiological stress induced analgesia: catecholamine mediated and naloxone reversible response. *Life Sci.*, 1980; **27**: 185–188.

35. Paalzow, G.H. and Paalzow, L.K. Separate noradrenergic receptors could mediate clonidine-induced antinociception. *J. Pharmacol. Exp. Ther.*, 1982, **223**: 795–800.

36. Bentley, G.A., Newton, S.H. and Starr, J. Studies on the antinociceptive action of α-agonist drugs and their interactions with opioid mechanisms. *Br. J. Pharmacol.*, 1983; **79**: 125–134.

37. Shankar, N., Varshaney, A., Bhattacharya, A. and Sharma, K.N. Electroacupuncture, morphine and clonidine: a comparative study of analgesic effects. *Indian J. Physiol. Pharmacol.*, 1996; **40**: 225–230.

38. Wall, P.D. and Gutnick, M. Ongoing activity in peripheral nerves; the physiology and pharmacology of impulses originating from a neuroma. *Exp. Neurol.*, 1974; **43**: 580–593.

39. Bhattacharya, N. Role of autonomic nervous system in nociception. Proceedings of 10th World Congress on Pain. 2002; San Diego IASP, Abstract 81–P77, p. 27.

Pain Updated: Mechanisms and Effects
Edited by R. Mathur
Copyright © 2006 Anamaya Publishers, New Delhi, India

10. Biochemical Correlates of Electrophysiological Ageing of the Brain

Rameshwar Singh,[1] Deepak Sharma,[1]
Sangeeta Singh[2] and Jaspreet Kaur[3]

[1]School of Life Sciences, Jawaharlal Nehru University, New Delhi-110 067, India

[2]Zoology Department, Bareilly College, Bareilly, India

[3]School of Graduate Medical Education, Neuroscience Research Center,
Seton Hall University, South Orange, New Jersey 07079-2689, USA

Abstract. Electrical activity is the functional basis of the nervous system. During the ageing of the nervous system there are alterations in its electrophysiological activity (action potentials, synaptic potentials, compounded wave forms such as the electroencephalogram etc.). For example, the inability to produce bursts of high frequency firing in aged tissue may reduce neurotransmitter release which may adversely affect synaptic plasticity and information processing. Multiple-unit activity (action potentials simultaneously derived from many neurons) represents an electrophysiological marker of cellular firing activity. An age-related decline in the spontaneous (basal) neuronal firing may be of interest as one of the neuronal indicators of electrophysiological ageing of the brain. The mechanism of age-related alterations in electrical activity arising from biochemical changes in the nervous tissue is an important aspect to consider. Age-related changes in biochemical parameters such as lipid peroxidation, and membrane sodium-potassium adenosine triphosphatase (pump) affect the membrane electrophysiology. It is therefore, of interest to study the interrelationship between the ageing-related alterations in biochemical and multiple-unit activity. Pearson's correlation analyses between multiple-unit activity decline and various biochemical parameters reveal direct correlation between electrophysiological decline and oxidative stress-producing mechanisms. Statistical correlation together with the available experimental data show that oxidative stress parameters significantly contribute to the electrophysiological ageing of the brain. Treatment with drugs countering the oxidative stress may augment neuroelectric activity and consequently cognitive functions.

Introduction

The normally ageing brain shows a variety of changes, namely, morphological (regionally-selective neuron loss, progressive loss of neuronal processes, declining synapse numbers, neurotransmitter receptors losses), biochemical (declining neurotransmitter levels, increased lipid peroxidation and lipofuscin accumulation, decline in protein synthetic ability, peroxidation of proteins), electrophysiological (altered action and synaptic potentials) and behavioural (loss in cognitive ability). These may be linked to various ageing-related brain dysfunctions. Neural electrophysiological signals such as the membrane potential, action potential, synaptic potentials, evoked potentials and the electroencephalogram (EEG) reflect various facets and status of neuronal physiological activity [1, 2]. Many types of electrophysiological signals are affected during ageing [3-9]. For example, the synaptosomal resting membrane potential appears to decrease [10, 11]. The overshoot of action potential, its after hyperpolarization, and duration increases [12], while the velocity of the nerve impulse tends to decrease in some restricted set of fibers [13]. The EEG tends to show altered frequencies and synchronization with ageing [9, 14]. Such age-related alterations in electrophysiological activity constitute the electrophysiological ageing of the nervous tissue. Multiple unit activity (MUA), that is, action potentials recorded simultaneously from a population of neurons, represents an electrophysiological marker of the cellular firing activity of the concerned neuronal population [5]. Its alterations may reflect the biochemical, physiological and behavioural changes of neurons [15, 16]. Age-related decline in spontaneous (basal) neuronal firing is of considerable interest as one of the neuroelectric indicators of the ageing brain. An age-related reduction in the spontaneous neuronal firing occurs in several brain areas, for example, the inferior and superior colliculi [3], locus coeruleus [17], forebrain [18], the parietal cortex [4], the hippocampal CA3 area, thalamus and striatum of rat [5, 19, 20].

The linkages between biochemical and electrical signals are of importance [21]. This contention is supported by the report that membrane lipid peroxidation and Na^+-K^+ ATPase (the membrane sodium pump) activity influence the generation of membrane electrical activity signals [19, 22], such as action potentials and may thus be involved in the electrophysiological ageing of the brain areas. It is, therefore, of interest to study the interrelationship between the ageing-related alterations in biochemical (lipid peroxidation and Na^+-K^+ ATPase) and MUA. Moreover, the action of antilipidperoxidative enzymes like glutathione peroxidase (GPx), glutathione-S-transferase (GST) may determine the lipid peroxidation status of a tissue. It will also be important to determine whether or not these age-related changes in these parameters also correlate with age-related changes in MUA.

The main objective of the present work has therefore been to determine statistical correlation between the age-related changes in multiple unit action potentials and the biochemical parameters: membrane lipid peroxidation, lipofuscin levels, Na^+-K^+ ATPase activity, GPx, GST activity with a view to gain insight into the biochemical substrates of the electrophysiological ageing of the brain tissue. Since brain regions differ in their vulnerability to ageing, we have selected the following regions to study these parameters: parietal cortex, hippocampus, striatum and thalamus [19, 23]. Age-related changes in the MUA were determined in the abovementioned brain regions of rats aged 6, 12, 18 and 24 months.

Materials and Methods

The experiments were performed on male Wistar rats of 6, 12, 18 and 24 months of age. Housing conditions and the record of health status of these rats has been reported elsewhere [5].

Multiple unit action (MUA) potentials and the EEG were recorded in free-moving conscious rats. Chronic cortical and intracranial electrodes were implanted stereotaxically in the parietal cortex, striatum, hippocampus and thalamus. Stereotaxic coordinates for the brain regions were: cortex 2.0 mm lateral to mid line and 2.0 mm posterior to bregma; striatum AP-0.3 mm, L3.3 mm, V4.5 mm, thalamus; AP-3.3 mm, L2.5 mm, V6.0 mm, and hippocampus AP-4.3 mm, L4.3 mm, V4.5 mm [24]. For recording MUA, composite extracellular signals were routed through a high impedance probe, amplified and filtered by AC preamplifiers (Grass Medical Instruments, Quincy, Massachussets, USA), electronically discriminated by using WPI window discriminators, displayed on a storage oscilloscope and simultaneously recorded on a polygraph. Recording sessions were limited to the awake immobile state as described in our previous reports [5, 19, 25].

At the end of the electrical recording session brains were immediately taken out and cooled in a deep freezer. The brain regions were rapidly dissected out according to stereotaxic coordinates [24]. For all the biochemical parameters chosen assays ($n = 5$ per parameter per age-group) were performed in the selected brain regions. Tissue samples were homogenized in 0.1 M phosphate buffer (pH 7.0). Lipofuscin concentration and lipid peroxidation levels were assayed in this homogenate according to the methods of Tappel et al. [26] and Rehncrona et al. [27], respectively. Crude synaptosomal and cytosol fractions were prepared by differentially centrifuging the homogenate [28]. Na^+-K^+ ATPase activity was determined by the method of Agakawa and Tsukada [29]. GST and GPx activities were assayed in cytosol by the method of Habig et al [30] and Flohe and Gunzler [31], respectively. To determine the effects of age, data was subjected to statistical analysis utilizing one way analysis of variance and to determine correlation between various parameters, utilizing Pearson's method [32]. Details of biochemical methods and statistical analysis are described in our previous reports [5, 19].

Results

Effect of Ageing

Ageing decreased the spontaneous multiple unit action potentials counts in all the four regions (ANOVA, $p < 0.01$) (Fig. 1). In the thalamus, the rate of MUA decline was lower than in the other three brain regions. The hippocampus appeared to show greater decline in MUA than other regions.

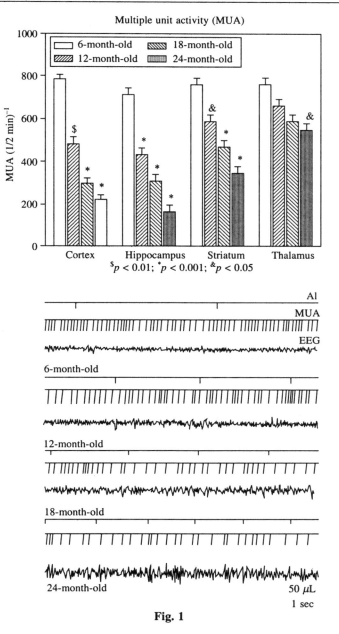

Fig. 1

Ageing elevated (ANOVA, $p < 0.01$) the levels of lipofuscin in all the selected brain regions while the lipid peroxidation levels were accentuated in cortex, striatum and hippocampus but not in the thalamus. GPx activity declined with age in all these regions whereas the Na^+-K^+ ATPase activity showed an age-related decline in the cortex, hippocampus and striatum but not in the thalamus. The GST activity declined in all these regions only during ageing from 12 to 24 months. A part of this data is described elsewhere [19, 20].

Correlation Between MUA and Na⁺-K⁺ ATPase Activity

Correlation Between MUA and Na⁺-K⁺ ATPase Activity
Pearson's correlation between the age-related decline in MUA and the age-related depression in Na⁺-K⁺ ATPase activity showed strong relationship (Fig. 2). The age-related decrease of Na⁺-K⁺ ATPase activity correlated significantly positively with the age-related decrease of MUA in the parietal cortex, $r = + 0.901, p < 0.01$, hippocampus $r = +0.925, p < 0.01$ and striatum, $r = + 0.971, p < 0.01$.

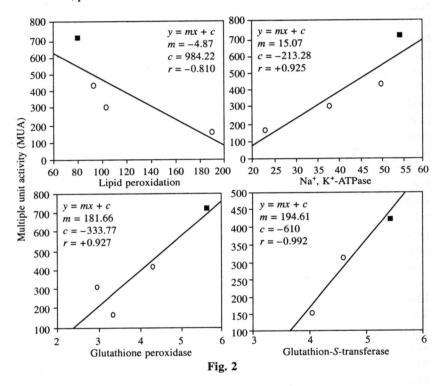

Fig. 2

Correlation Between MUA and Lipid Peroxidation, Lipofuscin Levels

Correlation Between MUA and Lipid Peroxidation, Lipofuscin Levels
The age-related increase in lipid peroxidation negatively correlated with the age-related decrease in MUA in the following regions: parietal cortex $r = -0.976, p < 0.01$, hippocampus $r = 0.810, p < 0.01$ and striatum $r = -0.964$, $p < 0.01$. A significant negative correlation was found between the age-related changes in MUA and those in lipofuscin levels in all the brain regions studied: cortex $r = -0.920$, hippocampus $r = -0.925$, striatum $r = -0.967$, and thalamus $r = -0.976$ ($p < 0.01$ in all regions).

Correlation Between MUA, GPx and GST

Correlation Between MUA, GPx and GST
The age-related decrease in GST activity was significantly correlated with

the age-related decrease in MUA in all the four brain regions studied: cortex $r = +0.952$, hippocampus $r = +0.992$, striatum $r = +0.999$ and thalamus $r = +0.999$ ($p < 0.01$ in all regions). The age-related decreases in GPx and MUA were also significantly correlated in all the four brain regions: cortex $r = +0.975$, hippocampus $r = +0.927$, striatum $r = +0.911$ and thalamus $r = +0.949$ ($p < 0.01$ in all regions).

Discussion

In this article we have considered the age-related MUA decline as a measure of electrophysiological ageing of the brain. The MUA decline, like other neurophysiological signals such as the EEG [2] can be considered as a measure of neuronal impairment. Of the four brain regions we investigated, the hippocampus and cortex showed greater age-related declines in MUA whereas the thalamus showed the lowest decline. This is consistent with the view that thalamus has a much lower age-sensitivity [19] and thus shows a lower level of age-related impairment in MUA. The hippocampus and cortex are known to show greater age-sensitivity [33] and therefore exhibit higher impairment in MUA. Our data on age-related decline in MUA although have been obtained from a cross sectional study, are consistent with data that have resulted from longitudinal studies on MUA [3].

The main objective of our study was concerned with the biochemical correlates of ageing related decline in electrophysiological activity. Our data showed that the age-related MUA decline was strongly correlated with age-related alterations in the five observed biochemical parameters, namely, lipid peroxidation, lipofuscin content, and the activities of Na^+-K^+ ATPase, GPx and GST.

Experimental data have shown that membrane lipid peroxidation significantly influences membrane electrophysiological activity. For example, lipid peroxidation can alter action potential production [34], and can also lead to generation of epileptiform electrical activity [25]. Membrane lipid peroxidation shows age-related elevation and is known to contribute to the ageing of membranes [22]. Therefore, the observed statistical correlation between the age-related decline in MUA and elevation in lipid peroxidation is indicative of a causal relationship between the two parameters.

The synaptosomal Na^+-K^+ ATPase activity also declines with ageing. And this age-related decline is also strongly correlated with the age-related decline in MUA. Experimental data have shown that changes in membrane Na^+-K^+ ATPase activity are associated with altered membrane electrophysiological activity [35]. For instance, decreased Na^+-K^+ ATPase activity in natural hypothermia results in an inhibition of neuronal firing [36]. Furthermore, increase in Na^+-K^+ ATPase activity have been reported to result in an increased neuronal electrical activity [37, 38]. It is of interest to note that decreased sodium pump activity will result in membrane depolarization [39]. Presynaptic afferent depolarization during synaptic neurotransmission results in a lowering of the frequency of action potentials generated at the post-synaptic neuron. Therefore, the statistical correlation between the age-related inhibition of Na^+-K^+ ATPase activity and the age-related decrease in MUA in various brain regions observed in our study reflects causal relationship.

The cause of inhibition of Na^+-K^+ ATPase activity with ageing may lie in the age-related increase in lipid peroxidation because the activity of this enzyme is known to be susceptible to elevation in lipid peroxidation and age-related depression in Na^+-K^+ ATPase have been found [19]. However, the age-related decline in this enzyme activity may also be due to several other causes: such as direct effects of free radicals [35], decrease in the availability of ATP consequent to age-related mitochondrial bio-energetic impairment [40, 41].

From the above discussion, it would appear that statistical correlation of MUA with both of these parameters, i.e. lipid peroxidation and Na^+-K^+ ATPase activity is because of biochemical interrelationship between the latter parameters.

Our data showed a strong correlation between the age-related MUA decline and age-related elevation of lipofuscin levels. Since, lipofuscin is mostly formed from lipid peroxidation and their products this correlation may be reflective of the correlation between the MUA and lipid peroxidation. The potential relationship of lipofuscin to disturbance in neuronal function (cellular function) remains controversial. Since lipofuscin granules contain increased amount of iron, it may sensitize the cell to oxidative injury. It has been thus reported "that lipofuscin may not only be a manifestation of ageing, but also a factor inducing cellular damage in old age leading to depletion of cell function" [42]. Therefore, lipofuscin may make its own contribution to oxidative stress, distinct from that resulting from the oxidative stress derived from other sources. Therefore, the correlation between the age-related elevation in lipofuscin and the age-treated decrease in MUA may include lipofuscin's own influence on electrical activity.

The statistical correlation of age-related decline in MUA with age-related decreases in GPx and GST observed in our study would basically reflect their antilipidperoxidant activity. These two enzymes showed age-related decline, which would favor an increase in lipid peroxidation. Elevated lipid peroxidation is associated with decreased MUA.

The results from Pearson's correlation analysis between the MUA decline and various biochemical parameters revealed direct correlation between electrophysiological decline and oxidative stress-producing mechanisms. The correlation suggests a link between the electrical activity decline and oxidative mechanisms. Therefore, these statistical correlations together with the available experimental data show that the oxidative stress parameters significantly contribute to the electrophysiological ageing of the brain. Our results are consistent with the findings showing that treatment with drugs countering the oxidative stress augments neuroelectrical activity [20, 43] and other cognitive functions [41]. It is of interest here to note that activity of the nervous system may be of central importance in the regulation of organismal ageing [44]. Therefore, therapeutic strategies aimed at countering the age-related oxidative stress, potential for neurodegenerative disorders and cognitive decline [45] in the brain by pharmacological means [46, 47] would constitute a promising approach for retarding ageing and senescence.

Acknowledgement

The senior author (RS) is supported by a University Grants Commission's (New Delhi) Emeritus Fellowship Award.

References

1. Malmo, H.P. and Malmo, R.B. Movement related forebrain and midbrain multiple unit activity in rats. *Electroencephalogr. Clin. Neurophysiol.*, 1977; **42**: 501–509.
2. Musha, T., Asada, T., Yamashita, F., Kinoshita, T., Chen, Z., Matsuda, H., Uno, M. and Shankle, W.R. A new EEG method for estimating cortical neuronal impairment that is sensitive to early stage Alzheimer's disease. *Clin. Neurophysiol.*, 2002; **113**: 1052–1058.
3. Malmo, H.P. and Malmo, R.B. Multiple unit activity recorded longitudinally in rats from pubescence to old age. *Neurobiol. Aging.*, 1982; **3**: 43–53.
4. Roy, D. and Singh, R. Age related changes in multiple unit activity of the rat brain parietal cortex and the effect of centrophenoxine. *Exp. Gerontol.*, 1988; **23**: 161–174.
5. Sharma, D., Maurya, A.K. and Singh, R. Age related decline in multiple unit action potentials of CA3 region of rat hippocampus: correlation with lipid peroxidation and lipofuscin concentration and the effect of centrophenoxine. *Neurobiol. Aging.*, 1993; **14**: 319–330.
6. Kolev, V., Yordanova, J., Basar-Eroglu, C. and Basar, E. Age effects on visual EEG responses reveal distinct frontal alpha networks. *Clin. Neurophysiol.*, 2002; **113**: 901–910.
7. Pfutze, E.M., Sommer, W. and Schweinberger, S.R. Age-related slowing in face and name recognition: evidence from event-related brain potentials. *Psychol. Ageing.*, 2002; **17**: 140–160.
8. West, R. and Covell, E. Effects of aging on event-related neural activity related to prospective memory. *Neuroreport*, 2001; **12**: 2855–2858.
9. McEvoy, L.K., Pellouchoud, E., Smith, M.E. and Gevins, A. Neurophysiological signals of working memory in normal aging. *Brain Res Cogn. Brain Res*, 2001; **11**: 363–376.
10. Frolkis, V.V., Stupina, A.S., Martinenko, O.A., Toth, S. and Timchenko, A.I. Ageing of the neurons in the molusc Lymnaea stagnalis-structure function and sensitivity to transmitters. *Mech. Ageing. Dev.*, 1984; **25**: 91–102.
11. Tanaka, Y. and Ando, S., Synaptic ageing as revealed by changes in membrane potential and decreased activity in Na^+-K^+ATPase. *Brain Res.*, 1990; **506**: 46–52.
12. Bunting, T.A. and Scott, B.S. Ageing and ethanol alter neuronal electric membrane properties. *Brain Research*, 1989; **501**: 105–115.
13. Aston-Jones, G., Roger, J., Shaver, R.D., Dinan, T.G., Moss, D.E. Age-impaired impulse flow from nucleus basalis to cortex. *Nature* (London) 1985; **318**: 462–464.

14. Duffy, F.H., McAnulty, G.B. and Albert, M.S. Effects of age upon interhemispheric EEG coherence in normal adults. *Neurobiol. Aging*, 1996; **17**: 587–599.

15. Mizumori, S.J.Y., Lavoie, A.M. and Kalyani, A. Redistribution of spatial representation in the hippocampus of aged rats performing a spatial memory task. *Behav. Neurosci*, 1996; **110**: 1006–1016.

16. Barnes, C.A., Suster, M.S., Shen, J., McNaughton, B.L. Multistability of cognitive maps in the hippocampus of old rats. *Nature*, 1997; **388**: 272–275.

17. Olpe, H.R., Steinmann, M. Age-related decline in the activity of noradrenergic neurons of the rat locus coeruleus. *Brain Res*, 1982; **251**: 174–176.

18. Jones, R.S. and Olpe, H.R. Altered sensitivity of forebrain neurones to iontophoretically applied noradrenaline in ageing rats. *Neurobiol. Aging*, 1983; **4**: 97–99.

19. Kaur, J., Sharma, D. and Singh, R. Regional effects of ageing on Na^+-K^+ATPase activity in rat brain and correlation with multiple unit action potentials and lipid peroxidation. *Indian J. Biochem. Biophy.*, 1998; **35**: 364–371.

20. Kaur, J., Sharma, D., Singh, R. Acetyl-L-carnitine enhances Na^+-K^+ ATPase glutathione-S-transferase and multiple unit activity and reduces lipid peroxidation and lipofuscin concentration in aged rat brain regions. *Neurosci. Lett.*, 2001; **301**: 1–4.

21. Katz, P.S. and Clemens, S., Biochemical networks in nervous system: expanding neuronal information capacity beyond voltage signals. *Trends Neurosci*, 2001; **24**: 18–25.

22. Mattson, M.P., Modification of ion homeostasis by lipid peroxidation : roles in neuronal degeneration and adaptive plasticity. *Trends Neurosci*, 1998; **21**: 53–57.

23. Arendt, T. and Bigl, V. Alzheimer's disease: a presumptive threshold phenomenon. *Neurobiol. Aging.*, 1987; **8**: 552–554.

24. Paxinos, G. and Watson, C., The rat brain in stereotaxic coordinates. Academic Press, New York, 1982.

25. Singh, R. and Pathak, D.N. Lipid peroxidation and glutathione peroxidase; glutathione reductase, superoxide dismutase, catalase and glucose-6-phosphate dehydrogenase activities in $FeCl_3$-induced epileptogenic foci in the rat brain. *Epilepsia*, 1990; **31**: 15–26.

26. Tappel, A.L., Fletcher, B. and Deamer, D. Effect of antioxidants and nutrients on lipid peroxidation fluorescent product and ageng parameters in the mouse. *J. Gerontol*, 1973; **28**: 415–424.

27. Rehncrona, S., Smith, D.S. and Akesson, B. Peroxidative changes in brain cortical fatty acids and phospholipids, as characterized during Fe^{2+} and ascorbic acid stimulated peroxidation *in vitro*. *J. Neurochem.*, 1980; **34**: 1630–1638.

28. Gray, E.G. and Whittaker, V.P. The isolation of nerve endings from brain: an electron microscopic study of cell fragments derived by homogenization and centrifugation. *J. Anatomy.*, 1962; **96**: 79–88.

29. Akagawa, K. and Tsukada, Y. Presence and characteristics of catecholamine sensitive Na^+-K^+ ATPase in rat striatum. *J. Neurochem*, 1979; **32**: 269–271.

30. Habig, W.H., Pabst, M.J., Jakoby, W.B. Glutathione-S-transferase. The first enzymatic step in mercapturic acid formation. *J. Biol. Chem.*, 1974; **249**: 7130–7139.

31. Flohe, L. and Gunzler, W.A. Assays of glutathione peroxidase. *Methods Enzymol.*, 1984; **105**: 114–121.

32. Downie, N.M., Heath, R.W. Basic Statistical Methods. Harper and Row, New York, 1984.

33. Amenta, F., Mignini, F., Ricci, A., Sabbatini, M., Tomassoni, D. and Tayebati,

S.K. Age-related changes of dopamine receptors in the rat hippocampus: a light microscope autoradiography study. *Mech. Ageing. Dev.*, 2001; **122**: 2071–2083.

34. Pellmar, T. Electrophysiological correlates of peroxide damage in guinea pig hippocampus *in vitro*. *Brain Res*, 1986; **364**: 377–381.

35. Lees, G.J. Inhibition of sodium-potassium-ATPase; a potential ubiquitous mechanism contributing to central nervous system neuropathology. *Brain Res Brain Res Rev*, 1991; **16**: 283–300.

36. Deboer, T. and Tobler I. Temperature dependence of EEG frequencies during natural hypothermia. *Brain Res*, 1995; **670**: 153–156.

37. Huttenlocher, P.P. and Rawson, M.D. Neuronal activity and adenosine triphosphatase in immature cerebral cortex. *Exp. Neurol.*, 1968; **22**: 118–129.

38. Riddle, D.R., Gutierrez, G.Z.D., White, L.E., Richards, A. and Purves, D. Differential metabolic and electrical activity in the somatic sensory cortex of juvenile and adult rats. *J. Neurosci*, 1993; **13**: 4193–4213.

39. Beal, M.F. Ageing, energy, and oxidative stress in neurodegenerative diseases. *Ann. Neurol.*, 1995; **38**: 357–366.

40. Tretter, L. and Adam-Vizi, V. Early events in free radical mediated damage of isolated nerve terminals: effects of peroxides on membrane potential and intracellular Na^+ and Ca^+ concentrations. *J. Neurochem.*, 1996; **66**: 2057–2066.

41. Martinez, M., Hernandez, A.I. and Martinez, N. N-acetylcysteine delays age associated memory impairment in mice: role in synaptic mitochondria. *Brain Res.*, 2000; **855**: 100–106.

42. Terman, A., Dalen, H. and Brunk, U.T. Ceroid lipofuscin-loaded human fibroblasts show decreased survival time and diminished autophagocytosis during amino acid starvation. *Exp. Gerontol.*, 1999; **34**: 943–957.

43. Kaur, J., Singh, S., Sharma, D. and Singh, R. Neurostimulatory and antioxidative effects of L-deprenyl in aged rat brain regions. *Biogerontology*, 2003; **4(2)**: 105–111.

44. Boulianne, G.L. Neuronal regulation of life span: clues from flies and worms. *Mech. Ageing. Develop.*, 2001; **122**: 883–894.

45. Poon, H.F., Calabrese, V., Scapagnini, G. and Butterfield, A. Free radicals: key to brain aging and heme oxygenase as a cellular response to oxidative stress. *J. Gerontol. Medical Sciences*, 2004; **59A**: 478–493.

46. Milgram, N.W., Head, E., Zicker, S.C., Ikeda-Douglas, C., Murphey, H., Muggenberg, B.A., Siwak, C.T., Tapp, P.D., Lowry, S.R. and Cotman, C.W. Long-term treatment with antioxidants and a program of behavioral enrichment reduces age-dependent impairment in discrimination and reversal learning in beagle dogs. *Exp. Gerontol.*, 2004; **39**: 753–765.

47. Grasing, K., He, S. and Li, N. Selegiline modifies the extinction of responding following morphine self-administration, but does not alter cue-duced reinstatement, reacquisition of morphine reinforcement, or precipitated withdrawal. *Pharmacological Res.*, 2005; **51**: 69–78.

Pain Updated: Mechanisms and Effects
Edited by R. Mathur

11. Alzheimer's Disease: Potential Therapies and Treatments in Discovery-Problem Still Unsolved

Y. Singh[1] and H.K. Mangat[2]

[1]School of Environmental Sciences, Jawaharlal Nehru University,
New Delhi-110 067, India

[2]Department of Zoology, Guru Nanak Dev University, Amritsar, India

Abstract. Alzheimer's disease (AD) is the single biggest unmet medical challenge in neurology. Amyloid plaques and neurofibrillary tangles are hallmarks of AD. The AD may disrupt thinking and memory by blocking messages between nerve cells. Amyloid hypothesis states that overproduction of β amyloid protein (Aβ) causes AD due to amyloid deposition and later hyperphosphorylation of tau protein may form neurofibrillary tangles inside neurons. Amyloid precursor protein (APP) may have role in long term memory formation. α, β and γ secretases cleave APP at different sites. Treating AD involves cholinesterase inhibitors, non-steroidal anti-inflammatory drugs (NSAID's), extracts of *Ginkgo biloba* leaves, anti-oxidants such as vitamin E, BACE inhibitors, hormone replacement therapy, beta peptide sheet breakers, anti-aggregation approaches, insulin degrading enzymes, immunotherapy and using calcium channel blockers. Modulators of signal transduction and statins (inhibitors of cholesterol synthesizing enzyme HMG-CoA reductase) may be used as therapies for AD treatment but some of them are in phase I or II trials.

Introduction

Alzheimer's disease was first described by Dr. Alois Alzheimer in 1906 who noticed changes in brain tissues of woman who died of unusual mental illness. He found abnormal clumps (amyloid plaques) and tangled bundles of fibers (called neurofibrillary tangles). These plaques and tangles in brain are considered hallmarks of Alzheimer's disease. AD is most common form of dementia among older people and occurs after age 60. It affects parts of brain that control thought, memory and language. It affects 12 million people worldwide and 4 million Americans today. AD may disrupt thinking and memory by blocking messages between nerve cells. It causes personality changes, decline thinking abilities, people think less clearly and are confused Later they may forget to do simple tasks such as dressing themselves, brushing their teeth, eat with proper utensils and may become anxious and aggressive or wander away from home.

AD puts heavy economic burden on society. A study estimated that annual cost of caring is $ 18408 for patient with mild AD; $ 30096 for patient with moderate AD; $36132 for patient with severe AD. The annual cost of caring for AD patients is estimated to be $ 100 million (Leon et al., 1998).

What Goes Wrong?

The current theory of AD etiology and pathogenesis is amyloid cascade hypothesis which states that overproduction of beta-amyloid protein (Aβ) or failure to clear this peptide leads to AD primarily through amyloid deposition, which produces neurofibrillary tangles; these are then associated with cell death and memory impairment, the hallmark of dementia [1, 3].

The major constituent of amyloid plaques is 42 amino acid peptide (Aβ42), which is cleaved from much larger precursor protein (APP). APP, a type one transmembrane (TM) protein, is known to be involved in neurite extension and also shares some of properties of cell-adhesion molecules [2]. Cell adhesion molecules have been implicated in synaptic structural changes that are involved in transfer of short term memory to long term memory. There appears to be deficit in this ability during early phases of Alzheimer's disease and support the evidence of APP's role in long term memory formation [2] (Fig. 1). Thus Aβ formation appears to be critical step in the development of AD. The normal ubiquitous pathway of APP metabolism in cell culture involves cleavage by alpha-secretase. In this step no Aβ formation occurs and no deposition.

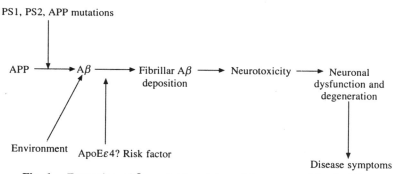

Fig. 1. Formation of β-amyloid protein and its neurotoxicity in AD.

The alternative β-secretase pathway prominent in cells derived from CNS, leads to cleavage of APP at N-terminus, generating a cell associated β-C-terminal fragment (β-CTF). This fragment is cleared in the TM domain by γ-secretase generating $A\beta_{1-40}$ (90%) and $A\beta_{1-42}$ (10%) [1]; $A\beta_{1-40}$ is major species secreted from cultured cells found in CSF of normal and Alzheimer's disease individuals, whereas the 42 amino acids long $A\beta_{1-42}$ is major component of amyloid deposition. Thus, it seems that $A\beta_{1-42}$ is essential early event in AD that leads to increased rate of amyloid deposition and neurodegeneration [5]. The enzyme cleaving the TM domain to generate the C-terminus of Aβ is γ-secretase. $A\beta_{1-42}$ is major pathological culprit in AD because it is more prone to aggregation and deposit [1]. Genes for gamma-secretase are presenilin 1 (PS1) and presenilin 2 (PS2). Since gene deletion of PS1 has shown its requirement for normal conversion of APP to $A\beta$ by γ-secretase, so it is clear that PS1 and PS2 are themselves γ-secretases; and their activity increase the production of highly amyloidogeneic $A\beta_{42}$ isoform [6, 7] (Fig. 2).

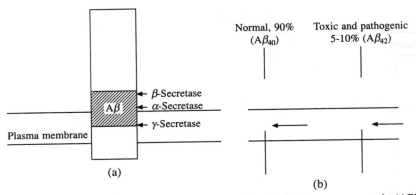

Fig. 2   (a) Sites of actions of α, β and γ secretases on amyloid precursor protein (APP) and (b) cleaving of APP and formation of normal and toxic β amyloid protein.

Besides amyloid plaques, NFTs (neurofibrillary tangles) are also found in brain of AD sufferers. NFT's are bundles of fibers found within neuronal cell bodies and consist of paired helical filaments. A major component of the paired helical filaments is abnormally hyperphosphorylated forms of protein tau (axonal microtubule associated protein) that enhances microtubule assembly [8, 11]. The normal function of tau protein is to bind and thus maintain the structure of neuronal microtubules. Tau is produced either indirectly or by $A\beta_{42}$, or directly in some forms of frontotemporal dementia by mutations in tau itself [3].

Research has shown that tau dysfunction can lead to neuronal damage and death resulting in pathological and clinical phenotype with similarities to AD.

Tau → Abnormal phosphorylation → Associated to form paired helical filaments
↓
Aggregate and become
↓
NFTs

Genetic Factors

Mutations in all three genes, viz. APP, PS1 and PS2, have one common pathogenic action that they alter APP processing and thus increased amount of 42 amino acid peptide $A\beta_{42}$ is produced. APP, PS1 and PS2 genes are associated with early onset of familial Alzheimer's disease (FAD) (Table 1). PS1 and PS2 alter gamma secretase activity to increase the production of highly amyloidogenic $A\beta_{42}$ isoform [9, 10]. Both, late onset and sporadic AD, have strong association with apolipoprotein E (ApoE), allele ε4, located on chromosome 19q [3]. Inherited mutation in presenilin or APP genes increased the production of $A\beta_{42}$ peptide, which has greater propensity to form fibrils than $A\beta_{40}$. Aβ fibrils initiate the neurodegeneration process and may induce tau hyperphosphorylation and later enhances neurotoxicity [11].

Table 1   Genes of Alzheimer's disease (AD)

Chromosome	Gene	Allele	Effects
21	APP	—	Early onset of FAD ↑ Aβ production
14	PS-1	—	Early onset of FAD ↑ Aβ production
1	PS-2	—	Early onset of FAD ↑ Aβ production
19	ApoE	ε4	↑ Risk of AD ↓ Age of onset of AD

↑ : increase; ↓ : decrease

Treatment

AD appears to be multifactorial disease that should be approached from many perspectives. It cannot be cured or prevented fully, however therapeutic treatments do exist. FDA have approved of two drug treatments. Cholinesterase inhibitors such as Cognex (tacrine) and Aricept (donepezil) show the cognitive decline in AD. Studies also show that estrogens reduces the risk of AD in women by impeding the deposition of Aβ. Non-steroidal anti-inflammatory drugs (NSAIDs) may also reduce symptoms of AD. Recently, rivastigmine (exelon) belonging to same class of drugs as donepezil and tacrine, may be used to cure AD but not fully. Galantamine (reminyl) may prevent some symptoms from becoming worse [12]. These drugs may help control behavioral symptoms of AD such as sleeplessness, agitation, wandering, anxiety and depression. Treating these symptoms often makes patient more comfortable and makes their care easier for caregivers. Developing new treatments for AD is an active area of research. Scientists are testing a number of drugs to see if they prevent AD, slow the disease, and help reduce behavioral symptoms. Two different types of NSAIDs which might slow progression of AD, viz. Rofecoxib (Vioxx) and Naproxen (Aleve) are currently being studied [13, 14].

Recent research showed that *Ginkgo biloba*, an extract made from leaves of ginkgo tree may be of some help in treating AD symptoms. There is no evidence that ginkgo will cure or prevent AD. The AD patients have very high levels of brain chemical glutamate, making brain cells insensitive to glutamate bursts that help in new memory development. Thus patient cannot remember. One drug that regulates glutamate has been approved in Europe. Currently there has been no proven way to prevent AD. A vaccine is being developed and early testing is underway. Medications like NSAIDs, antioxidant such as Vitamin E, estrogen replacement therapy and *Ginkgo biloba*; none are recommended because all have side effects and can interact with other medications. AD is a disease that turns parts of brain into sticky mess and thus inhibits its functions. Thus, the onset of disease has to be prevented or stopped early. Once the brain tissue is destroyed, it cannot be restored. The prevention of AD takes number of approaches, viz. prevent particles that may form plaques from forming; flush out brain particles that can accumulate and cause plaque; destroy the particles that may form plaque; and destroy the plaque [13, 14, 15].

Research Advancement and Potential Therapies: Taking New Steps

The Food and Drug Administration (FDA) has approved three medications for AD which inhibit acetyl cholinesterase, an enzyme that normally breaks down acetylcholine (a key neurotransmitter involved in cognitive functioning). This neurotransmitter is produced by one set of neurons whose function is gradually lost in AD. The first of these medications, approved in 1993 was tacrine (Cognex). The second approved in 1996 was donepezilhydrochloride (Aricept). Aricept is a drug most commonly used to treat mild to moderate AD. However, Cognex and Aricept does not stop or reverse the progression of AD, it appears to help only some AD patients for period ranging from months to about two years, so its utility is limited. In April 2000, FDA approved rivastigmine (exelon) for treatment of mild to moderate AD [14, 15]. In clinical trials involving more than 3900 patients worldwide, the drug improved patient's ability to carry out activities like eating and dressing. Patients also had fewer or lesser behavioral symptoms, like delusions and agitation, improvement in cognitive functions such as thinking, memory and speaking. However, like the other two drugs, exelon also does not stop or reverse AD [15].

Another strategy is to inhibit the production of Aβ peptide by inhibiting either or both of two enzymatic cleavage events which liberate Aβ from the full length APP precursor protein (i.e. inhibition of β- or γ-secretase) [16]. Alternate strategy is to inhibit the aggregation of Aβ peptide monomers into toxic fibrils. Much of AD research has been focused on amyloid cascade (Fig. 3). The cascade is initiated when large transmembrane protein APP is cleaved by proteases β- and γ-secretase [17].

Aβ_{42}, considered to be most pathogenic species, is secreted into extra cellular space where it aggregates or Aβ aggregates may also form within cells. Cofactors like Zn and glycosaminoglycans (GAGs) are proposed to enhance Aβ aggregation and their interaction with Aβ is targeted by certain aggregation inhibitors. The aggregates ultimately form signature plaques of

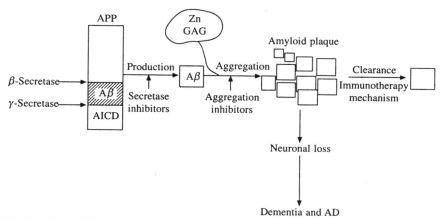

Fig. 3. Amyloid cascade events in production and aggregation of β-amyloid (Aβ) and its prevention from aggregation.

Alzheimer's disease [18]. As $A\beta_{42}$ generation is the first step in cascade, shutting down or reducing its production is desirable. Proteases have been successfully targeted for drug development. Hence, it was assumed that these enzymes were ideal targets from the therapeutic intervention. By 1992 numerous companies have synthesized potent γ-secretase inhibitor but not beta secretase inhibitor. In 2001, Bristol-Myers-Squibb announced that the first of these compounds had moved into phase two clinical trials [19].

In case of secretase inhibition, toxicity could arise from several sources. Another possible source of toxicity is reduction of other APP metabolites that may be important, e.g. the amyloid intracellular domain (AICD) may have signaling role (Fig. 3). The accumulation of APP metabolites resulting from secretase inhibition may lead to toxicity (for instance the C-terminal β-secretase cleavage product in case of β-secretase inhibition). Although, *in vitro* reconstitution of active enzyme has not been accomplished, it seems that β-secretase is complex of several proteins, which requires activity of presenilin 1 and other transmembrane proteins. Since, gene deletion of PS1 has shown its requirement for normal γ-secretase cleavage of APP to Aβ, PS1 is postulated to be either unique diaspartyl cofactor for γ-secretase itself, or an auto-activated intramembranous aspartyl protease. Proteins Aphl and Pen2 are required for notch pathway signaling, γ-secretase cleavage of APP and presenilin protein accumulation [20, 21]. A member of *C. elegans* presenilin family, sel-12 is facilitator of lin-12/notch signaling during determination of cell fate in development. PS1 can interact with novel neuron specific member of Armadillo family, δ-catenin, as in the yeast two hybrid system, both δ and β catenins co-immunoprecipitate with PS1 [21]. Knock out of PS1 is lethal, likely due to the role of γ-secretase in processing of notch, a molecule important for variety of cell fate decisions. This is major concern for γ-secretase inhibitors. But from drug development perspective, the γ-secretase has lost a lot of its appeal [22].

β-secretase initially received less attention in drug development because all potent compounds identified in the early cell based screens inhibited the γ-secretase pathway. This changed with β-secretase by solving of its structure [23]. Memapsin 2 (β-secretase) is membrane associated aspartic protease involved in production of β amyloid peptide in Alzheimer's disease and is major target for drug design. The β-secretase cleaves APP on the lumenal side of membrane and its activity is rate limiting step of Aβ production *in vivo* [23]. Human brain aspartic protease memapsin 2 or BACE is demonstrated to be β-secretase. This specific information has been used to design potent inhibitor against this enzyme. OM 99-2 and eight residue transition state inhibitor is used for this purpose. Two metallo proteases ADAM10 and Tace, are involved in cleavage of APP. It was not until very recently that the BACE (β site APP cleaving enzyme) was reported [24]. The cloning of human transmembrane aspartic protease BACE with all known characteristics of β-secretase is under way and could be used as drug targeting [26]. In addition BACE is expressed at higher levels in neurons than in glia. This result supports the idea that neurons are the primary source of extra cellular Aβ deposited in amyloid plaques. If BACE is long sought β-secretase, its inhibition may be successful with aspartic protease inhibitors and this may have important implications for the AD sufferers [25]. Potent peptidic β-secretase inhibitors have been featured in several publications, but due to large active site, the generation of the potent and specific drug like inhibitors is a major challenge. The large active site requires the identification of small organic molecules that contact the active site at several positions, similar to large peptidic inhibitors. Most companies have invested in preclinical trials on β-secretase inhibition [25, 26].

Removing Amyloid

The ways in which brain may destroy amyloid naturally is yet unknown. Certain kinds of scavenging microglia can engulf β amyloid, which suggests that they have potential for clearing amyloid from AD brain even without being activated by immune response against amyloid. It is shown that microglial uptake of β amyloid can be reduced by some forms of complement, a component of inflammation cascade that occurs in AD brain. More damaging fibrillar complement containing plaques may develop as AD progresses. These results suggest that mechanism that inhibits the inflammatory process may increase the capacity of certain types of microglia to engulf amyloid and may be of therapeutic value [27, 28]. One way to prevent amyloid plaque formation is to stop beta amlyloid production. It is shown that estrogens might reduce risk of developing AD by lowering β amyloid production, i.e. the cultured neurons treated with estrogen reduce secretion of β amyloid peptides. In other studies, testosterone also decreases secretion of β amyloid. Another way to prevent amyloid plaque formation is to break β amyloid into pieces once it is released from cells, and before it has chance to aggregate into insoluble plaques. An enzyme called 'insulin degrading enzyme' can do this in tissue culture. The enzyme regulate extra cellular amyloid levels, suggesting that it might do the same in brain. Finding ways to increase the activity of this enzyme could conceivably be therapy for AD [28].

Another approach taken to prevent plaque formation is to develop short peptides called 'β peptide sheet breakers', which inhibit β amyloid from forming plaques. A research shows that β peptide sheet breakers also reduce plaques formation when injected into brain of rats with amyloid plaques. The peptide breakers reduce plaques size, neuronal shrinkage and microglial activity around plaques and broke up amyloid deposits even after they were formed [28]. Presenilins may be important in their involvement in cell death pathways. In transgenic mouse models, neurons expressing presenilin 1 mutations carry AD in humans are more vulnerable to stress related cell death. Neurons in these mice can be rescued by treating them with inhibitors of programmed cell death (apoptosis) that worked through channels in the cell that transport calcium. Yet another function suggested for presenilin is that they are involved in cell-cell communication through maintaining synapses. The studies showed that presenilin 1 is located at synapses and that it may be necessary for proper connections between neurons. Presenilin mutations that cause AD could possibly affect presenilin function at the synaptic connections between brain cells. Further research on presenilin mutations can give us many treatment options in future [7, 21].

Anti-Aggregation Approaches

On theoretical grounds, anti-aggregation approaches are very attractive, as generation of Aβ is physiological event, aggregation of monomeric Aβ into oligomers and fibrils with β sheet structure is pathogenic and harmful [28]. However, this approach has failed. Some companies give advanced anti-aggregation programmes. NeuroChem Inc. has developed small molecule inhibitors of the interaction between Aβ and glycosaminoglycans, which is proposed to be involved in formation of amyloid deposits in AD. A safety trial is over and NeuroChem plans to move into phase II trials soon. Short peptide Aβ derivatives developed by Serono have also shown *in vivo* efficiency upon intra peritoneal injection in amyloid mouse. Chelating zinc reported to be critical for Aβ aggregation with antibiotic clioquninol lower amyloid burden *in vivo* [29]. This compound has been used in small phase II clinical trials and results were good. Anti-inflammatory drugs that interfere with aspects of microglial and astrocytic responses in the brain may be used and anti-oxidants, free radical scavengers, calcium channel blockers and modulators of signal transduction that could protect neurons from effects of accumulation of Aβ are other treatment options [30].

Immunotherapy and AD

Amyloid β peptide (Aβ) may be removed by using antibodies directed towards

Aβ. Such antibodies could be either passively administered or induced by immunization with Aβ as vaccine. To address this strategy a robust transgenic mouse model of Alzheimer's disease (TgCRND 8) mice has been generated which develops profuse cerebral deposition of Aβ into amyloid plaques, accompanied by cognitive impairment. It has been shown that immunization with Aβ$_{42}$ results in significant reduction in cerebral amyloid plaques and improvement in cognitive functions when administrated early in the course of disease. Immunization later in course of disease, when amyloid burdens are high, also results in improvement in cognitive function, but with slower time course [31, 32]. In contrast, immunization with irrelevant antigen (islet associated peptide) has no significant effect on cognitive function or cerebral amyloid plaque load compared to control mice. Indeed there are many mechanisms including F$_C$-mediated degradation by macrophages/microglia, peripheral sink effects; or inhibition of Aβ aggregation; and each vaccine may selectively induce only some of these effects [33].

However, use of Aβ$_{1-42}$ as vaccine in humans may not be appropriate as it crosses the blood brain barrier, forms toxic fibrils and can seed fibril formation. It is reported that immunization in transgenic mice (Tg 2576) for seven months with soluble non-amyloidogenic, nontoxic Aβ homologous peptides reduced cortical and hippocampal brain amyloid burden by 89 and 81%, respectively. Thus, immunization with non-amyloidogeneic Aβ derivatives represents a potentially safer therapeutic approach to reduce amyloid burden in Alzheimer's disease, instead of using toxic Aβ fibrils [34].

Anti-oxidants and AD

Aβ initiated inflammation and neurotoxic process include excessive generation of free radicals and cause peroxidative injury to proteins and other macromolecules in neurons. In this regard a therapeutic trial of antioxidant vitamin E seemed to result in slower clinical progression of disease. Among many possible metabolic consequences of Aβ accumulation and aggregation, altered ionic homeostasis particularly excessive calcium entry into neurons, could well contribute to neuronal dysfunction and cell death, based on studies of *in vitro* effects of aggregated Aβ. Oxidative processes have been suggested as elements in development of Alzheimer's disease, but whether dietary intake of vitamin E and other antioxidant nutrients prevents its development is a subject of debate. It is shown that increasing vitamin E intake from foods was associated with decreased risk of developing AD after adjustment for age, education, sex, race, ApoEε4 allele and length of follow-up. The protective association of vitamin E was observed only among persons who were ApoEε4 negative. Intake of vitamin C, β-carotene, vitamin E from supplements (not directly from food) was not significantly associated with risk of AD [35].

Recent Treatments Used

Non steroidal anti-inflammatory drugs provide some degree of protection from Alzheimer's disease. Epidemiological studies have documented a reduced prevalence of AD among users of NSAIDs. It is proposed that NSAIDs exert their beneficial effects in part by reducing neurotoxic inflammatory responses in brain. Drugs such as aspirin, ibuprofen, indomethacin and sulindac sulphide decrease the highly amyloidogeneic $A\beta_{42}$ peptide produced from variety of cultured cells by as much as 80%. This effect was not seen in all NSAIDs and seems not to be mediated by inhibition of cyclooxygenase (Cox) activity, the principal pharmacological target of NSAIDs [35, 36]. Furthermore, short term administration of ibuprofen to mice that produce mutant β amyloid precursor protein (APP) lowered their brain levels of $A\beta_{42}$. In cultured cells, the decrease in $A\beta_{42}$ secretion was accompanied in Aβ (1-38) isoform, showing that NSAIDs alter gamma secretase activity without significantly perturbing other APP processing pathways or notch cleavage. Hence, it is clear that NSAIDs directly affect amyloid pathology in brain by reducing $A\beta_{42}$ peptide levels independently of Cox activity [36].

It is proposed that at least part of AD phenotype is due to chronic brain inflammation. Based on this, large placebo-controlled trials of specific Cox-2 inhibitors in AD have been done. Epidemiological studies suggest that treatment with statins, i.e. inhibitors of cholesterol-synthesizing enzyme HMG-CoA-reductase, also protects from Alzheimer's disease. 3-hydroxy-3-methyl glutaryl co-enzyme A reductase (HMG-CoA-reductase) may directly affect $A\beta_{42}$ production although microvascular and endothelial effects of statins and other indirect mechanisms cannot be excluded [37, 38, 39]. Statins could influence treatment of AD before more direct amyloid therapy becomes available. Pfizer is initiating a placebo-controlled study using its cholesterol blocker, lipitor. If effect of statins on AD is due to $A\beta_{42}$ modulation, then inhibition of cholesterol-ester formation may be alternative approach for treating AD. Simvastatin also reduces amyloid burden in AD patients [40, 41]. Although there are many therapies for AD treatment but none is fully safe and have some side effects.

Conclusion

Alzheimer's disease is the single biggest unmet medical challenge and problem which still remains unsolved to date. It affects 12 million people worldwide. AD puts heavy economic burden on society. Its main cause is classic model in neurology, i.e. 'amyloid cascade hypothesis' according to which the overproduction of β-amyloid protein ($A\beta_{42}$) or failure to clear this peptide leads to AD. $A\beta_{42}$ peptide gets deposited as fibrils or could hyperphosphorylate tau protein, which may form neurofibrillary tangles (NFTs) inside neurons and cause toxicity. This could cause neuronal death and memory impairment by blocking messages between nerve cells. Loss of synapses and malfunctioning of synaptic proteins contribute to the progressive cognitive impairment in Alzheimer's disease. In this review an attempt has been made to discuss recent therapies and treatments available for AD patients. Although number of treatment options are being tested by biotechnology and pharmaceutical companies, if just one of them works fully the most frequent neurodegenerative disorder may be cured.

Acknowledgement
We thank Dr. Paul Raj R. for his useful comments and helpful suggestions while preparing this review. Thanks are also due to Mr. Balwant Singh for drawing the figures and typing assistance.

References

1. Sinha, S. and Lieberburg, I. Cellular mechanisms of β amyloid production and secretion. *PNAS* (1999): **96 (20)**:11049–53.
2. Rosenkranz, J.A. and Rose, S.P.R. Cell adhesion molecules, glucocorticoids and long term memory formation. *TINS* (1995): **18 (11)**: 502–505.
3. Hardy, J., Duff, K., Hardy, K.G., Perez-Tur, J. and Hulton, M. Genetic dissection of Alzheimer's disease and related dementias: amyloid plaque formation its relationship to tau. *Nature Neuroscience* (1998): **1(5)**, 355–358.
4. St. George-Hyslop, P.H. and Westaway, D.A. Antibody clears senile plaques. *Nature* (1999): **400 (6740)**: 116–117.
5. Neve, R.L. and Robakis, N. Alzheimer's disease: a re-examination of amyloid hypothesis. *TINS* (1998): **21 (1)**: 15–19.
6. Xia Weiming et al. Presenilin 1 regulates the processing of β amyloid precursor protein terminal fragments and the generation of β amyloid protein in endoplasmic reticulum and golgi. *Biochemistry* (1998): **37 (4)**: 16465–16471.
7. Wolfe, M.S. and Xia, W. Two transmembrane aspartases in presenilin 1 required for presenilin endoproteolysis and γ secretase activity. *Nature* (1999): **398 (6727)**: 513–517.
8. De Girolomi, U., Anthony, D.C. and Frosch, M.P. The central nervous system. In: Contran R.S., Kumar, V., Cellings, T., (editors) Robbins Pathologic Basis of Disease. 6th ed. Philadelphia: WB Saunders (1999): p. 1229–1332.
9. Hardy, J. The Alzheimer's family of diseases: many etiologies, or one pathogenesis? *PNAS* (1997): **94(6)**: 2095–2097.
10. Mayenx, R. et al. Plasma amyloid β peptide 1–42 and incipient Alzheimer's disease. *Annual Neurology* (1999): **46**: 412–416.
11. Yanker, B.A. New clues to Alzheimer's disease unraveling the roles of amyloid and tau. *Nature Medicine* (1996): **2(8)**: 850–851.
12. Vasser, R. et al. β-secretase cleavage of Alzheimer's amyloid precursor protein by transmembrane aspartic protease BACE. *Science* (1999): **286 (5440)**: 735–740.
13. Davis, K.L. and Samuels, S.C. In: Pharmacological management of neurological and psychiratric disorders (eds. Enna, S.J. and Coyle, J.T.) 267–316, McGraw-Hill, New York (1998).
14. Doody, R.S. Therapeutic standards in Alzheimer's disease. *Alzheimer Dis. Assoc. Diord.* (1999): **13**, 520–526.
15. Hardy, J. and Allsop, D. Amyloid deposition as the central event in the etiology of Alzheimer's disease. *Treands Pharmacol.* (1991): **12**, 383–388.
16. Joachim, C.L. and Selkoe, D.J. The seminal role of β amyloidal in the pathogenesis of Alzheimer's disease. *Alzheimer Dis. Assoc. Disord.* (1992): **6,7**–34.

17. Younkin, S.G. The role of β amyloid in Alzheimer's disease. *J. Physiol.* (Paris). (1999): **92**, 289–292.

18. Selkoe, D.J. Translating cell biology into therapeutic advances in Alzheimer's disease. *Nature* (1999): **399**, A23–A31.

19. Leung, D., Abbenante, G. and Fairlie, D.P. Protease inhibitors: current status and future prospects. *J. Med. Chem.* (2000): **43**, 305–341.

20. Francis, R. et al. Aph1 and pen-2 are required for notch pathway signaling, γ secretase cleavage of APP and presenilin protein accumulation. *Dev. Cell* (2002): **3**, 85–97.

21. Sisodia, S.S. and St. George-Hyslop, PH γ secretase, Notch, Aβ and Alzheimer's disease: Where do the presenilins fit in? *Nat. Rev. Neurosci.* (2002): **3**, 281–290.

22. Hardy, J. and Israel, J. In search of γ secretase. *Nature* (1999): **398 (6727)**: 466–467.

23. Hong, L. Structure of protease domain of memapsin 2 (β-secretase) complexed with inhibitor. *Science*, (2000): **290**, 150–153.

24. Lue, Y. et al. Mice deficient in BACE-1, the Alzheimer's β-secretase, have normal phenotype and abolished β amyloid generation. *Nat. Neuroscience.* (2000): **4**, 231–32.

25. Citron, M. β-secretase as target for treatment of Alzheimer's disease. *J. Neuroscience Res.* (2002), **70(3)**:373–379.

26. Sinha, S. Purification and cloning of amyloid precursor protein β secretase from human brain. *Nature* (1999): **402**, 537–540.

27. Hock, B.J. and Lamb, B.T. Transgenic mouse models of Alzheimer's disease. *Trends Genetics* (2001): **17**, S7–S12.

28. Soto, C. Plaque busters: strategies to inhibit amyloid formation in Alzheimer's disease. *Mol. Med. Today* (1999): **5**, 343–350.

29. Cherney, R.A. Treatment with copper-zinc chelator markedly and rapidly inhibits β amyloid accumulation in Alzheimer's disease transgenic mice. *Neuron* (2001): **30**, 665–676.

30. Bush, A. and Tanzi, R.E. The galvanization of β amyloid in Alzheimer's disease. *Proc. Natl. Acad. Sci. USA* (2002): **99**, 7317–7319.

31. Schenk, D. et al. Immunization with amyloid β attenuates Alzheimer's disease like pathology in PDAPP mouse. *Nature* (1999): **400**, 173–177.

32. Bord, F. et al. Peripherally administered antibodies against amyloid β peptide enter the central nervous system and reduce pathology in mouse model. *Nat. Med.* (2000): **6**, 916–919.

33. DeMattos, R.B. et al. Peripheral anti Aβ antibody alters CNS and plasma Aβ clearance AD decrease brain Aβ burden in mouse model of Alzheimer's disease. *Proc. Natl. Acad. Sci. USA* (2001): **98**, 8850–8855.

34. Steinberg, D. Companies halt first Alzheimer vaccine trial. *The Scientist* (2002): **16**, 22–23.

35. McGeer, P.L. and McGeer, E.G. Inflammation, auto toxicity and Alzheimer's disease. *Neurobiol. Aging* (2001): **22**, 799–809.

36. Weggen, S. et al. A subset of NSAIDs lower amyloidogenic Aβ42 independently of cyclooxygenase activity. *Nature* (2001): **414**, 212–216.

37. Wolozin, B., Kellman, W., Ruesseau, P., Celesia, G.G. and Siegel, G. Decreased prevalence of Alzheimer's disease associated with 3-hydroxy-3-methyl glutaryl coenzyme-A reductase inhibitors. *Arch. Neurol.* (2000): **57**, 1439–1443.

38. Jick, H., Zomberg, G.L., Jick, S.S., Seshadri, S. and Drachman, D.A. Statins and the risk of dementia. *Lancet* (2000): **356**, 1627–1631.

39. Fassbender, K. et al. Simvastatin strongly reduces levels of Alzheimer's disease

β amyloid peptides $A\beta_{42}$ and $A\beta_{40}$ *in vitro* and *in vivo*. *Proc. Natl. Acad. Sci. USA* (2001): **98**, 5856–5861.

40. Golde, T.E. and Eckman, C.B. Cholesterol modification as an emerging strategy for treatment of Alzheimer's disease. *Drug Discovery. Today* (2001): **6**, 1049–1055.

41. Puglielli, L. et al. Acyl-coenzyme A: cholesterol acyltransferase modulates the generation of amyloid β peptide. *Nat. Cell Biol.* (2001): **3**, 905–912.

12. Pain Assessment as a Marker for Alzheimer's Disease

R. Mathur, M. Tripathi*, R. Pal and T.N. Gopinath

Department of Physiology, All India Institute of Medical Sciences,
New Delhi-110029, India

*Department of Neurology, All India Institute of Medical Sciences,
New Delhi-110029, India

Abstract. Alzheimer's diesease (AD) patients have altered pain perception. It is not known whether it is due to actual impairment of pain experience or reporting of less pain. The aim of our study is to assess pain status in AD. Cases consisted of probable AD from Cognitive Disorder Clinic, AIIMS. Pain response was evaluated by the nociceptive flexion reflex (RIII) and visual analogue scale (VAS). All AD patients with MMSE scores ranging from 2 to 24 showed a complete attenuation of RIII reflex at all strengths of test current (1-11mA). Control subjects were age matched healthy volunteers. In these subjects an increase in the EMG response was seen with a similar increase in stimulus strength. We conclude that AD patients have decreased pain as indicated by RIII reflex and VAS. It is suggested that threshold of RIII reflex could serve as a marker for AD in dementia patients.

Introduction

Dementia increases exponentially as a function of age with a prevalence of 1% at 65 years, which doubles approximately every five years thereafter. The prevalence in excess of 25% by 85 years of age [1]. Dementia is a syndrome, a diagnostic entity characterized by a progressive decline in cortical functions including cognitive, behavioral and emotional aspects. The most common forms of dementia in the aged population are Alzheimer's disease and the vascular dementias. It seems likely that dementia will affect the cognitive, behavioral and emotional facets of pain since pain is a construct incorporating sensory/discriminative, cognitive/evaluative and affective/ motivational components [2].

Elderly individuals traditionally report less pain than their younger counterparts, despite the increased frequency of illness-related pain with advancing age [3]. Several studies have shown that pain perception is altered in dementia patients like the low use of analgesics in AD patients [4]; low incidence 2% [5] compared to 40% in normal elderly subjects [6], of post-lumbar puncture headache, decreased pain reports in patients with increasing severity of dementia [7] and more suffering during actual painful conditions than chronic affective situations [8]. It is not clear whether older adults experience less or report less pain. The issue is further complicated in demented persons because compromised cognitive and verbal skills confound interpretation of their subjective experiences. The methods utilized to record pain in most of these studies have added to the confusion. Further it is not known whether patients with dementia experience pain in the same way as cognitively normal adults.

Experimentally pain has been studied in AD patients. Porter et al [9] reported changes in heart rate, respiratory sinus arrhythmia, anxiety and pain in dementia patients (albeit of different severity), prior to, during and following venepuncture. Visual analogue scale was used to record pain. Benedetti et al. [10] reported increase in pain tolerance but no change in pain threshold while recording responses to electrical stimulation and arm ischemia. Scherder and Bouma [8] tested comprehension of visual pain scales (CAS, FAS and FPS) for pain assessment in AD patients (early and moderate) which were found to be better compared to verbal reports. All these studies have utilized patient's subjective reports, which may not be truly reflective of the pain experience, due to the impaired cognitive functions in the patients. It emerges from the afore said that there are difficulties in assessing pain, which range from the reliability of patient report to the contents and presentation of the actual scale used. It therefore, supports the need for further research utilizing more objective methods of evaluation including monitoring of physiological parameters. [11].

We have evaluated pain in AD patients by the nociceptive flexion reflex (NFR, RIII), which has been proposed as a good physiological correlate of pain. It is a physiological, polysynaptic reflex allowing for painful stimuli to activate an appropriate withdrawal response and has been shown to be a reliable and objective tool for measurement of an individual's pain experience [12].

Methods

Subjects

Patients: Eleven communicative patients of either sex, in the age range of 63-84 years suffering from Alzheimer's disease (AD) were recruited from the Cognitive Disorder Clinic, Neurology Department, All India Institute of Medical Sciences, New Delhi. In all the AD patients diagnosis was probable based on the NINCDS-ADRDA criteria [13] (Table 1). The severity of dementia in all the patients was assessed by MMSE score [14] and a battery of neuropsychological tests administered at the cognitive disorder clinic.

Controls: Six healthy subjects in the age range of 46-67 years were recruited from the relatives of the patients who had come to the Cognitive Disorder Clinic accompanying the patients. They were screened by the MMSE score.

Table 1   Age distribution and MMSE scores of control and AD patients

S. No.	AD patients			Control subjects		
	Age (yrs)	Sex	MMSE score	Age (yrs)	Sex	MMSE score
1	64	M	24	57	M	30
2	73	M	6	59	M	30
3	84	F	17	52	M	30
4	65	F	17	67	F	29
5	72	F	24	66	M	30
6	63	M	22	46	F	29
7	80	M	12			
8	72	F	6			
9	72	F	6			
10	55	M	2			
11	66	F	20			

An informed consent was obtained from the person accompanying the patient to the laboratory. The Institute of Human Ethical Clearance Committee approved the study.

Pain Stimulus and Nociceptive Flexion Reflex (NFR) Recording
Subjects were asked to report to the laboratory between 08:30 and 09:00 h after an overnight fast. They were explained about the procedure before recording the NFR(RIII). The subjects were asked to relax completely and were seated in a comfortable posture with the knee flexed at 130° and ankle at 90° to obtain complete relaxation of muscles [15, 16]. The temperature and humidity of the laboratory was maintained at 25-27°C and 50%, respectively. To stimulate the sural nerve, the skin over the retromalleolar aspect of the lateral malleolus was abraded using a scrubber, cleared with spirit and (Ag-AgCl) electrode cups were fixed with the conducting gel. Similarly, surface electrodes were placed over the biceps femoris to record the EMG response to the electrical stimulus. The electrode assembly was then connected to the Biopac Computer System (Model V_3 6.7; Biopac System, Inc.,California 93117, USA).

Before recording NFR, the subject was acquainted with the nature of the elecrical stimulus. The sural nerve was then stimulated with a train of 5 stimuli of 1 msec duration at 1 ms interval, generated by a computer controlled stimulator. The subjects received electrical stimuli of 1 through 11 mA in ascending steps of 2 mA at intervals of 5 min. The experiment was aborted if the subject reported of intolerable pain on visual analogue scale (VAS). The RIII response to the electrical stimulus was recorded, which is an objective measure of pain wherein the threshold of pain is similar to the threshold of RIII reflex [15]. The minimum intensity of stimulation eliciting the RIII in EMG response was considered the NFR threshold. The duration and amplitude of the RIII reflex response was calculated.

Results

The MMSE scores of Alzheimer's disease patients ranged from 2 to 24, while of control subjects from 29 to 30 (Table 1).

The amplitude of RIII reflex was analyzed by dividing the records into 12 bins of 20 ms each. The first three bins preceded the response, bins IV-VI contained the response and bins X-XII followed the response. The maximum amplitude of the response was analyzed in a bin wise manner. The EMG activity was found to be comparable (no statistically significant difference) in the bins I-III (pre-response basal EMG) and X-XII (post-response EMG), but was found to be significantly different during the bin IV (Fig. 1, Table 2).

Table 2   Maximum amplitude of RIII reflex in bin IV

Stimulus strength (mA)	Maximum amplitude (µV) (Mean ± SD)	
	Control subjects	AD patients
5	40.29 ± 1.49	7.58 ± 0.82***
7	37.75 + 1.93	7.62 ± 0.62***
9	45.68 ± 1.53	7.41 ± 0.50***

The mean maximum amplitude of the response in bin IV was lesser (7.58 ± 0.826 µV; $p < 0.001$) in AD patients than in the control subjects (40.29 ± 1.49 µV) with 5 mA stimulation strength. The maximum amplitude was 7.62 ± 0.622 µV in AD patients and 37.75 ± 1.93 µV ($p < 0.001$) in control subjects with 7 mA stimulation strength. At 9 mA, the maximum amplitude did not vary (7.41 ± 0.50 µV) in AD patients while it increased (45.68 ± 1.53 µV) in control subjects.

Discussion

Nociceptive flexion reflex (RIII) was used to access the pain status in AD patients. A complete attenuation of the RIII reflex was observed as a rule in AD patients.

The lower limb flexion reflex, elicited through electrical stimulation has been proposed as a good physiological correlate of pain. Specifically, the nociceptive (RIII) component of the flexion reflex has been found to have the same threshold as that of pain sensation [15]. It has also been shown that both flexion reflex and visual analogue scale (VAS) rating bore a direct linear relationship with stimulus intensity and with each other [17]. RIII is recorded by stimulation of the sural nerve, either on or through the skin. This elicits two different reflex responses in the biceps femoris. The first, RII is of short latency low threshold and corresponds to a tactile reflex. The second RIII is of longer latency and higher threshold, and corresponds to a nociceptive reflex. The threshold for RIII was found to be the threshold of pain sensation.

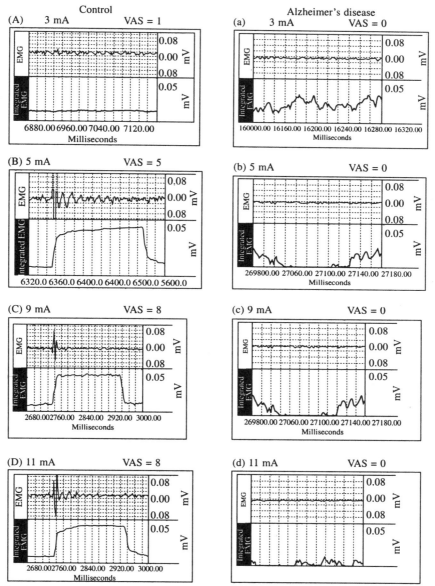

Fig. 1. Representative original tracings of nociceptive flexion reflex record in control subject and Alzheimer's disease patient. Series of records have been obtained when the stimulus strength was gradually increased from 3 to 11 mA. Simultaneously the subjective perception of the pain was obtained on visual analogue scale (VAS).

The RIII is believed to be mediated by group III afferents (Aδ) which subserve fast pain. The RIII has been used to understand the mechanisms of morphine [18] and hypnotic anagesia [19]. Morphine suppresses both the

RIII, pain reports [18] and hypnotic analgesia [19] indicating that a major component of its effects is related to inhibitory mechanisms at the spinal level.

Neuropathological changes in the brain are progressive and characteristic of AD. They are identified as the neurofibrillary tangles and the neuritic plaques in histopathology. There are three identifiable anatomical stages namely, entorhinal, hippocampal and neocortical during progression of the disease. These areas are incidentally involved in pain processing and therefore could possibly influence pain perception. Since thalamus and primary somatosensory cortex are not significantly involved a general sensory deficit is not the hallmark of AD. It is, therefore, possible to record evoked potentials although a functional interpretation of the stimulus is not possible by the patient. Moreover, loss in limbic structures such as hippocampus and prefrontal cortex may explain the affective, cognitive aspects of AD. The associated changes in orbital cortex, frontal cortex, hippocampus, amygdala and ventral hypothalamus [20, 21] have obvious implications for any motivational, arousal and affective reactions to pain. The emotional affective function is influenced due to the conspicuous neuronal and synaptic loss in the prefrontal and limbic regions [20, 21, 22].

It has been shown that supraspinal influences can affect the RIII reflex. Pain sensation and RIII reflex is reported to be affected by mental task and stress [12]. Some supraspinal descending systems influences from reticular or limbic structures can exert a global inhibitory or excitatory action on both ascending and reflex nociceptive messages, whereas others can have a predominantly inhibitory effect on nociceptive ascending paths while sparing the nociceptive reflexes [12]. Analgesia has been reported from microinjection of opioid agonists into amygdala, which is blocked by lidocaine inactivation [23] or opioid antagonist injection into the periaqueductal grey (PAG). The amygdala receives massive input from both the hippocampus and neocortex and is a major source of afferents to the PAG [24, 25] which is involved in supraspinal pain modulation.

Further, the somatosensory evoked potentials (SEPs) were shown to be significantly related to stimulation of noxious and non-noxious somatosensory processes [26] in a study on the sural nerve (compound action potential), the spinal withdrawal reflex RIII SEP. In central medial nucleus of amygdala lesion in rats, the threshold of vocalization after discharge increase significantly indicating a strong analgesia [27], whereas unilateral stimulation of central nucleus of amygdala, basolateral nucleus and medial amygdaloid nucleus, results in the reduction of the tonic (formalin induced) pain, indicating analgesia. The thresholds of SV and VAD were elevated whereas the threshold of TF is not affected significantly by unilateral amygdala stimulation. On the contrary, TFL was accentuated again indicating analgesia [28]. Animal studies have also shown that the stimulation of hypothalamic lateral area and ventromedial nucleus leads to strong analgesia, which is similar in magnitude and direction to that observed in amygdala (anesthetized rats and monkeys) [29, 30].

However, lesion of lateral hypothalamus does not lead to a diagonally opposite result in the thresholds of reflex motor responses mediated at the spinal cord, brain stem and limbic areas. The results reflext on analgesia to phasic stimuli and hyperalgesia to tonic formalin pain. Therefore, it is not true that the lesion of an area leads to an uniform increase of decrease in the pain response because even in the same area, there are different types of neurons having different thresholds, connectivity as well as receptors. On the basis of these behavioral and electrophysiological studies in animals (anaesthetized or behaving) it can be said that lesion or infarct in several limbic areas leads to a complex analysis of the sensory information. This may also hold true in AD patients as well, since they have multiple lesions in several limbic structures.

A complete attenuation of nociceptive flexion reflex was seen in our probable AD diagnosed patients. The method can be used clinically to support the diagnosis and differentiate AD from other types of dementias. The NFR recording (RIII) technique is a quick, simple, reliable and reproducible. It is therefore crucial to screen dementia patients for their responses to pain [31].

References

1. Jorm, A.F. and Henderson, A.S. The Problem of Dementia in Australia, Australian Government Publishing Service, Canberra, 1993.
2. Melzack, R. and Casey, K.L. Sensory, motivational and central control determination of pain. In: Kenshalo, D.R. (ed). The skin senses. Spring Field, Thomas 1968; pp. 423–442.
3. Farrell, M.J., Katz, B. and Helme, R.D. The impact of dementia on the pain experience. *Pain* 1996; **67** : 7–15.
4. Scherder, E.J. and Bouma, A. Is decreased use of analgesics in Alzheimer's disease due to a change in the affective component of pain? *Alzheimer Assoc. Disord.* 1997; **11(3)**: 171–174.
5. Blennow, K., Wallin, A. and Hager, O. Low frequency of post-lumbar puncture headache in demented patients. *Acta Neurologica Scand.* 1993, **88**: 221–223.
6. Knutz, K.M., Kokmen, E., Stevens, J.C., Miller, P. Offord, K.P. and Ho, M.M. Post-lumbar puncture headaches: experience in 501 consecutive procedure, *Neurology* 1992; **42**: 1884–1887.
7. Parmelee, P.A., Snith, B. and Katz, I.R. Pain complaints and cognitive status among elderly institution residents. *J. Am. Geriatrics. Soc.* 1993; **41**: 517–522.
8. Scherder, E.J. and Bouma, A. Visual analogue scales for pain assessment in Alzheimer's disease. *Gerontology.* 2000; **46(1)**: 47–53.
9. Porter, F.L., Malhotra, K.M., Wolf, C.M. Morris, J.C, Miller, J.P. and Smith, M.C. Dementia and response to pain in the elderly. *Pain,* 1996; **68**: 413–421.
10. Benedetti, F., Sergio, V., Cluadia, R., Elisabetta, L., Bruno, B., Lorenzo, P. and Innocenzo, R. Pain threshold and tolerance in Alzheimer's disease. *Pain* 1999; **80**: 377–382.
11. Kovach, C.R., Weissman, D.E., Griffic, J., Matson, S. and Muchka, S. Assessment and treatment of discomfort for people with late-stage dementia. *J. Pain Symptom Management* 1999; **18**: 412–9.
12. Sklijarevski, V. and R. Mandan, N.M. The nociceptive flexion reflex in humans: Review article. *Pain* 2002; **96**: 3–8.

13. McKhann, G., Drachman, D., Folstein, M., Katman, R., Price, D. and Stadlan, E.M. Clinical diagnosis of Alzheimer's disease. Report of the NINCDS-ADRDA Work Group under the auspices of Department of Health and Human Services Task Forces on Alzheimer's disease. *Neurology* 1984; **34**: 939–944.

14. Folstein, M.F., Folstein, S.E. and McHugh, P.R. 'Mini-mental state' a practical method for grading the cognitive state for the clinician. *J. Psychiatric Research* 1975; **12**: 189–198.

15. Willer, J.C. Comparartive study of perceived pain and nociceptive flexion reflex in man. *Pain* 1977; **3**: 69–80.

16. Sandrini, G., Ruiz, L., Capararo, M., Garofoli, F., Beretta, A. and Nappi, G., Central analogesic activity of ibuprofen. A neurophysiological study in humans. *Int. J. Clin. Pharmacol. Res.* 1992; **12(4)**: 197–204.

17. Chan, C.W. and Dallaire, M. Subjective pain sensation is linearly correlated with the flexion reflex in man. *Brain Res.* 1989; **479**: 145–150.

18. Willer, J.C. Studies on pain. Effect of morphine on a spinal nociceptive flexion reflex and related pain sensation in man. *Brain Res.* 1985; **331**: 105–114.

19. Kiernan, B.D., Dane, J.R., Philips, L.H. and Price, D.D. Hypnotic analgesia reduces RIII nociceptive reflex: further evidence concerning the multifactorial nature of hypnotic analgesia. *Pain* 1995; **60**: 39–47.

20 Mountjoy, C.Q., Roth, M., Evan, J.J. and Evans, H.M. Control neuronal counts in normal elderly control and demented patients. *Neurobiol. Aging.* 1983; **(4)**: 1–11.

21. Hyman, B.T., Van, H.G.W., Damasio, A.R. and Barnes, C.L. Alzheimer's disease: cell-specific pathology isolates the hippocampal formation. *Science* 1984; **225**: 1168–1170.

22. Scheff, S.W. and Price, D.A. Alzheimer's disease related synapse loss in the cingulate cortex. *J. Alzheimer Dis.* 2001; **3**: 495–505.

23. Helmstetter, F.J., Tershner, S.A., Poore, L.H. and Bellgowan, P.S. Antinociception following opioid stimulation of the basolateral amygdala is expressed through the periaqueductal gray and rostral ventromedial medulla. *Brain Res.* 1998; **779(1-2)**: 104-18.

24. Amaral, D.G., Price, J.L., Pitkanen, A. and Carmichael, S.T. Anatomical organization of the primate amygdaloid complex. In: Aggleton, J.P. (ed), 1992, The Amygdala. Wiley-Liss, New York, pp. 1-66.

25. Gray, T.S. and Magnuson, D.J. Peptide immunoreactive neurons in the amygdala and the bed nucleus of the stria terminalis project to the midbrain central gray in the rat. *Peptide* 1992; **13**: 451–460.

26. Dowman, R. Spinal and supraspinal correlates of nociception in man. *Pain* 1991; **45**: 269–281.

27. Jain, S., Mathur, R., Sharma, R. and Nayar, U. Neural tissue transplant in the lateral hypothalamic lesioned rats: Functional recovery pattern. *Neurobiology* 1999; **7(4)**: 421–430.

28. Mena, N.B., Mathur, R. and Nayar, U. Amygdalar involvement in pain. *Indian J. Physiol. Pharmacol.* 1995, **39(4)** 339–349.

29. Mathur, R. and Nayar, U. Role of ventromedial hypothalamus in pain modulation. In : Pain Updated: Mechanisms and Effects, Mathur, R. (ed), 2006, Anamaya Publishers, New Delhi, pp. 32–65.

30. Jain, S., Narasaiah, M., Nayar, U. and Mathur, R. Amygdalar Influences on Pain. In: Pain Updated: Mechanisms and Effects, Mathur, R. (ed), 2006, Anamaya Publishers, New Delhi, pp. 82–94.

31. Pickering, G., Jourdan, D. and Dubray, C. Acute versus chronic pain treatment in Alzheimer's disease. *Eur. J. Pain*, 2005 (in press).

13. Pain Assessment in Syndrome X Patients

R. Mathur and S. Pande

Neurophysiology Laboratory, Department of Physiology,
All India Institute of Medical Sciences, New Delhi-110 029, India

Introduction

Ever since this term was first introduced by Kemp [1] in 1973 to describe episodic chest pain with non-specific ST depression in ECG, a positive stress test but normal coronary angiographic studies, syndrome X remains a diagnostic and therapeutic puzzle. Even though long term prognosis in terms of mortality or major cardiac events remain favourable in these patients, the recurrent and prolonged episodes of chest pain impair the quality of life significantly [2]. Moreover, as the chest pain is severe enough to warrant repeated hospital admissions and investigations, a major economic burden is imposed on both, the family and health care system. The considerable social and economic morbidity associated with this syndrome is therefore a cause for concern, making it a topic for intense research for the past three decades.

The chest pain in patients has been ascribed by various studies [3-8] to several abnormalities ranging from myocardial blood flow, opioid status, information processing, myocardial tissue, blood vessels and nerves but a satisfactory explanation for the pathogenesis of pain remains elusive (Table 1). Nevertheless, the distinct aspects of this syndrome are that a chest pain typical of angina is reported by less than half the patients while the patients are predominantly postmenopausal females. In most cases, pain is often atypical in location, unrelated to exertion, more prolonged, unrelieved by rest and the conventional anti-anginal medication. The metabolic markers of ischemia, namely, trans-myocardial lactate production, coronary sinus oxygen saturation, a decrease in pH have not been demonstrated consistently in these patients [9, 10]. Moreover, trans-esophageal echocardiography has also failed to demonstrate regional wall motion abnormalities consistent with ischemia in most cases. These findings have led investigators to question not only the ischemic, but even cardiac origin of pain in syndrome X. Recently, the possibility of aberrant pain perception as the principal cause of pain in these patients is being evaluated. Pain is experienced spontaneously without accompanying changes in ECG.

Table 1   **Postulated causes for abnormal pain in syndrome X**

S. No.	Postulated causes
1	Dysfunction in coronary microvasculature
2	Impaired endothelial function resulting from decreased nitric oxide and estrogen
3	Increased endothelin-1
4	Diminished coronary reserve causing dynamic alteration in coronary blood flow in situations of increased demand
5	Alterations in Na-H co-transport mechanism
6	Autonomic nervous system imbalance

Characteristics of Pain

The characteristics of pain have been studied utilizing various methods. Pain sensitivity to experimental noxious stimuli is evaluated by tourniquet test (ischemic pain), cold pressor test, electrical stimulation of skin nociceptive afferents [11], and boluses of normal saline intra-atrially [12] in syndrome X patients. They reported a lower threshold for forearm ischemia and skin stimulation as compared to the chronic stable angina patients, supporting the contention of an enhanced pain perception albeit to the cutaneous stimuli. A cutaneous hypersensitivity to noxious stimuli cannot be extrapolated to cardiac tissue, till established. Therefore, recently a relation between cardiac and cutaneous sensitivity, was studied. The effect of ventricular pacing, thermal sensitivity in syndrome X patients was compared with the hypertrophic cardiomyopathy, coronary artery disease and valvular disease patients [13]. They reported that pacing indeed reproduced chest pain and the cutaneous threshold was higher in syndrome X patients as compared to the other groups. However, a definite relation between cardiac and cutaneous sensitivity could not be established.

Moreover, the probability of behavorial factors contributing towards chest pain was evaluated by utilizing positive and negative (absence of electrical stimulus) pacing in syndrome X patients [14]. They complained of pain even in the absence of true pacing, which occurred at a lower threshold and greater severity. It is suggested that besides enhanced perception of potentially painful stimuli, subjective psychological factors also contribute to reporting of pain specially in the absence of true stimulus.

Factors Leading to Abnormal Pain

Dynamic PET has provided a new insight into the abnormal processing of pain information in these patients during rest and dibutamine infusion [15]. It was found that anterior insula was activated in syndrome X patients unlike coronary artery disease patients. They proposed this syndrome to be a cortical pain syndrome, a 'top down' process resulting from ineffective gating by the thalamus, which leads to extensive cortical activation in the absence of discernible myocardial pathology.

It is proposed that an abnormal function of afferent cardiac sympathetic nerve endings may be the cause of enhanced pain perception on the basis of [I] Metaiodobenzylguanidine uptake in syndrome X patients as compared to the uptake in controls [16].

The abnormal pain in syndrome X patients is also attributed to an aberration in endogenous opioids as reflected by the neuroendocrine approach [17]. There is an attenuated leutinizing hormone release after naloxone administration in these patients as compared to controls. The authors suggest the a lower central endogenous opioid activity contributes to the increased pain perception in these patients. The contention receives further support by the improvement in condition by training these patients [18]. It is reported that there is an increase in exercise capacity with eight weeks of training including an 100% increase in time for onset of pain and a rightward shift of the pain response to exercise curve whereas, the severity of pain remained unaltered. It implies that the underlying pain mechanism remains unaltered by physical training but the deconditioning associated with this chronic pain syndrome, postulated to be responsible for decrease in the threshold of pain on exertion was certainly significant. It is possible that the effect is due to an increase in the opioid status of the individual since exercise is known to increase β-endorphin secretion.

Current Working Hypothesis

Ongoing research by both schools of thought (ischemic versus pain perception disorder) has led to the current working hypothesis that intermittent ischemia in small myocardial regions induce functional alterations in afferent cardiac adrenergic fibers which may increase their sensitivity to cardiac stimuli and the micro vascular events (Fig. 1). These stimuli/events usually are unable to trigger ·pain in normal individuals but are perceived as painful by these patients.

Future Directions

It is essential to decipher whether or not the enhanced pain perception is generalised or restricted cardiac phenomenon. Although these studies have given us reason enough to believe that aberrant pain perception is indeed the major putative mechanism responsible for chest pain, it remains to be resolved whether the opioid status and neural processing add to the cause of the syndrome.

Presently, it appears that deviation in pain perception, cortical information processing and opioid secretion from the normal are the underlying causes for the abnormal pain in syndrome X patients (Table 1). However, the consensus is against the abnormal cortical information processing because the study lacks appropriate controls. Besides, the issue is complex because we are ignorant about the interaction amongst various neural sites involved in pain processing let alone about the identification of the sites. This is further

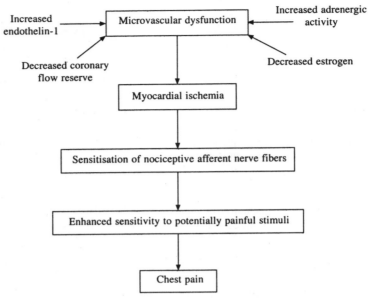

Fig. 1. Proposed working hypothesis.

complicated by a differential processing of somatic and visceral afferent information, and the responses initiated. On the other hand, there are contentious reports regarding the general somatic versus cardiac hyperalgesia in these patients. It is probable that the studies regarding pain perception have utilized different types of noxious stimuli, which may have led to the controversy in the literature. It is well known that the response to noxious stimuli is determined by the stimulus characteristics besides the other micro- and macro-environmental influences. We, therefore, propose that the responses to various noxious and non-noxious stimuli on the opioid release to assess opioid status should be studied more systematically in these patients. This will also provide a simple economical albeit confirmatory test for the diagnosis and management of syndrome X in addition to understanding of the underlying pathophysiology. It is expected that with the advancement in the technology, more studies on animals and syndrome X patients will be able to provide the answer.

Till the time a consensus is reached regarding the exact pathogenesis and consequently, the management of syndrome X, the establishment of generalized hyperalgesia as the major cause of chest pain in most patients would aid in assuring patients of a 'normal cardiac status' and favorable prognosis. Moreover, it would alleviate their anxiety considerably. Additional research for evaluation of mechanisms of increased pain sensitivity is, therefore, recommended. Angiography, however, remains the gold standard for conclusive exclusion of coronary disease.

References

1. Kemp, H.G. Left ventricular function in patients with anginal syndrome and normal coronary arteriograms. *Am J. Cardiol.*, 1973; **32**: 375–376.
2. William, L. Proudfit, Bruschke, A.V.G., Sones, P.M. Clinical cause of patients with normal or slightly or moderately abnormal coronary arteriograms: 10 year follow up of 521 patients. *Circulation*, 1998; **62**: 712–717.
3. Cannon, R.O., Epstein, S.E. "Microvascular angina" as a cause of chest pain with angiographically normal coronary arteries. *Am J Cardiol*, 1988; **61**: 1338–1343.
4. Quyyumi, A.A., Cannon, R.O., Panza, J.A., Diodati, J.G., Epstein, S.E. Endothelial dysfunction in patients with normal coronary arteries. *Circulation*, 1992; **86**: 1864–1871.
5. Camici, P.G., Gistri, R., Lorenzoni, R., Sorace, O., Michelassi, C., Bongiorni, M.G., Salvadori, P.A., L'Abatte A. Coronary reserve and exercise ECG in patients with chest pain and normal coronary angiograms. *Circulation*, 1992; **86**: 179–186.
6. Rosano, P., Panikowski, S., Adamopoulos, S., Collins, P., Poole- Wilson, P.A., Coats, A.J.J., Kaski, J.C. Abnormal autonomic control of the cardiovascular system in syndrome X. *Am J Coll Cardiol.* 1994; **73**: 1174–1179.
7. Gaspardone, A., Ferri, C., Crea, F., Versaci, F., Tomai, F., Santucci, A., Chiariello, L., Gioffre, P.A. Enhanced activity of sodium-lithium counter transport in patients with cardiac Syndrome X : a potential link between cardiac and metabolic syndrome X. *J Am Coll Cardiol.*, 1998; **32**: 2031–2034.
8. Rosano, G.M., Collins, P. Kaski, J.C., Lindsay, D.C., Sarrel, P.M., Poole-Wilson, P.A. Syndrome, X. in women is associated with estrogen deficiency. *N Engl J Med.* 1997, **337(26)** : 1920.
9. Nihoyannpolous, P., Kaski, J.C., Crake, T., Maseri, A. Absence of myocardial dysfunction during stress in patients with syndrome X. *J. Am Cell Cardiol* 1991; **18**: 1463–1470.
10. Camici, P.G., Marracini, P., Lorenzoni, R., Buzzi, Goli, G., Pecesi, N., Perissinotto, A., Ferrannini, E., Labbate, A., Marzilli, M. Coronary hemodynamics and myocardial metabolism in patients with syndrome X : response to pacing stress. *J Am Cell Cardiol*, 1991; **17**: 1461–1470.
11. Turiel, M., Galasi, A.R., Glazier, J.J., Kaski, J.C., Maseri A. Pain threshold and tolerance in women with syndrome X and women with stable angina pectori. *Am J. Cardiol*, 1987; **6**: 503–507.
12. Shapiro, L.M., Crake, T., Poole-Wilson, P.A. Is altered cardiac sensation responsible for chest pain in patients with normal coronary arteries? Clinical observation during cardiac catheterisation. *BMJ*, 1988; **296**: 190–191.
13. Cannon, R.O., Quyummi, A.A., Schenke, W.H., Fananpazir, L., Tucker, E.E., Gaughan, A.M., Gracely, R.H., Cattau, E.L., Epstein, S.E. Abnormal cardiac sensitivity in patients with chest pain and normal coronary arteries. *J Am Coll Cardiol* 1990; **16**: 1359–1366.
14. Pasceri, V., Lanza, G.A., Buffon, A., Montenero, A.S., Crea, F., Maseri, A. Role of abnormal pain sensitivity and behavioral factors in determining chest pain syndrome X. *J Am Coll Cardiol.*, 1998; **31**: 62–66.
15. Rosen, S.D., Pauelesu, E., Wise, R.J.S., Camici, P.G. Central neural contribution to the perception of chest pain in cardiac syndrome X. *Heart*, 2002; **87**: 513–519.
16. Lanza, G.A., Giordana, A.G., Pristipino, C., Calcagni, M.L., Guido, M., Trani, C., Franceschini, R., Crea, F., Troncone, L., Maseri, A. Abnormal cardiac adrenergic nerve function in patients with syndrome X detected by [123I] Metaiodobenzyl guanidine myocardial scintigraphy. *Circulation*, 1997; **96**: 821–826.

17. Fedele, F., Agati, L., Pugliese, M., Cerevellini, P., Beneditti, G., Magni, G., Vitarelli, A. Role of central endogenous opiate system in patients with syndrome X. *Am. Heart J*, 1998; **136**: 1003–1008.

18. Eriksonn, B.E.,Tyni-Lenne, R., Svedenberg, J., Hallin, R., Urstad, K.J., Urstad, M.J., Bergman, K., Sylven, C., Syndrome X: Physical training counteracts deconditioning and pain in syndrome X. *J AM Coll Cardiol*, 2000; **36**: 1619–1625.

Pain Updated: Mechanisms and Effects
Edited by R. Mathur

14. Neuroprotective Effect of GDNF Against 6-OHDA in Young and Aged Rats

Shalini Singh, Riyaz Ahmed and Bal Krishana

Department of Physiology, Maulana Azad Medical College, New Delhi-110 002, India

Abstract: Glial derived neurotrophic factor (GDNF) caused significant restoration in dopaminergic neurons against 6-hydroxydopamine (6-OHDA) in young rat. The present study was undertaken to determine if GDNF would provide similar protective effects in aged rats. 6-OHDA was injected in to the lateral sector of the rat striatum. Intrastriatal administration of GDNF injection significantly changed apomorphine induced rotations from 155 ± 10 to 210 ± 14, staircase test from 70% to 53%, stepping test from 8 ± 2 steps to 6 ± 1 steps and initiation time from 10 ± 1 s to 12 ± 1 s in young and aged animals respectively. These results indicate that GDNF are an effective neuroprotective agent for young as well as aged dopaminergic neurons in rat model of Parkinson's disease. However, the extent of protection is less in the aged animals.

Introduction

Glial cell line-derived neurotrophic factor (GDNF) is a member of the transforming growth factor-β (TGF-β) which induces the closely related molecules neuroturin, artemin/neublastin and persephin. These GDNF family ligands bind to heterodimeric receptor complexes consisting of high-affinity ligand-binding proteins, the GPI-anchored GDNF receptor α components, and a c-RET receptor tyrosine kinase mediating signal transduction [1]. Since its discovery, GDNF has been shown *in vitro* and *in vivo* to function as a trophic factor for midbrain dopamine (DA) neurons. Previous studies have reported that 6-OHDA induced the loss of the dopaminergic phenotype in substantia nigra neurons of the rat, which can be reversed by GDNF administration [2]. If GDNF is administered after inducing lesions with 6-OHDA or 1-methyl-4-phenyl-1,2,3,6-tetrahydropyridine (MPTP), partial histochemical, neurochemical and behavioral recovery have been reported in both rodents and monkeys. GDNF is a potent survival factor for transplanted embryonic dopaminergic neurons. When infused into oculotransplants of fetal ventral mesencephalic tissues, it stimulates the growth of transplanted dopaminergic neurons [3]. It also enhances the survival and fiber outgrowth from fetal ventral mesencephalic transplants after pre-incubating the transplant with GDNF or infusing GDNF into the transplant site intermittently or chronically [4]. Continuous release of low levels of GDNF into a perinigral region protects nigral dopaminergic neurons against axotomy-induced lesion and improves pharmacological rotational behavior by non-dopaminergic mechanisms [5]. Further more intermittent injections of GDNF into a perinigral region prevents 6-OHDA induced degeneration of nigral dopaminergic neurons [6] and delivery of GDNF to peripheral regions using viral vectors has been shown to halt 6-OHDA induced degeneration of dopamine neurons [7-8]. Similar protective effects of GDNF have been reported against the DA depleting effects of MPTP and methamphetamine. These studies, as well as several others, emphasize the trophic effects of GDNF on DA neurons and suggest that GDNF may have therapeutic potential for treating diseases such as Parkinson's disease.

The abovementioned studies focused on the use of young adult animals to examine the *in vivo* effects of GDNF. However, since the degeneration of substantia nigra DA neurons that occurs in Parkinson's disease is more often than not confined to elderly individuals, it is of interest to determine whether the protective effects of GDNF against 6-OHDA in young adult rats can be extended to aged animals. To further define the extent of protection offered by GDNF, the present study examined the 2 h time point between GDNF and 6-OHDA administration in 3 and 24-month-old Sprague Dawley rats. These experiments were designed to evaluate the scope of GDNF neuroprotection in aged animals against intrastriatal 6-OHDA lesions by evaluating various behavior and histological tests.

Methods

Fortyeight male Sprague Dawley rats, weighing 200-250 g at the beginning of the experiment, were housed and treated in compliance with the regulation, policies and principles of the Institutional Animal Ethical Committee. They had free access to food pellets and water. They were kept in an airconditioned room with a regular 12 h light-12 h dark cycle. All efforts were made to reduce the number of animals used and their suffering. The rats received the treatment as given in Table 1.

Table 1   The groups of rats on the basis of treatment received

Groups	Treatment	Number of rats
1	Control rats	12
2	6-OHDA-lesioned rats with 2 µl GDNF vehicle (10 mM citrate buffer with 150 mM NaCl, pH 5) into lateral striatum only	12
3	6-OHDA lesioned young rats with GDNF 10 µg dissolved in 2 µl vehicle into lateral striatum only	12
4	6-OHDA lesioned aged rats with GDNF 10 µg dissolved in 2 µl vehicle into lateral striatum only	12

6-OHDA Lesioning

Unilateral lesion was produced by stereotaxic injection of 8 μg 6-OHDA in to the striatum. For this all the animals were anaesthetized with pentobarbital (40 mg/kg ip) and placed in David Kopf stereotaxic frame [9]. The coordinates were 0 mm anterior-posterior, 3.5 lateral, 5.5 mm dorso ventral to the dura with the tooth bar setting at 3.3 mm below the interaural line [10].

Rotational Behavior

At 4 weeks after lesion surgery, apomorphine (0.05 mg/kg) induced rotations was observed [9]. The left and right full-body turns were monitored for 30 min. Net rotational asymmetry score was expressed as full-body turns per minute in the direction ipsilateral or contralateral to the lesion.

Staircase Test

This test was assessed using the staircase adopted from Montoya [11]. The rats were placed on a restrictive food diet of about 12 g per rat each day to maintain 90% of their initial weight. Paw reaching training was started 5 days after food restriction in plexiglass test box and their ability to reach and grasp for pellets was measured. Six pellets were placed on both sides of every step, giving a total of 30 pellets available on each side. The test score corresponds to the number of pellets taken and eaten. Analysis was then performed using the results of the last 3 days during the performance plateau. The success rate, i.e. the number of pellets eaten divided by the number of pellets taken, was also calculated in all rats.

Stepping Test

At four weeks post-lesion, forelimb akinesia was examined in a sidestepping test wherein the number of adjusting steps for both directions (left and right) and both fore paws are counted by the method described by Schallert et al [12]. Two days before the experiment, the examiner becomes familiar with the grip used to handle the rat during the test. On the day of the test, the "blind" examiner fixed the hind limbs of the rat with one hand while holding the rat; the forelimb which is not to be monitored with the other hand; and the unrestrained forepaw was touching the table. The numbers of adjusting steps taken by the unrestrained forepaw were counted while the rat was slowly moved sideways (0.9 m in 5 sec) along the table surface by the examiner. The movement was conducted first in the forehand and then in the backhand direction. The test was performed for each forelimb in both movement directions. It was repeated twice a day on three consecutive days, and the average of the six subtests was calculated.

Initiation Time

The time to actively initiate a forelimb movement was determined in the same test session as for the stepping test. The rats were pretrained for two days to turn up a wooden ramp (1.1 m) into their home cage. During the test, the rat was held as described for the stepping test and placed with its unrestrained paw (the one to be monitored) on the bottom of the ramp. The time elapsed before the rat actively initiated movement with the unrestrained forelimb and started to step forward along the ramp towards the home cage was recorded. One hundred eighty seconds was used as a break off point for initiation of stepping. The test was performed once a day for each forelimb on three consecutive days and the mean of the three test sessions was calculated [13-15].

Histological Evaluation

After the completion of behavior test, all the rats were anaesthetized with lethal dose of sodium pentobarbital. The rats were perfused with 4% paraformaldehyde in 0.1 M, pH 7.4 phosphate buffer solution (PBS). The brains were removed and placed in the same fixative for 24 h. Then they were transferred to 15% sucrose in 0.1 M PBS until they sank. Brain sections (5 μm cryostat coronal sections) were cut using a microtome. They were stained with Haematoxylin and Eosin and observed for neurons under light microscope [16-17].

Statistical Analysis

Comparisons between lesioned and nonlesioned sides within the same group were performed using paired Student's t-test. Statistical significance level was set at $p < 0.05$ for all tests [18].

Results

Groups 2, 3 and 4 rats showed contra lateral rotations when stimulated by apomorphine after 5 weeks of 6-OHDA lesions. Rotations began almost immediately after apomorphine (0.05 mg/kg, s.c.) injection and were studied for 30 min (Table 2, Fig. 1). Control rats did not show statistical significant rotation response ($p > 0.1$). The post lesion p value for group 2, 3 and 4 were statistically significant (< 0.001).

Table 2   Effect of apomorphine injection in rats pre-and post-6-OHDA lesion

Groups	Number of rotations in 6-OHDA lesion rats	
	Before apomorphine injection	After apomorphine injection
1	10 ± 1	12 ± 2
2	12 ± 1	258 ± 16
3	11 ± 2	155 ± 10
4	10 ± 2	210 ± 12

Skilled forelimb tests revealed a significant treatment effect in young and aged rats (Figs. 2 to 4). We found that rats in all groups performed equally

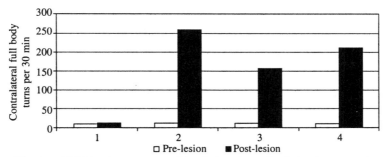

Fig. 1. GDNF reduces apomorphine-induced rotation behavior scores in young and aged rats.

well on the side ipsilateral to the lesion, i.e. they were taking close to 30 (of 30) pellets and eating 27 of them ($p > 0.1$). In contrast, on the side contralateral to the lesion, the 6-OHDA-lesion only rats showed a significant impairments in performance. Group 2 rats took 12 ± 3, eaten 4 ± 1 pellets compared to 27 ± 3 taken and 25 ± 2 eaten in Group 1; 20 ± 2 taken and 14 ± 2 eaten in Group 3; 15 ± 2 taken and 8 ± 3 eaten in Group 4 on the contra lateral side. The success rate was significantly reduced to approximately 33% in Group 2, 70% in Group 3 and 53% in Group 4 compared to 93% in Group 1 rats.

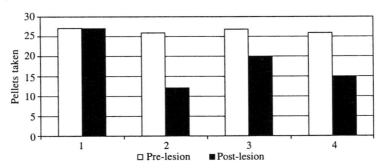

Fig. 2. GDNF induce behavioral recovery in young and aged rats. Staircase test (pellet taken)

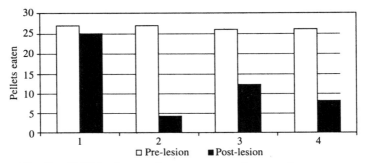

Fig. 3. GDNF reduces pellets eaten scores in the staircase test.

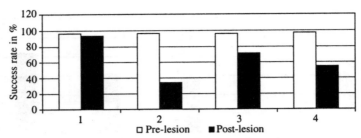

Fig. 4. GDNF increases the success rate in staircase test.

Comparison of stepping test among all the groups also revealed a statistically significant effect in young and aged rats on the contralateral side to the lesion. The 6-OHDA lesion did not affect the performance of the ipsilateral side which is comparable to the control group of rats ($p > 0.1$). Number of steps was found 12 ± 2 in Group 1, 3 ± 1 in Group 2, 8 ± 1 in Group 3 and 6 ± 2 in Group 4 contralateral to lesion in forehand direction (Fig. 5). The number of steps were 13 ± 2, 4 ± 1, 9 ± 1 and 6 ± 2 in Groups 1 to 4, respectively in backhand direction (Fig. 6). Aged rats (Group 4) showed less behavioral recovery than young rats (Group 3) in these tests.

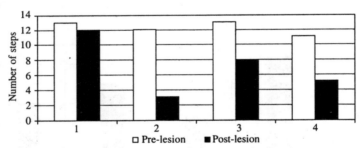

Fig. 5. GDNF induces behavior recovery in stepping test.

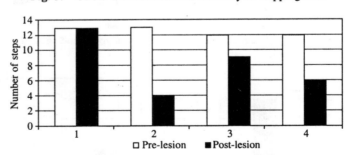

Fig. 6. GDNF increases behavioral recovery in stepping test.

Initiation of movement on the forelimb ipsilateral to the 6-OHDA lesion was immediate and not different from the normal controls ($p > 0.1$). We observed statistically significant initiation time of movement on the forelimb contralateral to lesion. We found initiation time to be 2 ± 1, 15 ± 2, 10 ± 2

and 12 ± 2 in Groups 1 to 4, respectively (Fig. 7). Initiation time was markedly increased in Group 2 while it was significantly reduced in GDNF treated young rats (Group 3) and aged rats (Group 4).

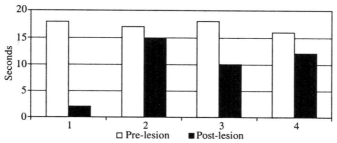

Fig. 7. Initiation time is increased by GDNF treatment.

We performed histological evaluation of brain sections in all the groups of rats. There was an almost complete loss of dopaminergic neurons in Group 2 whereas, the neurons were partially protected in the striatum of the GDNF treated rats (Groups 3 and 4). Histological analysis supported the behavioral data, i.e. the intrastriatal injection of GDNF protected dopaminergic neurons from the 6-OHDA neurotoxicity. On similar lines the aged rats showed less restoration in cell loss than young rats.

Discussion

The results of present study demonstrate that the administration of GDNF prior to an intrastriatal 6-OHDA injection protects striatal DA neurons in young and aged rats. However, there was less protection in aged rats compared to young rats.

The performance of the rats in the rotational behavior, staircase test, stepping test, initiation time and histological tests were highly correlated with the amount of DA in the lesioned striatum, thus demonstrating that these tests provide highly sensitive measures of the extent of denervation in the lateral part of the caudate-putamen [13]. Olsson et al [13] reported that rotation and forelimb akinesia might have similar underlying mechanisms, i.e. tonic activation of DA receptors in striatum and/or substantia nigra. The behavior tests indicate that the recovery of function by GDNF in the 6-OHDA lesion model is critically dependent on restoration of DA neurotransmission in the denervated striatum.

GDNF ameliorated significant rotational behavior induced by apomorphine in 6-OHDA treated young and aged rats. Earlier studies have reported a significant increase in DA turnover as well as an augmentation of the rotational behavior after a single injection of GDNF [19-20]. In the intact nigrostriatal system, DA is known to release from the axon terminals in the striatum where it may play an important role in the modulation of basal ganglia function through the striato-nigral output pathway [20]. Previous pharmacological studies in rodents have shown that the effects of DA-releasing agents like amphetamine and DA receptor agonists such as apomorphine on motor behaviors such as rotation and locomotion are mediated in part by activation of DA receptors in the SN [20-21], thus raising the possibility that DA released within the nigra itself could compensate for the loss of striatal innervation in the 6-OHDA rats. In support of this possibility, Hoffer et al [22] and Nikkhah et al [23] have observed reduced apomorphine-induced rotation associated with increased DA levels of TH-positive cells and fibers in the SN after either intranigral GDNF injection or intranigral DA neuron transplants in 6-OHDA-lesioned rats.

The results of the present study strongly demonstrate the neuroprotective effect of GDNF against 6-OHDA induced dopaminergic neurotoxicity in hemiparkinsonium rat. However, the extent of protection is less in aged rats. It may be due to neurochemical and cellular changes in the nigrostriatal dopaminergic changes during aging. There are reductions in striatal levels of DA as well as DA receptors [24]. Neuronal loss in the substantia nigra reaches about 50% by the ninth decade in humans [25]. Reduction in high affinity DA uptake sites [26], DA transporter messenger RNA [27] and TH messenger RNA [27] also become evident as individuals age. It has been postulated that free radicals play a major role in the neuronal degeneration that occurs during aging as well as in many neurodegenerative diseases such as Parkinson's disease. It is possible that GDNF is eliciting its protective effect by enhancing or maintaining the synthesis of free radical scavenging enzymes. Indeed, it has recently been reported that intrastriatal GDNF leads to an upregulation of the antioxidant enzymes glutathione peroxidase, superoxide dismutase and catalase [28]. Furthermore, in primary cultures of rat mesencephalon, GDNF can suppress the production of reactive oxygen species [6]. Therefore, the protection of DA neurons in the present experiments may be due to the upregulation of expression and/or activity of antioxidant enzyme systems [29]. The naturally occurring decrease in these enzymes with age may in part explain why the 24-month-old rats were least protected by the GDNF. To elucidate the exact mechanism of action of GDNF, further study is needed.

Acknowledgment

The authors are grateful for the financial support from Indian Council of Medical Research, New Delhi.

References

1. Baloh RH, Enomoto H, Johnsons EM, Milbrandt J. The family ligands and receptors: implication for neural development. *Curr. Opinn. Nerobio* 2000; **10(1)**: 103–110.
2. Bowenkamp KE, Hoffman AF, Gerhardt GA, Henry MA. Glial cell line derived

neurotrophic factor supports survival of injured mid brain dopaminergic neurons. *J. Comp. Neurol* 1991; **355**: 479–489.

3. Stromberg I, Bjorklund L, Johansson M, Tomae A, Collins F, Olson L, Hoffer B, Humpel C. Glial cell line-derived neurotrophic factor is expressed in the developing but not adult striatum and stimulates dopamine neurons in vivo. *Exp. Neurol* 1993; **124**: 401–412.

4. Apostolides C, Scanford E, Hong M, Mendez I. Glial cell line derived neurotrophic factor improves intrastriatal graft survival of stored dopaminergic cells. *Neuroscience* 1998; **83**: 363–372.

5. Aaetge LT, Zurn AD, Achischer P. GDNF reduces drug-induced rotational behaviour after medial forebrain bundle transaction by a mechanisms not involving striatal dopamine. *J Neuroscience* 1997; **17**: 325–333.

6. Sauer H, Resenblad C, Bjorklund A. Glial cell line-derived neurotrophic factor but not transforming growth factor β3 prevents delayed degeneration of nigral dopaminergic neurons following striatal 6-hydroxydopamine. *Proc Natl Acad Sci USA* 1995; **92**: 8935–8953.

7. Lundberg DLC, Lin Q, Chang Y, ChiangYL, Hay CM, Mohajeri H, Davidson,BL, Bohn MC. Dopaminergic neurons protected from degeneration by GDNF gene therapy. *Science* 1997; **275**: 838–841.

8. Deumens R, Blokland A, Prickaerts J. Modeling Parkinson's disease in rat : an evaluation of 6-OHDA lesion of the nigrostiatal pathway. *Expel Neurol* 2002; **175**: 303–317.

9. Ungerstedt U. Postsynaptic supersensitivity after 6-hydroxydopamine induced degeneration of the nigrostriatal system in the rat brain. *Acta Physiol Scand Suppl* 1997; **367**: 69–93.

10. Paxinos G, Watson C. The rat brain in stereotaxic coordinates. Academic Press, San Diego. CA. 1982.

11. Montoya CP, Campbell-Hope L J, Pemberton KD, Dennett S B. The "staircase test": a measure of independent forelimb reaching and grasping abilities in rats. *Journal of Neuroscience Methods* 1991; **36**: 219–228.

12. Schallert T, Ryck M, Whishaw IQ, Ramirez VD, Teitelbaum P. Excessive bracing reactions and their control by atropine and L-dopa in an animal analog of parkinsonism. *Exp.Neurol* 1979; **64**: 33–43.

13. Olsson M, Nikkhah G, Bentlage C, Bjorklund. A. Forelimb akinesia in the rat Parkinson model: Differential effects of dopamine agonists and nigral transplants as assessed by a new stepping test. *J. Neurosci* 1995; **15**: 3863–3875.

14. Winkler C, Sauer H, Lee CS, Bjorklund A. Short-term GDNF treatment provides long-term rescue of lesioned nigral dopaminergic neurons in a rat model of Parkinson's disease. *J. Neurosci* 1996; **16**: 7206–7215.

15. Schallert T, Hall S. Disengage' sensorimotor deficit following apparent recovery from unilateral dopamine depletion. *Behav. Brain Res* 1998; **30**: 15–24.

16. Saji M, Blau AD, Volpe BT. Prevention of transneuronal degeneration in the substantia nigra reticulata by ablation of the subthalamic nucleus. *Expl Neurol* 1988; **141**: 120–129.

17. Sahd JL, Lara MC, Cabrera GM, Echavarria AV. Histological and ultrastructural characterization of interfascicular neurons in the rat anterior commissure. *Brain Research* 2002; **931**: 81–91.

18. Subbakrishna DK. Statistics for neuroscientists. *Annals of Indian Academy of Neurology* 2000; **3**: 55.

19. Hudson J, Granholm A-C, Gerhardt GA, Henry MA, Hoffiman A, Biddle P, Leela NS, Mackerlova L, Lile JD, Collins F, Hoffer BJ. Glial cell line-derived neurotrophic

factor augments midbrain dopaminergic circuits *in vivo*, *Brain Res. Bull* 1995; **36**: 425–432.

20. Robertson HA. Dopamine receptor interactions: some implications for the treatment of Parkinson's disease. *Trends Neurosci* 1992; **15**: 201–206.

21. Cheramy A, Leviel V, Glowinski J. Dendritic release of dopamine in the substantia nigra. *Nature* 1981; **289**: 537–542.

22. Hoffer BJ, Hoffman A, Bowenkamp K, Huettl P, Hudson J, Martin D, Lin LF, Gerhardt GA. Glial cell line-derived neurotrophic factor reverses toxin-induced injury to midbrain dopaminergic neurons *in vivo*. *Neurosci Lett* 1994; **182**: 107–111.

23. Nikkhah G, Bentlage C, Cunningham MG, Bjorklund A. Intranigral fetal dopamine grafts induce behavioral compensation in the rat Parkinson model. *J Neurosci* 1994; **14**: 3449–3461.

24. Kish SJ, Shannak K, Rajput A, Deck JH, Hornykiewiez O. Aging produces a specific pattern of striatal dopamine loss: implications for the entiology of idiopathic Parkinson's disease, *J Neurochem* 1992; **58**: 642–648.

25. Horvath TB, Davis KL, Central nervous system disorders in aging. In: E.L. Schneider, J.W. Rowe (Eds.), Handbook of the Biology of Aging, 3rd Edition, Academic Press, San Diego 1990; pp. 306–329.

26. Allard P, Marecusson JO. Age-correlated loss of dopamine uptake sites labeled with [3H]GBR 12935 in human putamen, *Neurobiol. Aging* 1989; **10**: 661–664.

27. Bannon MJ, Poosch MS, Xia Y, Goebel DJ, Cassin B, Kapatos G. Dopamine transporter mRNA content in human substantia nigra decreases precipitously with age, *Proc. Natl. Acad. Sci. USA* 1992; **89**: 7095–7099.

28. Chao CC, Lee EH, Neuroprotective machanism of glial cell line-derived neurotrophic factor on dopamine neurons: role of antioxidation. *Neuropharmacology* 1999; **39**: 913–916.

29. Kearns CM, Gash DM. GDNF protects nigral dopamine neurons against 6-hydroxydopamine *in vivo*. *Brain Res* 1995; **672**: 104–111.

Pain Updated: Mechanisms and Effects
Edited by R. Mathur

15. Pain in Neonates

N.B. Mathur and D. Mathur*

Professor of Pediatrics, Incharge Referral Neonatal Unit, *Department of Physiology,
Maulana Azad Medical College, Lok Nayak Hospital, New Delhi, India

Abstract. In the past, it was felt that neonates were unable to feel pain and that even if they could, they would not remember it. These views were based on the belief that the neural pathways involved in nociception were immature at birth and infants' behavioral responses to painful stimuli seemed erratic and inconsistent. This lead to ignoring analgesia in the newborn which would be regarded as inhuman now. In the recent years, the neurophysiology of pain in the newborn has received considerable attention. Pain receptor density in newborn skin is similar to that of adults. The central connections of these are complete by 30 weeks of gestation. Nociceptive stimuli can be carried in unmyelinated or thinly myelinated nerve fibres. The neuropeptides, monoamines and catecholamines implicated in pathways in adults are present in fetal life. The assessment of severity of pain in the newborn is difficult due to limited and nonspecific response of the neonate. The areas used to provide measures of neonatal pain are: (a) behavioral, (b) physiological and (c) biochemical and metabolic. Behavioral scoring systems have been evolved involving features like facial expression, body posture, withdrawal response, muscle tone and restlessness to constitute a pain score. Physiological parameters altered by pain include heart rate, blood pressure and cutaneous blood flow. Pain is associated with altered levels of corticosteroids and biochemical markers of protein catabolism. However, it is inevitable that on occasions our assessment of pain can be difficult and fallacious. While pain is associated with restless or agitated behavior, on occasions, some infants with severe pain will remain immobile.

Introduction

The infant's response to pain results in a number of adverse physiological changes. These include elevations in heart rate, blood pressure and fall in oxygenation. In the sick preterm neonates such fluctuations are known to be associated with complications. Infants treated for pain during and after surgery have a reduced incidence of post-operative thrombotic complications and an increased incidence of intraventricular haemorrhage and necrotising enterocolitis. The release of glucagon, catecholamines and corticosteroids leads to catabolic state and is associated with an increased incidence of post-operative disseminated intravascular coagulation. Management of pain in neonate is required in clinical situations like post-operative period, septic arthritis, peritonitis and during mechanical ventilation and procedures.

Pain Experience in Neonates

Pain is defined as an unpleasant sensory and emotional experience associated with actual or potential tissue damage or described in terms of such damage [1]. In the past neonates have not been given analgesia because of the controversy over whether they feel pain and are stable enough to tolerate the effects of analgesics. There is increasing evidence that neonates including preterms have a CNS that is more mature than earlier thought [2-5]. Pain pathways are myelinated in the fetus in the second and third trimester and are completely myelinated by 30-37 weeks. Even thinly or nonmyelinated fibres carry pain stimuli. Incomplete myelination implies slower transmission which is offset by the shorter distance the impulse has to travel in the neonates. The infant's capacity for memory is far greater than earlier thought [3, 6, 7] and a neuropsychologic complex of altered pain threshold and related behavior has been identified [8-11].

Pathophysiology

Neonates have a developing, incompletely myelinated nervous system at birth. However, all the components of the nociceptive (pain) pathways are present [4, 5] Pain receptor density in newborn skin is similar to that of adults. The central connections of these are complete by 30 weeks of gestation. Nociceptive stimuli can be carried in unmyelinated or thinly myelinated nerve fibers. The neuropeptides, monoamines and catecholamines implicated in pathways in adults are present in fetal life.

Peripheral Nervous System

Pain receptors (nociceptors) are the A-δ fibers and C fibers that are widely spread in the superficial layers of the skin, periosteum, fascia, peritoneum, joints, muscles, pleura, dura and tooth pulp. Most visceral tissues have fewer nociceptors, and these transmit to the spinal cord through the sympathetic, parasympathetic and splanchnic nerves. Tissue damage and inflammation cause the release of arachidonic acid and other chemicals that can sensitise nerve endings and cause vasodilatation and plasma extravasation. This causes pain, swelling and hyperalgesia [12, 13].

A-delta fibers are myelinated and therefore capable of fast impulse conduction. These nerves are responsible for 'fast' or 'first' pain. They are also known as high threshold mechanoreceptors because they respond to strong pressure or tissue injury. The C fibers (polymodal nociceptors) are unmyelinated, conduct impulses more slowly, and are the main nociceptors for transmitting chemical, thermal and mechanical noxious stimuli to the spinal cord [14]. The A-delta fibers seem to develop ahead of the C fibers in the skin and the spinal cord. They start to function at initially lower thresholds than when they mature. Thus, less stimulation is required for conduction of what may be perceived as pain. Complete myelination occurs during the second and third trimesters. Lack of myelination had been thought to indicate the inability of a neonate to perceive pain. However, incomplete myelination leads only to slower conduction, which is offset by the shorter distances traversed in the infant [4].

Reflex responses to somatic stimuli begin at $7^1/_2$ post-conceptual weeks in the perioral skin and continue to develop in the palms of the hands before finally reaching the hind limbs by $13^1/_2$ to 14 weeks [4]. It is likely that both touching and pinching are transmitted by δ fibers in the human fetus. In rat pups the C fibers stimulate dorsal horn cells by the end of the first post-natal week and continue to mature for several weeks. This correlates with the third trimester and the early neonatal period in humans [4, 5].

Spinal Cord

Once a noxious stimulus is detected by the nociceptors, the signal is transmitted to the dorsal root ganglia and thence to the dorsal horn of the spinal cord [12]. Neurotransmitters and their receptors amplify or attenuate the signal in the dorsal horn before sending the signal to the brain [13]. Excitatory neurotransmitters such as SP and other neurokinins are increased after acute inflammation and may be required for the transmission of painful stimuli to the brain. Glutamate and aspartate are amino acids that appear to be involved in central hypersensitivity and 'wind up' [12]. Wind up is a phenomenon where by repetition of the same noxious stimulus leads to an exaggerated response. This response can continue even after the stimulus has been stopped and may contribute to the development of chronic pain syndromes. Wind up may also be responsible for converting a low level, pain related activity to a high level pain related activity [12]. An additional factor in the development of hypersensitivity and hyperalgesia is the presence of nociceptive specific receptors, which respond only to pain. In the presence of peripheral inflammation, the threshold of these receptors is decreased so that they are capable of responding to non-noxious stimuli [12]. Thus, an infant whose heel has been repeatedly pricked may demonstrate pain behavior when the heel is merely touched.

The spinal cord also contains inhibitory neurotransmitters GABA and glycine which are activated by descending neural pathways and decrease the intensity of pain transmission [5]. Descending inhibition modulates the pain response, yet allows specific pain response like limb withdrawal. Lack of inhibition produces exaggerated generalized responses to pain like body wriggling, facial grimacing and excessive crying. These pathways are not fully developed at birth in rat pups and probably humans [5].

SP and glutamate in the developing nervous system are not necessarily located in the areas normally found in adults. This may contribute to the unorganized, generalized responses noted with pain stimuli in the newborn.

Brain

Little is known about the development of the pathways to the higher brain centers, such as the hypothalamus and cortex. Evidence indicates immaturity of the inhibitory pathways [4, 5]. Cutaneous responses are exaggerated, occur at much lower thresholds, and reflex contractions last longer in newborns when compared with adults [4]. Newborn's nervous system is probably also capable of remembering noxious stimuli. Development in the human cortex continues for many years after birth.

Physiological Responses to Pain

Pain in neonates is associated with increased sympathetic stimulation, heart rate, respiratory rate, blood pressure, cardiac output, myocardial oxygen consumption, peripheral resistance, anxiety, emotional distress, hormonal imbalance and greater morbidity and mortality [15]. Both premature and full term infants express the same physiologic responses to pain and noxious stimuli as adults (Table 1). These responses can be attenuated with the use of analgesics.

Table 1   Neonatal pain responses

Behavioral	

(a) Vocalizations
  1. Crying—high pitched, tense and harsh
  2. Whimpering
  3. Moaning
	(b) Facial expressions
	  1. Grimacing
	  2. Furrowing of the brow
	  3. Quivering chin
	  4. Eye squeeze

(c) Body movements
  1. General diffuse body activity
  2. Limb withdrawal
  3. Swiping, thrashing
  4. Touch aversion
  5. Tone—hypertonicity, fisting, flaccidity
	(d) States
	  1. Altered sleep wake cycle
	  2. Difficult to comfort
	  3. Altered activity level
	  4. Feeding difficulties
	  5. Disrupted interaction with parents

Physiologic responses	

(a) Increase in:
  1. Heart rate
  2. Blood pressure
  3. Intracranial pressure,
    Intraventricular haemorrhage
  4. Respiratory rate
  5. Mean airway pressure
  6. PCO_2
	(b) Decrease in :
	  1. Depth of respiration (shallow)
	  2. Oxygenation—leading to apnea
	(c) Pallor/flushing
	(d) Diaphoresis
	(e) Dialated pupils

Hormonal/catabolic stress response	

(a) Increase in:
  1. Plasma renin activity
  2. Catecholamine levels
  3. Aldosterone
  4. Cortisol
  5. Growth hormone
  6. Glucagon
  7. Nitrogen excretion
	(b) Increase in serum:
	  1. Glucose
	  2. Lactate
	  3. Pyruvate
	  4. Ketones
	  5. Nonesterified fatty acids
	(c) Decrease in:
	  1. Insulin secretion

Etiology of Pain

Pain in neonates is frequently produced during invasive procedures in the neonatal intensive care unit (Table 2). One study found the number of invasive procedures in 54 neonates to be 3283. The commonest was heelstick (56%) followed by endotracheal suctioning (26%) and intravenous cannula insertion (8%) [16]. Analgesics were rarely used for intravenous cannula insertion, venipuncture, suprapubic bladder aspiration, urinary bladder catheterization, arterial line placement, lumbar puncture and paracentesis. Analgesics were used only in 60% of the time for placement of chest tubes, central lines and bone marrow aspirations.

Table 2 Common causes of pain in neonates

Invasive procedures	Surgical procedures	Others
1. Intravenous cannula	1. Central line placement	1. Fracture rib, clavicle
2. Venipuncture	2. Patent ductus arteriosus ligation	2. Extremity fracture
3. Heelstick	3. Tracho-oesophageal fistula repair	3. Necrotizing enterocolitis
4. Endotracheal suctioning	4. Gastroschisis repair	4. Bowel obstruction
5. Intramuscular injection	5. Omphalocoele repair	5. Improper position
6. Arterial line	6. Congenital diaphragmatic hernia repair	
7. Bladder aspiration	7. Inguinal hernia repair	
8. Urinary bladder catheterization	8. Cardiac surgery	
9. Insertion of chest tubes	9. Circumcision	
10. Lumbar puncture		
11. Paracentesis		
12. Mechanical ventilation		

Clinical Features

Assessment of pain in neonates is difficult as they cannot verbalise pain. There are four objectives in the assessment of pain, viz. detection of the presence of pain; impact of pain; pain relieving interventions and effectiveness of interventions [17, 18].

The following criteria have been used to assess neonatal pain, viz. behavioral, physiological, biochemical and metabolic. Behavioral scoring systems have been evolved involving features like facial expression, body posture, withdrawal response, muscle tone and restlessness to constitute a pain score. Physiological parameters altered by pain include heart rate, blood pressure and cutaneous blood flow. Pain is associated with altered levels of corticosteroids and biochemical markers of protein catabolism. Physiological parameters indicating pain are a result of sympathetic stimulation (Table 1). However, it is inevitable that on occasions our assessment of pain can be difficult and fallacious. While pain is associated with restless or agitated behavior, on occasions, some infants with severe pain will remain immobile. Pain responses may be delayed, cumulative or absent. Critically ill and premature neonates may have exhausted their energy to respond to pain. A more immature neonate may manifest disorganized and ineffective responses that make it more difficult to assess pain [19, 20, 21]. He may manifest alterations in sleep wake cycles and habituate to the overwhelming stimuli of the Neonatal Intensive Care Unit.

Pain Management in Neonates

Pain management of neonates continues to be inadequate despite convincing evidence supporting infants' capabiiity to perceive and respond to painful events at birth [22] and despite documentation of detrimental post-surgical outcomes following inadequate analgesia [23]. Studies indicate a lack of awareness among health care professionals of pain perception, assessment and management in neonates [24, 25]. When analgesics were used in infants, they often were administered on the basis of perception of health care professionals or family member. In addition, health care professionals often focussed on treatment of pain rather than a systemic approach to reduce or prevent pain [26, 27]. Therefore, the use of reliable and valid measures to minimize pain, maximize coping and minimize infant risk must be developed. The most effective management of pain in the neonates is by either preventing, limiting, or avoiding noxious stimuli [27]. Modifying the environment and providing anxiolytics for circumstances expected to be stressful also may be useful. The environment should be as conducive as possible to the well being of the neonate and family [28, 29].

Unnecessary noxious stimuli (acoustic, visual, tactile, vestibular) of neonates should be avoided. Simple comfort measures such as swaddling, non-nutritive sucking and positioning should be used whenever possible for minor procedures [30, 31]. Consideration of least painful method is important [32, 33, 34]. Skillful placement of peripheral, central or arterial line reduces need of repeated intra-venous puncture or intramuscular injections. In some cases, the risk benefit balance may favor the more invasive in dwelling catheter [32, 33, 34].

Fear of adverse reaction and toxic effect often contributed to inadequate use of analgesics. Absorption metabolism distribution and clearance of drugs in the neonate differs from the older child and adults as summarized in Table 3. Analgesics and sedatives used in neonates are summarized in Table 4.

Table 3 **Pharmacologic implications of physiological deviations in neonates from adults**

Parameter affected and its cause	Pharmacological effect
(a) Altered gastric acidity due to presence of alkaline amniotic fluids at birth, immature gastric mucosa and alkaline milk	Variable drug absorption
(b) Decreased gastric emptying time	Increased absorption of some drugs
(c) Decreased protein binding due to lower levels of albumin due to increased competition for binding sites by bilirubin	Increased level of free drug (opiods, local anesthetics)
(d) Increased volume of distribution due to larger volume of body water	Larger initial dose for effect (neuromuscular blocking agents, local anesthetics)
(e) Decreased drug metabolism due to immature liver enzymes	Prolonged effect of medication (morphine, fentanyl, neuromuscular blockers)
(f) Decreased drug clearance due to immature renal system and decreased glomerular filteration	Prolonged effect of medication (morphine)

Table 4 **Analgesics and sedatives used in neonates**

Drug	Dosage
(a) Systemic administration	
1. Morphine	(a) IV, IM, SC 0.05-0.2 mg/kg/dose; 2-4 hrly (b) Continuous IV infusion 10-15 µg/kg/hr
2. Fentanyl	(a) IV or SC 1-5 µg/kg/dose; 1-2 hrly (b) Continuous IV infusion 1-5 µg/kg/hr
3. Sufentanil citrate	(a) 0.5-1 µg/kg/dose; every 30 min-1 hr
4. Acetaminophen	(a) PO or PR 10-15 mg/kg/dose; every 4-6 hr
5. Ibuprofen	(a) PO 4-10 mg/kg/dose; every 6-8 hr
(b) Local	
1. Lidocaine	(a) 0.5-1% solution, maximum upto 50 ng/kg
2. Bupivicaine	(a) One time epidural dose 2.5 mg/kg (b) IV infusion, maximum upto 0.2 mg/kg/hr
3. EMLA (Lidocaine and Prilocaine)	(a) 2.5-5 g

IM: Intramuscular route; IV: Intravenous route; SC: Subcutaneous route; PO: Peroral route; PR: Per rectal route.

References

1. Mersky H. Clarification of chronic pain: disruption of chronic pain syndromes and definition of pain terms. *Pain* 1986; **3** (suppl) : 51.
2. American Academy of Pediatrics, Committee on Fetus and Newborn, Committee on Drugs, Section on Anaesthesiology and Section on Surgery; Neonatal Anaesthesia, *Pediatrics* 1987; **80**: 446.
3. Anand KJ, Hickey PR. Pain and its effect in the human neonate and fetus. *N Engl J Med* 1987; **317**: 1321–1329.
4. Fitzgerald M, Anand KJ. Developmental neuroanatomy and neurophysiology of pain. In: Schecter N, Bende C, Yaster M, editors, Pain in infants, children and adolescents, Baltimore.1993, Williams & Wilkins.
5. Fitzgerald M. Neurobiology of fetal and neonatal pain. In: Wall P, Melzad R, editors: Textbook of pain. Edinburgh, 1994, Churchhill Livingstone.
6. Herzog JM. A neonatal intensive care syndrome: a pain complex involving neuroplasticity and psychic trauma. In: Galenson E, Tyson RL, editors, Frontiers in infant psychiatry, New York, 1983, Basic Books.
7. Roove-Collier C, Hayne H. Reactivation of infant memory: implications for cognitive development. *Adv Child Dev Behav* 1987; **20**: 185–238.
8. Grunau R et al. Extremely low birth weight (ELBW) toddlers are relatively unresponsive to pain at 18 mo. Corrected age compared to larger birth weight children. Abstracts 18, Proceedings of the Neonatal Society, 1993.
9. Grunau RV, Whitfield MF, Petrie JH. Pain sensitivity and temperament in extremely low birth-weight premature toddlers and preterm and full term controls. *Pain* 1994; **58**: 341–346.
10. Grunau R, Whitfield MF, Petrie JH, Fryer EL. Early pain experience, child and family factors, as precursors of somatization: a prospective study of extremely premature and full term children. *Pain* 1994; **56**: 353–359.
11. Taddio A, Goldbach M, Ipp M, stevens B, Koren G. Effect of neonatal circumcision on pain responses during vaccination in boys. *Lancet* 1995; **345**: 291–292.
12. Devor M. Pain mechanism and pain syndromes. In: Campbell J, editors, Pain 1996. An updated review, Seattle,1996, IASP Press.
13. Dickenson A. Pharmacology of pain transmission and control. In: Campbell J, editors, Pain 1996. An updated review, Seattle,1996, IASP Press.
14. Meyer R, Campbell J, Raja S. Peripheral neuromechanisms of nociception. In: Wall P, Melzack R, editors, Textbook of pain, Edinburgh, 1994, Churchill Livingstone.
15. Cousins M. Acute and postoperative pain. In : Wall P, Melzack R, editors, Textbook of pain, Edinburgh, 1994, Churchill Livingstone.
16. Barker DP, Rutter N. Exposure to invasive procedures in neonatal intensive care unit admissions. *Arch Dis Child Fetal Neonatal Ed.* 1995; **72**: F47–48.
17. Lepley M et al. High-risk obstetrical care. In, Gardner S, Hagedorn M, edotors: Legal aspects of maternal child nursing practice, Menlo Park, Calif,1997, Addison-Wesley.
18. Porter F. Pain assessment in children and infants. In: Schecter N, Bende C, Yaster M, editors, Pain in infants, children and adolescents, Baltimore.1993, Williams & Wilkins.
19. Als H. Toward a synactive theory of development: promise for the assessment and support of infant individuality. *Infant Mental Health Journal* 1982; **3**: 299.
20. Craig KD, Whitfield MF, Grunav RV, Linton J, Hadjistavropouls HD. Pain in the preterm neonate: behavioral and physiological indices. *Pain* 1993; **52**: 287–299.

21. Van Cleve L, Johnson L, Andrews S, Hawkins S, Newbold J. Pain responses of hospitalised neonates to venipuncture. *Neonatal Netu* 1995; **14**: 31–36.
22. Anand KJ. The applied physiology of pain. In: Anand KJ, McGrath PJ, editors, Pain in Neonates. Amsterdam, Elsevier; 1993; pp 39–66.
23. Anand KJ, Hickey P. Halothane-morphine compared with high-dose sufentanil for anesthesia and postoperative analgesia in neonatal cardiac surgery. *N Engl J Med* 1992; **326**: 1–9.
24. Burokas L. Factors affecting nurses' decisions to mediate pediatric patients after surgery. *Heart Lung* 1985; **14**: 373–379.
25. Purcell-Jones G, Dormon F, Sumner E. Pediatric anesthetists' perceptions of neonatal and infant pain. *Pain* 1988; **33**: 181–187.
26. Clinical Practice Guideline AHCPR Publication No 92-0032. Acute Pain Management: Operative or Medical Procedures and Trauma. Rockville, MD: Agency for Health Care Policy and Research, Public Health Service, US Department of Health and Human Services; 1992.
27. Schechter NL, Blankson V, Pachter LM, Sullivan CM, Costa L. The ouchless place: No pain, children's gain. *Pediatrics* 1997; **99**: 890–894.
28. Sauve R, Saigal S. Optimizing the Neonatal Intensive Care Environment. Report of the Tenth Canadian Ross Conference in Pediatrics, GCI Communications; Abott Laboratories; Montreal, Canada, 1995.
29. American Academy of Pediatrics, Committee on Drugs. Guidelines for monitoring and management of pediatric patients during and after sedation for diagnostic and therapeutic procedures. *Pediatrics* 1992; **89**: 1110–1115.
30. Corff K, Seideman R, Venkataraman PS, Lutes L, Yates B. Facilitated tucking: A non-pharmacologic comfort measure for pain in preterm infants. *J Obstet Gynecol Neonatal Nurs.* 1995; **24**: 143–147.
31. Gunnar MR, Fisch RO, Malone S. The effects of pacifying stimulus on behavioral and adrenocortical responses to circumcision in the newborn. *J Am Acad Child Psychiatry* 1984; **23**: 34–38.
32. Shah VS, Taddio A, Bennett S, Speidel BD. Neonatal pain response to heelstick vs venepuncture for routine blood sampling. *Arch Dis Child* 1997; **77**: F143–F144.
33. Larsson BA, Tannfeldt G, Lagercrantz H, Olsson GL. Venipuncture is more effective and less painful than heel lancing for blood tests in neonates. *Pediatrics* 1998; **101**: 882–886.
34. Shah V, Ohlsson A. Venipuncture versus heel lance for blood sampling in term neonates. In: The Cochrane Library, Issue 4, 1999, Oxford Update Software.

16. Extremely Low Frequency Electromagnetic Field Phenomena in Biology

J. Behari

School of Environmental Sciences, Jawaharlal Nehru University,
New Delhi-110067, India

Abstract: Low level electromagnetic field phenomena in biological systems at extremely low frequencies is as yet most controversial, owing to a variety of reasons. The first and foremost mechanism of interaction is dependent upon a number of uncontrollable parameters. At extremely low frequencies electric E and magnetic H fields are uncoupled and quasi static approximation is therefore valid. The incident fields are those present without the presence of the object and the internal fields are those present in presence of the body. There is a difference in the degree of attenuation of the electric field and the magnetic field, the latter being transparent to the biosystems. The time dependent magnetic fields induce eddy currents and voltage in the body, which compete with the internal voltages and currents. The time dependent electric field (50 Hz), on the other hand, though offers a large value of the permittivity, there is a substantial concentration of electric field lines on the surface. Since these frequencies and their hormonics are present in the human body, their effect on biosystems is a matter of serious debate. However, the beneficial effect of modulated radio frequency fields (in treatment of bone fracture healing and osteoporosis) is now well accepted. It is suggestive of a cell dependent effect, the mechanism of which is yet to be fully understood.

Introduction

Since existence, living objects have constantly been the target of interaction by exogenous electric and magnetic fields, though their actual role in controlling these processes is still not understood. Static electric fields (100 V/m) arise due to the negatively charged ionosphere, and the earth has its own magnetic field (50 µT). According to the Poynting theorem the maximum average electromagnetic energy P_{em} deposition in a living system is given by

$$P_{em} = 1/2 \, [\varepsilon E_{rms}^2 + \mu H_{rms}^2]$$

where E_{rms} and H_{rms} are the electric and magnetic field (rms) intensities, respectively, and ε and μ are the dielectric constant and magnetic permeability of the biological medium, respectively. In the extremely low frequency region the fields to which the body is exposed could be geomagnetic field, ac magnetic fields, and electric fields and currents induced on or in the body may affect biological processes. The exact mechanisms by which these potential effects are produced have not yet been fully identified. Since the EMFs are intermixed it is impossible to identify which component constitutes the dose. The description of the relationship between the external fields and those currents induced in the body is called dosimetry.

Wherever electricity is generated, transmitted, or used, electric and magnetic fields (EMF) are created, due to the presence and motion of electric charges. Generally, these fields are time-varying vector quantities characterized by a number of parameters, including their frequency, phase, direction, and magnitude.

An electromagnetic field is composed of two components, the electric and the magnetic fields. The electric field is created by the presence of an electric charge. It describes the magnitude and direction of the force it exerts on a positive electric charge. The magnitude of the electric field depends on the difference in potential between charge-carrying bodies, including conductors, regardless of the amount of current that is flowing in them. In contrast, a magnetic field is created by the motion of electric charges. Typically, this motion is represented by a flow of charge in the form of an electric current, which gives the number of charges per second passing through the conductor. The magnetic field acts only on other electric charges in motion. Thus, a magnetic field is created by an electric current and describes the magnitude and direction of the force exerted on a nearby current (moving charges). The magnitude of the magnetic field is proportional to the current flow in a conductor, regardless of the voltage present.

In the extremely low frequency region the size of the object is much smaller than the wavelength of the source and this is an approximation in electric-circuit theory. The approximation in this range is the quasi-static EM field theory. An important gain of this approximation is that the electric E and the magnetic B fields are independent of each other, or they may be treated as uncoupled. E can be produced by either the time varying magnetic field or by distribution of charges or both. However, in static case $\frac{\partial \vec{B}}{\partial t}$ is zero and will not contribute to the E. Because E and B are uncoupled at low frequencies, the internal field can be computed by finding the internal E and B due to the internal B alone.

The role of extremely low frequency magnetic fields in affecting biological processes has been a matter of recent concern. Presently we are concerned with the effect on magnetic fields but will include electric fields when possible because of their inherently close association with electric power systems. Voltage and current determine the magnitude of the electric and the magnetic fields at a location, respectively, with the source geometry and distance from the source to the measurement location. The strength of an electric field is usually measured in volts per meter (V/m) or sometimes in kilovolts per meter (1 kV/m =1000 V/m). Magnetic fields can be designated by either magnetic flux density B or magnetic field strength H; both are proportional to the magnitude of the current. B is measured in the centimeter-gram-second unit, the gauss (G), or the unit of the System International (SI), the tesla (T); 1 mG = 1×10^{-3} G = 0.1 T. H is measured in SI units of amperes/m (A/m). B and H are related by the equation

$$B = \mu_0 H$$

where μ_0 = 1.26×10^{-6} Henry/m is the magnetic permeability of a vacuum. To a close approximation, μ_0 remains the same for air and body tissues, and only one of the variables, B or H, need be measured. In practice, B is the usual measured quantity and magnetic field refers to the magnetic flux density in microtesla (μT) (1 μT = 1×10^{-6} T). Unless otherwise stated, all voltage, current, and magnetic flux values are rms (root mean square).

EMF can be arranged in an orderly fashion in an electromagnetic spectrum, according to their frequency f or wavelength λ, where $\lambda = c/f$ and c is the velocity of light. The electromagnetic spectrum spans an enormous range of frequencies (Fig. 1), more than 15 orders of magnitude. Presently we focus

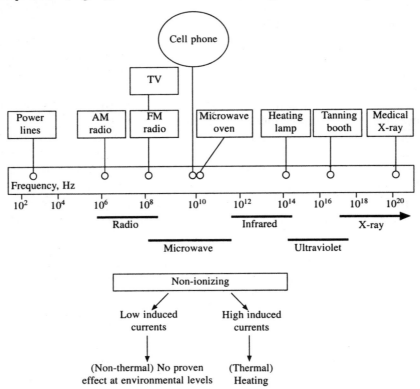

Fig. 1.   In terms of the electromagnetic spectrum, cell phones fall between microwave ovens and TV transmitters.

principally on EMF resulting from the use and distribution of electric power, allowing a great deal of simplification as these fields vary rather slowly over time. The frequency of EMF depends on the power-line source. In North America, power systems operate at a frequency of 60 Hz, while in India it is 50 Hz. These power-line fields fall in the extremely low frequency (ELF) region of the electromagnetic spectrum, which is defined by frequencies from dc to 300 Hz [1]. The alternating current flowing in the electric power system as dominant sinusoidal voltage and current waveforms; however, although 50 Hz is the predominant fundamental frequency, humans are exposed to a mixture of frequencies, and much higher frequencies (extending upto microwaves) are also possible (Fig. 2). For example, switching events can generate abrupt spikes in voltage and current waveforms, leading to high frequency 'transients', which can extend into radio frequencies above several megahertz (1 MHz = 10^6 Hz). Nonlinear characteristics in electrical devices can generate harmonics at integer multiples of the fundamental frequency extending upto several kilohertz (1 kHz = 10^3 Hz). EMF frequencies from some electronic equipment, like televisions and visual display terminals (VDT), can extend upto 50 kHz.

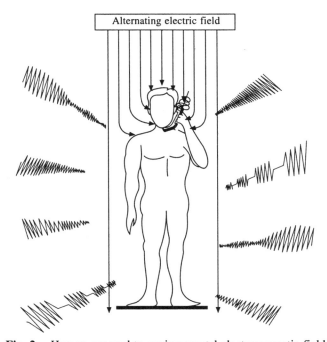

Fig. 2. Human exposed to environmental electromagnetic field.

Most devices that have electric wires, e.g. electric motors, electric equipment such as electric power lines, residential appliances, and industrial equipment, are potential sources of EMF. Residential exposures are dominated by ELF sources but also include exposure to microwave sources.

Unlike the fields from power lines and other alternating current sources, the earth's fields are largely 'static', that is they do not change over time. In contrast, EMF from power lines and other alternating current sources have a periodic component. The earth's magnetic field has a magnitude of about 50 μT over most of the USA and is oriented toward magnetic north; the vertical field component accounts for about two-third of the total vector magnitude. Devices that operate on direct current (dc) also produce static magnetic fields, and some occupational environments, such as aluminum smelting, can have extremely strong static fields.

Basis of Biological Effects

Extremely low frequency (ELF) electric fields at relatively high intensities can have acute biological effects. Nerve and muscle stimulation results in an immediate behavioral response in humans and other vertebrates [2, 3]. Extremely strong electric fields can permanently or transiently damage cell membranes [4] and produce burn injuries [5]. Stimulation of peripheral nerves at power frequencies in humans generally requires electric current densities in muscle tissue of the order of 1.0 A/m^2, which corresponds roughly inside tissues with an electric conductivity σ of 1 S/m to internal electric fields of the order of 1.0 V/m. Production of such currents inside living tissue at 60 Hz requires either direct, electrically conductive contact with a source of electric power or the presence of an electric field in the surrounding air of the order of several 100 kV/m. This requirement is a consequence of the physical laws of conservation of electric charge and continuity of electric displacement. In the case of steady-state sinusoidal electric fields of frequency f at a plane boundary between 'semi-infinite' media, the ratio of the internal electric field E_{int} over the external field E_{ext} is described by the relation [6]

$$(E_{int}/E_{ext}) = 4(10^{-8}) \tag{1}$$

Since for dry air the dielectric permittivity 8.84×10^{-12} F/m, the ratio given by eq. (1), which describes the attenuation of an external electric field relative to the apparent field inside the body, is roughly 100 million. Distortion of the field in air by the presence of a 'conducting' body, air moisture, contact with an electrically conducting earth, and variation of σ within the body, can reduce this ratio somewhat, but it will never be much less than 10 million. Details of current and field distributions that take into account body orientation and in homogeneity are given in [7] and [8].

Typical 60 Hz electric fields in homes rarely exceed 100 V/m [9] and are not more than 10 kV/m near ground level directly underneath a very high-voltage (~ 500 kV) transmission line. It is clear that the only person who will experience internal electric fields of the order of even 10^{-3} V/m due to an external electric field are utility workers in the immediate vicinity of high-voltage wires.

Time-varying magnetic fields induce electric fields into any material, according to Faraday's law

$$V = \oint E \cdot dl - \iint (\partial B / \partial t)\, ds \qquad (2)$$

where V is the induced voltage.

Left-hand side of eq. (2) indicates the electric field integrated over a closed boundary while right-hand side is the integral of the rate of change of the magnetic flux density B perpendicular to and integrated over the area enclosed by the contour designated on the left-hand side. The integral is also called *magnetic flux* ϕ. For a reasonably long, cylindrical body of radius r, eq. (2) leads to [6]

$$E = \pi f B r \qquad (3)$$

where B is the magnetic flux in tesla and r is in meters, which is frequently used to estimate the average electric field induced by a time-varying magnetic field. This equation can be used to calculate electric fields in the biological bodies, under the assumption that these are cylindrical. Further, since the left-hand side of eq. (3) gives only the induced electric field summed over a closed contour, this applies only to an electrically homogeneous medium. However, in electrically inhomogeneous tissue, this induced field can vary locally, giving rise to much larger or smaller values than the average [10].

The magnetic permeability μ of living tissue (with very few, localized exceptions) is practically equal to that of free space. Consequently, the magnetic flux density inside the body is nearly equal to that outside (free space). Eq. (3) then indicates that a 60 Hz field of 100 μT oriented along the head-to-feet axis of a human, with an average radius of 15 cm, will induce near the periphery of the body an average electric field of 2.8×10^{-3} V/m. In comparison, the average electric field near the rim of a petri dish, with a radius of 3 cm, induced by a vertical 60 Hz, 100 μT magnetic fields will be about 0.56×10^{-3} V/m.

These magnetically induced internal electric fields are very much larger than those due to a 100 V/m external electric field in air. A 100 V/m electric field represents the upper limit of those found in typical homes; though induced electric fields are much smaller than internal electric fields associated with nerve and muscle stimulation. The average electric field induced by a 0.3 μT, 60 Hz field near the surface of a human with a 15 cm radius is only 8.5×10^{-6} V/m. Thus, typical magnetic fields encountered in epidemiological studies of residences induce internal currents and electric fields that are roughly one million times smaller than the currents required producing acute nerve and muscle stimulation.

Since the induced voltage is proportional to the time rate of change of the H field, implying a linear increase with frequency (eq. (3)), we would expect that the ability of a time varying H field to induce currents deep inside a conducting object would increase with increase in frequency indefinitely. This is not true, because the displacement current density $\partial \bar{D}/\partial t$ ($\mathbf{D} = \varepsilon\,\mathbf{E}$), also becomes important as the frequency increases. At the sufficiently high frequencies the effects of both external E and H fields are limited by reflection losses as well as by skin effect.

Eq. (1) provides a rough approximation of the electric fields inside and outside an individual subjected to an external electric field. An electric field that is initially uniform becomes distorted in the immediate vicinity of a biological body (Fig. 3). If an individual is grounded or is standing on an insulating platform also will significantly affect the field distribution. For human exposure, the interest is usually not in the average electric field intensity in the body but rather in the field and current density distribution within parts of the body. The inhomogeneity of electric properties (e.g. bone vs muscle conductivity) and variations in the cross section of the limb and trunk determine the exact current density distribution. The maximum current densities in a human standing on electrically conducting ground in a 10 kV/m, 60 Hz electric fields are 0.03 A/m^2 in the leg and 0.04 A/m^2 in the neck [7, 11].

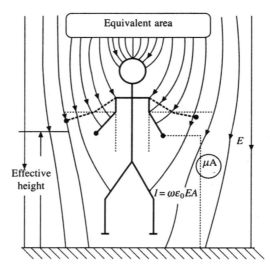

Fig. 3. Current flow through the human body located near ground in an electric field. The magnitude of current depends upon the location of the hand [25].

Fig. 4 shows various rat positions in which different current and voltages are induced inside various organs of the body. This arises not only because of the inhomogeneity of the body tissues and the cross section, but also the difference in the orientation of the body with respect to the incident field. In addition to the above, body size will also result in substantial differences in induced electric field intensity with equal exposure to external electric fields. Thus, rats in a cage must be exposed to a 30 kV/m, vertical, 60 Hz electric field in order to obtain roughly the same electric densities within the rat body as inside a human standing upright in a 10 kV/m, 60 Hz field [12].

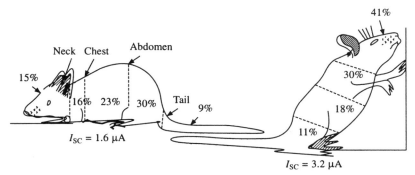

Fig. 4. Grounded rat exposed to vertical 60 Hz, 10 kV/m electric field. Rat body is divided into various segments, viz. head, neck, chest, abdomen and tail. Fractions of total short circuit current originating within each of five sections are shown as percentages [26].

Magnetic Fields Induced in the Body by External Magnetic Fields

The ELF magnetic flux density $B(t)$ inside living tissues is approximately equal to the external field. This relationship is a consequence of two conditions. First, the magnetic permeability of tissues and cells is approximately equal to that of free space. Second, the relatively low electric conductivity (~ 1 S/m) of living matter, in comparison with that of metallic structures (~ 10^7 S/m), guarantees that the magnitude of the secondary magnetic field produced by the induced eddy currents is negligible [13]. Therefore, the applied magnetic field can be measured externally without need to correct for the presence of an individual in the field.

The basic laws derived from 'classical' physics, which can operate either directly or indirectly and at either the macroscopic or the microscopic (molecular) level in field-biosystems interactions, are summarized below.

Forces and torques are given for both electric fields and magnetic flux densities. Individual electric charges, electric dipoles, and magnetic dipoles or magnetic moments are considered. These equations indicate that stationary or moving individual electric charges will undergo translatory motion in the direction of an applied electric field. In comparison, only charges that are already moving at some velocity v will be subjected to a magnetic or 'Lorentz' force $\vec{F} = e(\vec{E} + \vec{v} \times \vec{B})$ in a magnetic flux density B that is perpendicular to both v and B (as indicated by the cross-product). This perpendicular force on electric charges in a magnetic field leads to a circular motion and the 'cyclotron resonance' phenomenon results [14], which will appear only when the probability of collisions with stationary or randomly moving particles is extremely small [15]. The appearance of torques, producing rotation, requires either the pre-existence of dipole moments or their generation by an applied field. This includes phenomena at the atomic level, where the nuclear magnetic moment and nuclear angular momentum are responsible for nuclear magnetic resonance at frequencies determined by an applied dc magnetic field.

Various biophysical mechanisms have been proposed to account for the effects of EMF. Some mechanisms predict a strong (or weak) depending on the frequency content, magnitude, or spatial direction of the fields. Some mechanisms proposed for the interaction of magnetic field with tissues suggest a response from both the time-varying and static-field components or specify a unique combination of the static and time-varying field vectors for a particular target molecule. Also, the possible role of the state of the biological system, for example, awake, moving or sleeping, make the timing and duration of exposure important. There are great variety of possible exposure factors and, therefore, the exact nature of calculations becomes impossible. There the measurement of EMF for the purposes of health assessment is critical.

Fields Induced in Biological Systems

In the power distribution system, the line voltage or current is usually designated by the rms value. To compute the rms value, the instantaneous values are squared, averaged and the square root taken. Mathematically, the rms magnetic flux density is given by

$$B_{rms} = \sqrt{\frac{1}{T} \int_{t=0}^{t=2} B(t)^2 \, dt} \qquad (4)$$

where $B(t)$ is the instantaneous magnetic flux density and T the time for an integral over a number of periods of the fundamental frequency.

For a pure sinusoidal waveform, the rms value is related to the instantaneous peak value by a factor of $\sqrt{2}$, i.e. $B_{peak} = \sqrt{2} \, B_{rms}$. Similar formulae apply for computing the rms voltage and currents.

The measurements of EMF used in most studies are records of the magnitude of the field; they do not retain information on the directional orientation in space or changes in direction over time. This is accomplished by measuring the rms value of three orthogonal spatial components (x, y and z), and then combining these three values to find the magnitude of the rms. This value, sometimes referred to as the rms resultant, is computed as

$$B_{rms} = \sqrt{B_x^2 + B_y^2 + B_z^2} \qquad (5)$$

where B_x, B_y and B_z are the orthogonal magnetic flux density spatial components. As noted above, the magnitude does not depend on the direction of the field vector in space. Therefore, B_{rms} provides an isotropic measure that does not depend on the orientation of the coordinate system for the measuring device. This is a convenient property for personal exposure meters, in which the spatial orientation constantly changes as the subject moves about.

In many studies, instruments have been used to measure or estimate the time-weighted average (TWA) magnitude of the magnetic field. The TWA is computed from the equation

$$B_{rms} = \frac{1}{T} \int_0^1 B(t)\, dt \qquad (6)$$

where T is the averaging time.

Note that for a series of measurements uniformly spaced over time, the TWA reduces to the simple average (mean) of the values over T, the time interval. The TWA is by far the commonest exposure metric. It represents a measure of field magnitude, averaged overtime.

The electric power system in most of the countries is arranged in a series of building blocks or segments, with power lines connecting generating stations via a network of transmission lines, intermediate substations, and switching points to the local distribution lines, and ultimately to utility customers. By design, the voltage in a given portion of the system remains nearly constant; large transmission lines typically operate at > 35 kV (1100 kV) and primary distribution line separate at about 4-35 kV. These higher voltages on the transmission lines are stepped down at local substations by transformers to produce the voltages for the primary distribution lines. The primary distribution lines are further reduced by transformers at other points to a correspondingly lower voltage and higher current for residential or commercial use. Typically, residential service operates at 120/240 V. Roughly speaking, the power delivery in each segment of the electric system is the product of the voltage and current load. Thus, power is delivered by creating high voltage at moderate current in the transmission segments and transforming this into high current at moderate voltage for residential distribution. An important consequence of this distribution system is that transmission lines are usually larger sources of electric fields, because of the high line voltage. In most cases, transmission lines carry larger load currents than primary distribution lines but are located farther away from residences; however, in some cases transmission lines carry load currents similar to those of primary distribution lines. Thus, overall, commercial and residential power distribution systems can be a more significant source of magnetic fields than transmission lines but are usually not a very significant source of large electric fields.

In the normal situation, the voltage in a given segment of the power system remains roughly constant; the current in each portion could be highly variable over time, depending on the changing demand for electric power. As a result, in the absence of other changes (such as introducing shielding materials) at locations near power lines, electric fields remain fairly constant, while magnetic fields generally vary significantly over time. Interestingly, residential measurements of magnetic fields show appreciable morning and evening peaks [16] and a seasonal component, which varies by geographic region and closely follows the electrical use patterns of urban residents. Consequently, the timing of measurements during a day or season can lead to systematic bias in estimates of 24 h or annual average exposures [17].

Point charge and replacement of the original charge element by a charge of equal magnitude but opposite sign creates an electric dipole. A magnetic dipole represents the basic element that describes the magnetic field from a current loop, though uncontrollable parameters. The magnitude of the magnetic field decreases fairly rapidly with movement away from an isolated source; the magnitude falls at least inversely with distance and often with the square of distance or more. A worker standing next to a magnetic field source such as a small motor might experience a field magnitude of 100 T, but by moving a few feet away the magnitude may fall to background levels of <0.1 T. Naturally, the decrease in field strength with distance depends on the magnetic field source, and the pattern is different for a small motor and for a power line. A small motor or computer monitor is essentially a point source, in that the fields originate from a small-defined area. In contrast, a power line is a line source, which may decrease in strength much more slowly with distance and contribute exposure over a much larger area. Field strength of the source is only one consideration in assessing the exposure level while the others are the individual's proximity to the source and the time spent. Together, these factors determine the individual's total exposure to magnetic fields.

Human Exposure to Electropollution

The term electropollution is often used to describe the emissions caused by the non-ionizing portion of electromagnetic spectrum by a variety of appliances e.g. electrical power lines, power stations, transformers, electrical appliances for domestic and industrial use, microwave towers, radio TV and commercial terminals, electrical blankets, steel pipes, reinforcement bars that conduct an electrical current and underground transport systems. Preece et al [18] have showed that the ambient UK homes had a mean value of 0.06 µT, as measured by 24 h sampling in the main occupied rooms. These are, however, low when compared with US homes [16, 19]. The maximum current density induced in man by extra high voltage electrical field is 10^{-8} A/cm^2 and by *seafarer* magnetic field is 10^{-9} A/cm^2. These levels of fields are believed to be necessary to generate sensory effects. We are continuously exposed to these fields and in addition immersed in the earth's magnetic field, which has a typical flux density of around 50 µT. The biological body is however totally diamagnetic. Presently we are concerned with the large wavelength size as compared to the length of the human body. It is thus possible to treat electromagnetic fields by electric and magnetic fields separately. This approach is in contrast to high frequency fields where the electric and magnetic fields are intimately related.

In a typical urban environment the background 60 Hz fields range from 1 to 20 V/m and may be considerably larger near appliances where they may range upto 250 V/m [20] (Table 1).

Table 1   Representative electric fields and currents from household appliances

Items	Fields	Induced currents
Electric blanket	250 V/m	7-27 µA
Hair dryer	40 V/m, 10-25 G	
Electric train	60 V/m, 0.01-0.1 G	
Food mixer	50 V/m, 1-5 G	
Leakage currents		
Color TV	30 V/m, 1-5 G	
Vacuum cleaner	16 V/m, 0.1-1.0 G	
Clock	15 V/m	
Coffee mill	380 µ A	
Refrigerator	60 V/m, 40 µA	
Sewing machine	36 µA	
Coffee pot	30 V/m, 6 µA	
Heating pad		18 µA

It is apparent from Table 1 that the emitted electric and magnetic fields vary over a wide range. Preece et al [21] have reported that sources found in home with significant magnetic field of over 0.2 µT at 1 m include microwave ovens, washing machines, dishwashers, some electric showers and can openers. Out of these, washing machines and dishwashers are likely to be in use for considerable length of time. Hair dryers and vacuum cleaners have lightweight, completely unshielded motors and when in use is brought close to the body.

Comparison of Electric and Magnetic Field Exposure

Lovely et al [22] have concluded that rats exposed to 60 Hz magnetic fields (3.03 µT) would produce body currents generally equivalent to currents induced by exposure to a 160 kV/m, 60 Hz electric field. Therefore, it can be extrapolated that the biological responses in the rats exposed to the above electric field should also be shown by magnetic field of above intensity. However, there are two basic differences. First, the magnetically induced current densities will be greatest near the surface of the torso, while in the later case such maxima will appear at the center [23, 24]. Secondly, very strong current enhancements will occur in the legs and the feet of the grounded rats exposed to the electric fields [12], while no such enhancement is produced by magnetic field exposure. Voltage equivalence of the magnetic field induced currents does not lead to equivalence in anatomical distribution. This is manifested in difference in biological effects due to exposure to the strong electric and magnetic fields (Fig. 5).

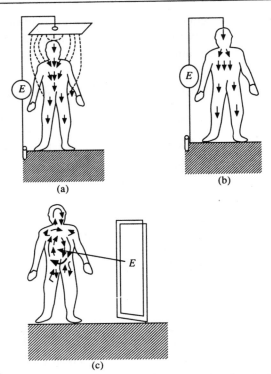

Fig. 5. Internal current density distribution for an errect primate. (a-c) Direction of arrows indicate the approximate direction of the internal body current flow and the width of the arrow are suggestive of the current densities. Paths for displacement current flow are shown by the dashed lines. (a) Electric field induced flow; (b) conduction case; (c) magnetic field induced flow [27].

It can be mentioned that the existence of static and dynamic EMF in the environment will result in the induction of magnetic and electric fields in the body. Because of the low permeability of the living tissues, both static and dynamic magnetic fields within the body will be similar to the magnetic fields outside the body.

Paradox

There are various experimental data, which cannot be easily explained. The puzzle is mainly concerning the low-level field effects. While these are often implicated as cancer promoter, such fields are also being used for bone fracture healing and decelerating osteoporosis. The field effects are dependent on the following parameters: frequency, polarization, duration (chronic, acute), nature of the wave shape, local environment (placement of the body with respect to the surroundings) and may be many others. Also the response of given cell types is dependent on one or more of these parameters. Needless to say that any attempt to control these parameters in a predetermined manner is an impossible demand, and hence, the controversy. A glaring example is the use of mobile phones. While it is generally accepted that the use of digital phones is a better option, the orientation of the head with respect to the phone and the distance are the critical parameters. Obviously to know the values of the induced field is a daunting task. The controversy therefore persists as to the nature of EMF-biointeraction. While the controversy persists the interest continues.

References

1. Poole C., Ozonoff D. Magnetic fields and childhood cancers. *IEEE Engineering in Medicine and Biology*, 1996; **15**: 41–49.
2. Malmivuo J., Plonsey R. Bioelectromagnetism: Principles and Applications of Bioelectrric and Biomagnetic Fields. Oxford University Press: New York, 1995.
3. Reilly J.P. Electrical stimulation and electropathology. Cambridge: Cambridge University Press, 1992.
4. Weaver J.C., Chizmadzhev Y. Electroporation. In : Handbook of Biological Effects of Electromagnetic Fields. Polk C., Postow E. (eds). CRC Press, Inc. 1996: 247–274.
5. Tropea B.I., Lee R.C. Thermal injury kinetics in electrical trauma. *Journal of Biomechanical Engineering*, 1992; **114**: 241–250.
6. Polk C. Introduction. In: CRC Handbook of Biological Effects of Electromagnetic Fields, pp. 1-24. CRC Press, Inc.: Boca Raton, F.L., 1986.
7. Kaune W.T., Forsythe W.C. Current densities measured in human models exposed to 60 Hz electric fields. *Bioelectromagnetics*, 1985; **6**: 13–32.
8. Dawson T.W., Caputa K., Stuchly M.A. Organ dosimetry for human exposure to 60 Hz electric or magnetic fields. In: The Annual Review of Research on Biological Effects of Electric and Magnetic Fields from the Generation, Delivery and Use of Electricity. San Antonio, T.X., 1996: 26–27.
9. Barnes F., Wachtel H., Savitz D., Fuller J. Use of wiring configuration and wiring codes for estimating externally generated electric and magnetic fields. *Bioelectromagnetics*, 1989; **10**: 13–21.
10. Polk C. Dosimetry of extremely-low-frequency magnetic fields. *Bioelectromagnetics* 1992c; **13**: 209–235.
11. Dawson T.W., Caputa K., Stuchly M.A. High-resolution organ dosimetry for human exposure to low-frequency electric fields. IEEE Transactions on Power Delivery, 1997: 1–8.
12. Kaune W.T., Phillips R.D. Comparison of the coupling of grounded humans, swine and rats to vertical, 60 Hz electric fields. *Bioelectromagnetics*, 1980; **1**: 117–129.
13. Polk C. Electric fields and surface charges induced by ELF magnetic fields. *Bioelectromagnetics*, 1990; **11**: 189–201.
14. Liboff A.R. Geomagnetic cyclotron resonance in membrane transport. *J. Biol. Phys.* 1985; **13**: 99–102.
15. Durney C.H., Rushforth C.K.., Anderson A.A. Resonant AC-DC magnetic fields: calculated response. *Bioelectromagnetics*, 1988; **9**: 315–336.
16. Dovan T., Kaune W.T., Savitz D.A. Repeatability of measurements of residential magnetic fields and wire codes. *Bioelectromagnetics*, 1993; **14**: 145–159.
17. Bracken T.D.., Kheifets L.I., Sussman S.S. Exposure assessment for power

frequency electric and magnetic fields (EMF) and its application to epidemiologic studies. *Journal of Exposure Analysis and Environmental Epidemiology*, 1993; **3**: 1–22.

18. Preece A.W., Grainger P., Golding J., Kaune W.T. Domestic magnetic field exposure in Avon. *Phys. Med. Biol.* 1996; **41**: 71–81

19. Kaune W.T., Zaffanella LE. Assessing historical exposures of children to power-frequency magnetic fields. *J. Expo. Anal. Environ. Epidemiol.* 1994; **4**: 149–170.

20. Barnes F.S. Interaction of DC electric fields with living matter. In : Handbook of Biological Effects of Electromagnetic Fields, Polk, C., Postow, E. (eds). Boca Raton, FL: CRC Press, Inc. 1986; 99–119.

21. Preece A.W. et al. Magnetic fields from domestic appliances in the UK. *Phys Med Biol.* 1997; **42**: 67–76.

22. Lovely R.H., Creim J.A., Kaune W.T., Miller M.C., Phillips R.D., Anderson L.E. Rats are not aversive when exposed to 60 Hz magnetic fields at 3.03 μT. *Bioelectromagnetics*, 1992; **13**: 351–362.

23. Miller D.L. Miniature-probe measurements of electric fields and currents induced by a 60 Hz magnetic field in rat and human models. *Bioelectromagnetics*, 1991; **1**: 157–171.

24. Kaune W.T., Forsythe W.C. Current densities induced in swine and rat models by power frequency electric fields. *Bioelectromagnetics*, 1988; **9**: 1–24.

25. Sheppard A.B., Eisenbud M. Biological effects of electric and magnetic fields of extremely low frequency. New York University Press, New York 1977.

26. Kaune W.T. Power-frequency electric fields averaged over the body surfaces of grounded humans and animals. *Bioelectromagnetics*, 1981; **2**: 403–406.

27. Bridges J.E., Preache M. Biological Influences of Power Frequency Electric Fields: A Tutorial Review from a Physical and Experimental Viewpoint. *Proceedings of the IEEE*, 1981; **69**: 1092–1106.

17. Pain Responses in Rats Exposed to 50 Hz Magnetic Field for Varied Durations

R. Mathur, L. Dhawan and R. Upadhyay

Department of Physiology Laboratory, All India Institute of Medical Sciences,
New Delhi-110029, India

Abstract. The ELF-MF interact with the bio system through alteration in neurotransmitters and membrane properties. A series of experiments were conducted to elucidate the cumulative effect of ELF-MF (50 Hz, 17.9 μT) in progressively increasing sessions. The study was aimed to explore opioid mediated-noxious stimulus initiated pain responses: its modulation by a palatable food-drink and stress, learning, memory and aggression. The data suggest a potent analgesia to phasic and tonic noxious stimuli although the former are more susceptible (significant analgesia 2 h/d × 15 in contrast to latter in 2 h/d × 30 group of rats). Palatability modulated analgesia (tail flick latency, threshold of tail flick, tonic pain) did not potentiate MF-analgesia, rather it decreased the threshold of pain which was statistically insignificant with control group. Similarly, instead of stress-analgesia noted in control rats, hyperalgesia was noted in MF rats. Sucrose ingestion during stress alleviated stress-analgesia in both groups of rats. In MF exposed rats the foot-shock induced aggression is significantly and notably absent, which is due to increase in 5-HT activity 5-HT is also reported to be affected by MF. It is suggested that the interaction involves opioids as well as serotonin.

Introduction

Endogenous and exogenous opioids have been implicated in responses to noxious stimuli, stimulation produced-analgesia, stress induced-analgesia [1, 2] and biointeraction with magnetic fields (MF) [3] by several researchers utilising different models. Opioid activate these analgesic mechanisms by interacting mainly with μ receptors located on neurons in the dorsal cord, which has been reviewed by Lipp [4] and Millan [5] and/or by hyperpolarizing GABA-ergic cells in the Periaqueductal Gray (PAG) thereby inactivating GABA inhibition. This allows the "off cells" within the PAG to activate the spinal adrenergic analgesic systems and the nucleus raphe magnus (NRM) serotonergic (5HT) system, which in turn activates systems within the dorsal horn that depress the transmission of pain sensations to the brain leading to analgesia. Opiates have also been shown to exert direct effects on the sensitivity of pain fibers. Endogenous analgesic system can be activated by either pain or non-painful sensations arriving from the periphery or by supraspinal sites.

μ and δ opiates have been suggested to decrease a voltage dependent calcium conductance and/or produce a membrane hypopolarization by increasing potassium conductance.

The physiological and molecular mechanism underlying bio-effects of MF involves opioids [3]. It is hypothesised that it may possibly relate to alteration in the opioid receptor number, their activation, sensitivity and dynamics, coupled with similar changes in other opioid modulated neurotransmitters and their synthesizing agents [6]. Kavaliers and Osenkopp [7] have recently suggested that the MF (weak rotating 50 Hz) differentially inhibit various opiate-induced analgesias, viz. μ, δ and κ opiate-induced analgesia while sparing the sigma opiate-directed analgesic responses in mice. Thus, any alteration in the binding, distribution, fluxes and intra-or extra-cellular levels of central calcium (Ca^{2+}) by magnetic stimuli could alter opiate systems and their effects. The calcium channel blocker (like Diltiazen and Verapamil) or calcium chelator, EGTA, reverse the inhibitory actions of the magnetic stimuli on opiate-induced effects, while the calcium ionophore, A21387 potentiate the MF effects. These results provide support for Ca^{2+} involvement in mediating MF effects [8]. The effects of Ca^{2+} may arise either from alteration in neurotransmitter release and binding, or the effects of opioids on excitable cell membranes, as well as from alterations in opiate receptor binding [9, 10]. MF, therefore, may also interfere with second messenger pathway, where calcium oscillations might be an integral component.

The entire activity of the central nervous system is the result of the dynamic interaction of the processes of inhibition and excitation within and between the neuronal subsystems, which are governed by neurotransmitters gamma-amino butyric acid (GABA) and glutamate, respectively, and any inadequacy therein may lead to pathological processes. It has been reported that the cell membranes are the main target for the extremely low frequency of magnetic field (ELF-MF) and they may also exert their effects by causing alteration in the membrane characteristics, neurotransmitter/neuromodulator release, receptor ligand binding and ionic fluxes [11]. The exposure to ELF for short duration (few minutes to hours) has been reported to decrease the affinity at GABA-ergic synapses and increase at glutamatergic synapses [12].

Therfore, there is sufficient evidence to say that MF influences brain activity in a subtle albeit significant manner via their effect on almost all the underlying neuro physiological processes. Nonetheless, opioids are the most frequently reported mediator of MF effects [3, 13, 14, 15]. Besides other effects, MF predominantly influences the response to pain. Several group of workers have reported analgesia to noxious stimuli [16, 17] while others to hyperalgesia (in human, pigeons etc.) and still others have reported no effect after exposure to MF. Such a spectrum of responses is not surprising because of factors residing in the biological system and inherent in the stimulus itself. In reference to former the physiological state of the individual including various types of opioid receptors, their concentration dictate the response, while the characteristics of fields, duration and time of exposure of the latter affect the response. Opioids have both excitatory and inhibitory effects depending on whether they open or close various types of potassium or calcium channels [18]. Therefore, the direction of change mediated by opioids is based on the neuron affected, receptor site and the "state" of the cells. A reduction in the inhibitory effects to opioids through increased Ca^{2+} explains a reduction in analgesia, whereas a potentiation of these inhibitory effects through a decrease in Ca^{2+} flux explains hyperalgesia [19, 20]. Moreover, an increase in K^+ flux is consistent with reductions in the excitatory effects of opioids, which leads to the potentiation of analgesia [18, 21].

Opioids have been implicated in MF bio-interaction on the bases of either blocking or substituting them. The pain responses to either acute thermal (latency of response) or tonic/chronic pain (constriction injury of sciatic nerve, formalin induced pain) have been studied in different species including humans [15]. The studies have been designed although primarily to determine the mechanism of MF bio-interaction utilising several animal models, and stimulation parameters. Therefore, we are ignorant about the effects of specific MF on the handling of noxious stimuli under different physiological states of the organism viz. stress, satiated and exposure durations. We have studied systematically the MF effect on pattern of pain responses that are primarily mediated by opioids. We report here the pattern of responses in MF exposed (17.9 μT) rats to: (i) a variety of noxious stimuli and durations since each influences a specific mechanism, (ii) noxious stimuli after ingestion of palatable food such as sucrose which modulates pain via ventromedial hypothalamus (VMH) and (iii) the chronic repeated stress which produces strong analgesia.

Materials and Methods

Groups
Rats were exposed to electromagnetic fields (17.9 μT, 50 Hz, each day) for either 7 h/day for 8 days or 2 h/day for 15 or 30 or 60 or 4 h/day for 180 days and were grouped as I through V, respectively. The control group of rats were similarly treated except for switching on the power supply of the chamber.

Magnetic Field Chamber
The equipment comprises electromagnetic (EM) coils mounted on a stand along with a movable platform for the rat cage and a current regulator that maintains a constant current through the EM coils [22]. EM coils are wound on circular formers at a diameter of 1000 mm, the two outer coils are wound with 18 turns each and two inner coils with 8 turns each. All coils are connected in series and provide a uniform MF of 17.9 μT, 50 Hz in the central area of the axis, where there is a platform for placing the rat cage. The polypropylene cage (38 $\times$24 $\times$ 15 cm) was specially designed to expose 6 rats simultaneously. The cage was divided into six chambers with a sufficiently ventilated wooden cover thereby partially restraining the rats.

Parameters Recorded

1. Nociceptive Responses

Latency of pain: The rat was partially restrained in a rat restrainer. The latency of motor response of the tail to the noxious thermal stimulus was noted utilising tail flick analgesia meter (Coulbourn Instruments, PA 18106, USA). The cut-off values for temperature and latency were preset at 45° C and 30 sec, respectively.

Threshold of pain: The threshold of pain was determined by stimulating nociceptive afferents. The current strength required for elicitation of motor responses mediated at spinal, brain stem and limbic areas were noted. Two needle electrodes were inserted intradermally into the tail, to stimulate by an alternating electric current of 40 Hz, biphasic square wave pulses, 1.5 ms duration and varying current strength of 200 ms (Grass Stimulator S4-G, USA). The current strength was increased in steps of 200 μA till the motor response of the tail (TF), vocalisation limited to stimulus (SV), vocalisation beyond the stimulus (VA) occurred.

Tonic pain : Freshly prepared algogen, formalin solution (5%, 50 μl) was subcutaneously injected into the plantar surface of the paw. Pain produced by formalin was quantified by observing the test paw of the rat as compared to the control paw [23]. The behavioural categories were assigned values of 0 through 3 which reflected a graded increase in pain intensity. Category 0: when all the paws were equally bearing the body weight; Category 1: when the test paw was groomed by the rat, or it was partially resting; Category 2: when the test paw was elevated or tucked under the body or Category 3: when the treated paw was vigorously shaken or bitten. Behavioural scores were continuously entered into the personal computer for 60 min. At the end of each time block of 5 min the program calculated the duration and frequency of each behavioural category. The mean pain rating during a block was then obtained using the formula $(T_1 + 2 \times T_2 + 3 \times T_3/t)$, where t is the duration of the block in seconds, and T_1-T_3 represents the number of seconds spent in Categories 1-3, respectively.

2. Stress Schedule

Pain response to stress: The stress included both physiological and psychological components. Different nociceptive stimuli elaborate either sensory discriminative dimension or affective, motivational components. The former can be elaborated in reflex and the latter in vocalization nociceptive responses. The stress comprises various types and intensities of noxious stimuli and restrain, which were received repeatedly by the rat at unexpected time. This schedule was repeated in six sessions during a period of 58 h with a rest of 32 h [23]. Each session lasted for 4 h followed by a rest in the home cage for 2 h. On day 1 the session began at 05:00, 11:00 and 17:00 h followed by a rest of 32 h and on day 3, the sessions IV through VI began at 05:00, 09:00 and 15:00 h, respectively.

Each of these stress stimuli were repeated thrice at 5 min interval. In each session the rat was subjected to the thermal noxious stress to the paws followed by the same to the tail (52.5 and 45°C respectively) and; the electrical stimulation of nociceptive afferents in the tail to determine the thresholds of TF, SV and VA. The sucrose fed group of rats received sucrose solution ad libitum after session I through IV in addition to the food pellets and tap water. The rest of the procedure remained same.

Pain Stress Related Aggressive Behaviour

Two rats (randomly picked up from either control or MF exposed groups) at a time were placed in a Behaviour Chamber (Coulbourn Instruments PA 18001, USA) having grid floor, which can deliver electric shock. Shock induced aggression was tested in them by giving 1/sec, 0.5 sec duration, 1 mA shock. Observations were repeated after gradually increasing the current in steps of 0.2 mA till the rats took up mutual upright fighting posture. Incidences and latencies of various degrees of aggressive behaviours and postures in relation to current level were noted and analysed. In brief, with the onset of shock the rats immediately began running and squeaking (Categories 1 and 2). Within seconds their respiration rate also increased (Category 3). In addition to these behaviours there was lifting up of their tails with continuing foot shock (Category 4). The rats soon stood up against each other on their hind feet and growled at each other (Category 5). While the foot shock still continued, the rats physically caught each other by neck, and thrashed (Category 6). The experiment was terminated by switching off the shock either at preset cut-off time (20 sec) or when they reached Category 6. The rats were categorised as Category 1 when they preferred to avoid shock rather than fight with each other. They either stood on hind legs quietly on one of the metallic bars or jumped repeatedly, jumped and sat on the house light, or the bar to avoid the shock.

Pain Stress Related Learning and Memory

Active avoidance: One-way shuttle box was used to test the learning and memory (recent) using active avoidance task. On the first day of experiment the rat was allowed to explore the box for 5 min. The door was then lowered down with the rat in the unsafe compartment (C2, where the rat will get the foot shock after the conditioned stimulus). After 20 sec the light and buzzer (conditioned stimulus, CS) was switched on in the C2. Five seconds later the rats received foot shock (25 Hz, 2 mA) (unconditioned stimulus, US) in C2 compartment until the rat escaped to the other compartment (C1) or for a maximum of 10 sec. If the rat crossed to the safe compartment during the conditioned stimulus an avoidance response was recorded otherwise no response was recorded. After an intertrial interval of 45 sec, the rat was shifted to the unsafe (C2) compartment and the session was repeated. The rats were given 50 trials. The test for memory was conducted after 48 h [24].

Passive avoidance: A wooden platform ($15 \times 10 \times 7$ cm) was placed in the center of the Behaviour Chamber whose floor has electrifiable grid (Coulbourn Instruments, PA, USA). The rat was placed in the wooden platform and covered by a same dimension perspex cover. The cover was suddenly removed. The latency to descend to grid floor was noted. After 10 sec of exploration the rat was returned to home cage. The procedure was repeated 3 times at 30 min interval. Immediately after the rat had descended from the wooden block on the third trial a 50 Hz, 1.5 mA shock was applied to the grid floor for 1 sec. The rat was returned to the home cage immediately. The test was repeated at the end of 24 h for retention of the foot shock experience and the performance on learnt task was studied similarly.

Results

1. Pattern of Pain Responses in a Variety of MF Exposure Conditions
Adult rats were exposed to MF (17.9 μT, 50 Hz for either 7 h/day $\times$ 8 or 2 h/day $\times$ 15 or 30 or 60 or 4 h/day $\times$ 180) and they were thus divided into 5 groups (groups I-V) on the basis of exposure duration. Their responses to pain were studied.

The latency of pain responses was significantly increased in all the groups of MF exposed rats except group I as compared to their controls (Fig. 1A). The thresholds of TF, SV and VA were significantly higher in all groups of rats except group I (Fig. 1 B-D). The results indicate analgesia in both the latency and threshold of phasic pain in our chronic MF exposed groups II-V, while prolonged exposure each day for fewer days (7 h/day $\times$ 8) (group I) was ineffective.

The response to tonic pain was also studied in groups II and III. The analgesia was progressive unlike phasic pain (Fig. 2 a, b). Area under the curves of Categories 0, 1 and 2 were statistically significantly increased while for Category 3 decreased (Fig. 2 c, d; Fig. 3; Table 1).

Effect of Naloxone
When anti-opioid (naloxone, Nx) was injected systemically to the rats it led to a decrease in the threshold of TF, SV and VA indicating hyperalgesia. However, when the same dose was given to MF exposed group I rats (7 h/d $\times$ 8 days) prior to exposure there was an increase in the thresholds, reversing the effect of MF.

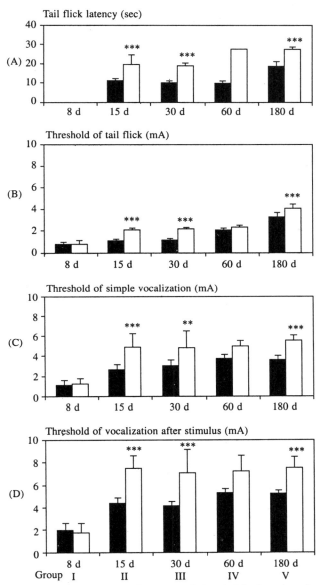

Fig. 1. Effect of MF exposure on latency and threshold of nociceptive responses to phasic stimuli as a function of exposure duraton. Rats were exposed to 7 h/d × 8 days (group I), 2 h/d × 15, 30, 60 days (groups II-IV, respectively) and 4 h/d × 180 days (group V). ***: statistical significant difference between MF exposed groups and their control group **$p < 0.01$ and **$p < 0.001$.

When naloxone pre-treated rats were exposed to MF for 15 or 30 days (groups II and III) the MF induced analgesia was reversed in tonic pain (Fig. 2 a, b, c, d).

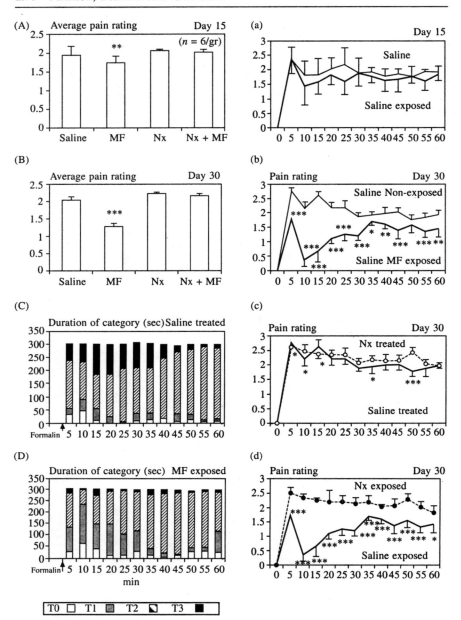

Fig. 2.   Effect of MF exposure on nociceptive responses to tonic stimulus as a function of exposure duration and opioids (groups II and III). The effect is compared in terms of pain rating during each block (5 min) of the observation period (60 min) in (a) through (d) and (A), (B), respectively. Duration of each category of pain rating (T_0-T_3) in control and MF exposed (group III) rats is shown in (C) and (D). The analgesia in MF exposed rats progresses with exposure duration ((a) versus (b), (A) versus (B) and (C) versus (D)), and attenuates by naloxone pre-treatment ((c) versus (d), (A) and (B)). *$p < 0.05$, **$p < 0.01$ and ***$p < 0.001$.

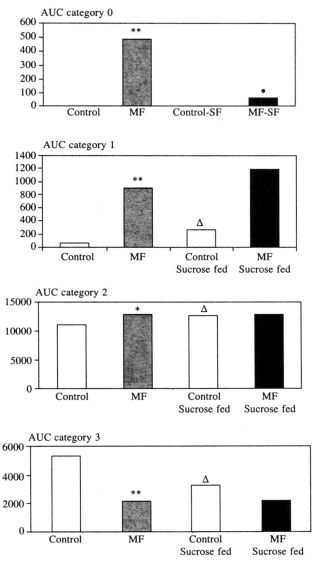

Fig. 3. Effect of MF exposure and sucrose ingestion (ad libitum from 2 through 4 weeks) on tonic pain in Group II rats. The area under the curve of categories 0 through 3 has been calculated for comparison amongst various groups. Analgesia by MF is depicted which was attenuated by sucrose ingestion (MF-SF). *: Comparison between control and MF exposed groups, Δ: comparison between control and control-sucrose fed, •: comparison between MF and MF-sucrose fed. One sign corresponds to $p < 0.05$ while two correspond to $p < 0.01$.

2. Effect of Ingestion of Palatable Food (Sucrose) on Pain Behaviour

The effect of ingestion of sucrose as a palatable substance provided ad libitum in addition to food and water for 8 or 15 days was studied on nociceptive

Table 1 **Area under the curve of various categories of formalin pain in group III rats**

Area under curve	Control median (range)	MF exposed median (range)
Category 0	1.475 (0.7–13.4)	486.25 (156.9–812.2)**
Category 1	61.025 (35.8–259.7)	905.675 (562.9–1830.7)**
Category 2	11103.99 (8699.1–12609.0)	12864.3 (12255.8–13243.4)*
Category 3	5340.938 (3623.5–7763.6)	2183.525 (1600.2–3018.9)**

responses in control and MF exposed group of rats (Fig. 5). The latter group of rats received it prior to and after the exposure each day. In the control rats the threshold and latency of spinally mediated motor responses were increased significantly post-sucrose ingestion while, threshold of the responses mediated via brain stem and limbic system (SV, VA respectively) were not affected. In MF exposed rats the trend was similar for only tail flick latency, while the threshold of tail flick was spared.

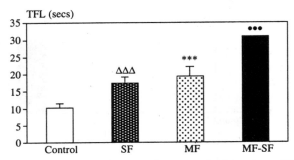

Fig. 4. Effect of MF exposure and sucrose ingestion for 2 weeks on TFL in group III rats. The MF analgesia is potentiated by sucrose ingestion. *: Comparison between control and MF exposed groups, Δ: Comparison between control and control-sucrose fed, •: Comparison between MF and MF-sucrose fed. Three signs denote $p < 0.001$.

The results of experiment indicate that in control rats sucrose ingestion let to analgesia only in the spinally mediated latency and threshold of motor response (TFL and TF), whereas in MF exposed rats it (sucrose) potentiated MF induced analgesia only in the tail flick latency and not in the thresholds. Instead, there was a trend towards return to normal.

The responses to tonic stimulus also revealed the same trend. In control rats the area under the curves of Categories 1 and 2 were increased while that for Category 3 was decreased indicating sucrose fed analgesia (Fig. 3). In MF group of rats area under the curves of Category 0 and 1 were increased while 2 and 3 were not altered, indicating a trend towards reversal of MF analgesia (Fig. 3).

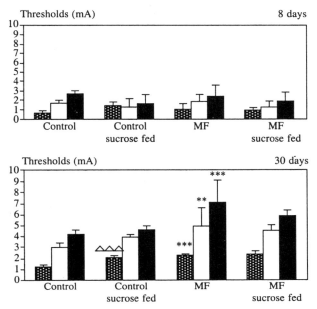

Fig. 5. Effect of MF exposure and sucrose ingestion on threshold of phasic pain in groups I and III rats. The threshold of TF increases after sucrose ingestion in intact rats, while the threshold of TF, SV and VA increase in group III rats after MF exposure. Sucrose ingestion in MF exposed rats did not affect their thresholds. *: Comparison between control and MF exposed group while triangles denote comprised between control and sucrose fed groups of rats. Single sign represents $p < 0.05$ and triple sign $p < 0.001$.

3. Effect of Stress in Pain Responses

The MF and control rats underwent a prolonged stress schedule of receiving a variety of noxious stimuli repeatedly for 58 h at unpredictable time and interval in six sessions (6, 12, 48, 52 and 58 h starting at 05:00 h on the day of experiment). The results of control rats indicate a stress induced analgesia whereas, in the MF group of rats there was hyperalgesia (Figs. 6 and 7).

4. Effect of Sucrose Ingestion on Stress-induced Pain Responses

Effect of sucrose ingestion only for 2 weeks (day 15 to 30) during 60-day exposure schedule (group IV) on the stress induced pain modulation in MF rats (Fig. 6). The stress-induced analgesia observed in control rats was reduced after sucrose ingestion (it remained limited to the last session only) whereas in the MF exposed group the stress-induced hyperalgesia was significantly reduced.

The result of our experiments 3 and 4 suggest that stress produces hyperalgesia in MF exposed rats in contrast to analgesia in control rats and ingestion of sucrose for a short duration (2 week during the two months of MF exposure) inhibited the effect of MF as well as the effect of stress in both

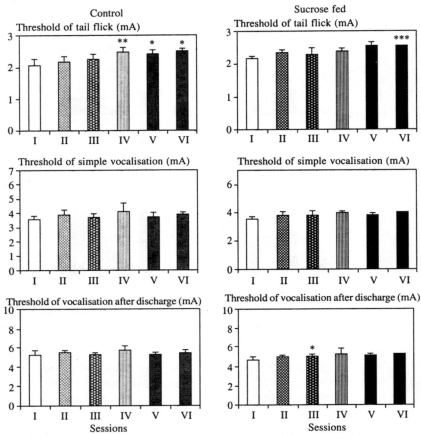

Fig. 6.   Effect of sucrose feeding on repeated, chronic stress (sessions I to VI) modulated-pain responses in group III rats. In control rats stress produced analgesia in TF while sucrose feeding alleviated it. Increase in threshold is statistically significant in relation to session I. *$p < 0.05$, **$p < 0.01$ and ***$p < 0.001$.

the groups. It appears that the sucrose ingestion attempts to antagonise the effect of stress.

5. Pain Stress Related Aggressive Behaviour

The study was conducted on rats exposed for 30 and 60 days, however the results of only latter are presented here.

The control rats invariably engaged themselves in a fighting posture (Category 5) or actual fights (Category 6) on receiving foot shock (Fig. 8). The latency to attain this posture varied from 19 to 1 sec (19, 15, 5, 1 sec) depending on the strength of current 1.2 to 2.0 mA (1.2, 1.4, 1.6, 1.8, 2.0 mA, respectively). As the strength of stimulation increased the latency to attain fighting posture decreased, whereas in the MF exposed group of rats the pattern of response was different. The rats proceeded from Category 4 to

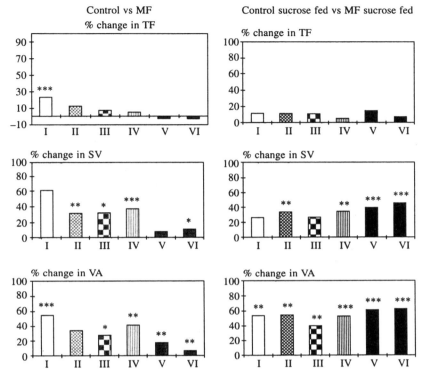

Fig. 7. Effect of sucrose feeding on stress response in MF exposed group of rats (group III). The bars represents the % mean difference in that session between the control and MF exposed groups. Sucrose feeding has potentiated MF induced analgesia. *: Statistically significant compared to session I. *$p < 0.05$, **$p < 0.01$ and ***$p < 0.001$.

escape/retreat (Category 1). This behaviour was characteristically and uniformly noted in all the rats ($n = 20$ rats). This was in steep contrast to the behaviour observed in the control group of rats.

The results are suggestive of an increase in the behaviours supporting escape from the noxious agent vis-à-vis the foot shock in MF exposed rats.

6. Pain Related Learning and Memory

Active avoidance task: The control group (III and IV) of rats learnt the task to actively avoid the shock by running to the safe compartment on receiving the signal in 50% or more of the trials after the initial 30 trials. All of them learnt the task without any error during block V. On the contrary, the exposed group of rats could perform the task with 50-80% error even after 50 trials (Table 2). The learning deficit is not significantly evident in initial trials.

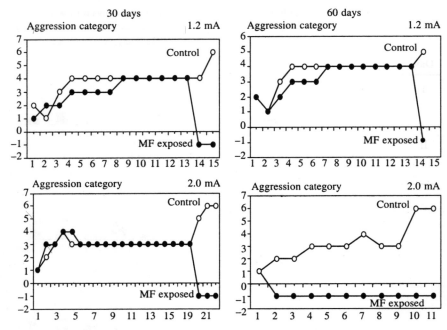

Fig. 8. Effect of MF on foot-shock (noxious stimulus) induced aggression in control and MF exposed rats (groups III and IV). Aggression categories are plotted against latency (sec). The MF exposed rats consistently escaped the noxious stimulus while the conrol rats engaged into mutual fight posture.

Table 2 Percent avoidance (mean ± SD) of the control and MF exposed rats

Block	30 Days		60 Days	
(10 trials)	Control	MF exposed	Control	MF exposed
I	24.0 ± 5.47	30.0 ± 18.70	18.33 ± 35.44	25.0 ± 20.70
II	26.0 ± 8.94	28.0 ± 25.88	33.33 ± 19.66	25.0 ± 24.20
III	26.0 ± 8.94	40.0 ± 22.36	30.0 ± 12.64	36.60 ± 21.60
IV	46.0 ± 11.40	54.0 ± 29.66	51.60 ± 17.22	48.30 ± 29.94
V	100.0 ± 0.0	58.0 ± 2.80**	100.0 ± 0.0	53.30 ± 23.38***

Passive avoidance task: The results indicate that MF exposed rats could not learn the task of avoiding the foot shock by avoiding to step down (Table 3). The latency to step down in trial I through III on day 1 of experiment was maintained on day 2 also in MF group, whereas the foot shock increased the latency to step down in control group on day 2 indicating that they retained this memory with fear as reflected in the latency to get down from platform in the day 2 trials.

Table 3   Passive avoidance latency (Mean ± SD sec) to step down

Day	Trial number	Foot shock	Latency (sec) Control	Latency (sec) MF exposed
I	1	No	32.50 ± 15.72	100.50 ± 112.53
	2	No	91.67 ± 104.43	155.50 ± 123.11
	3	No	77.50 ± 86.62	184.17 ± 133.77
		Shock		
II	1	No	168.67 ± 103.06	156.67 ± 116.22
	2	No	241.67± 73.53	161.92 ± 152.57***
	3	No	247.50 ± 58.20	202.50 ± 114.44***

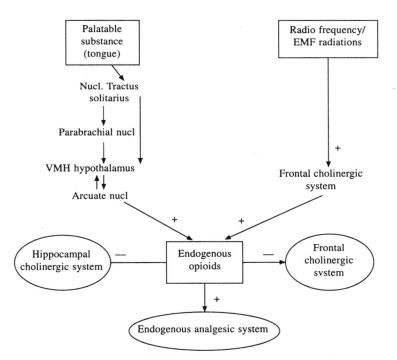

Fig. 9. Probable interaction of EMF radiations and palatable food substances via endogenous opioids in the mediation of their responses. Both the factors independently lead to analgesia in phasic and tonic pain responses.

Discussion

The results of our experiment 1 suggest that MF exposure (17.9 μT, 50 Hz) for 7 h/day × 8 days was ineffective in influencing nociceptive behaviour; 2 h/d × 15 days produced analgesia to phasic noxious stimuli and 2 h/d × 30 days produced analgesia to tonic noxious stimuli also. The effect on threshold of phasic noxious stimuli attained a maximum effect in group II rats

(2 h/d × 15 days), which did not progress in pari passu with increase in the exposure sessions. The analgesia was opioid mediated since it was attenuated by naloxone (anti-opioid) pre-treatment. The results suggest that there is a stepwise involvement of various underlying processes and a variation in the susceptibility of structures involved in their elaboration as well as in their modulation. Such a phenomenon is well known for several responses by the same insult/deviating factor (hypoxia, alcohol, anaesthetic agents, malnutrition); as well as for the same stimulus of different parameters. In addition, nociceptive responses are stimulus specific involving a set of neuro-chemical processes, some of which may be common, while others are specific to it. Suffice to say that MF interacts with the mechanisms underlying both the phasic and tonic pain responses although the latter are more resistant to it. We studied the effect of MF on opioid-mediated pain related behaviours, namely, nociceptive response to phasic and tonic noxious stimuli; pain modulation by palatable food and stress, learning, memory, and aggression.

The pattern of brain activity during tonic pain suggests a dynamic, delicate balance between the nociceptive and antinociceptive mechanisms [25]. Therefore, we systematically studied the chronic effect of MF on tonic pain in groups II and III rats. This was based on the following criteria:

Our preliminary studies indicating a statistically significant effect on tonic pain after several exposure sessions extending over 2 weeks [26]; the noxious stimulus (formalin inj.) leads to prolonged pain (several hours) [27]; and the algogen activates endogenous opioidergic system (EOS) to alleviate it. It is known that β endorphin (BEP) is released into the brain by painful stimulation [28], has a potent analgesic effect [29] and increases self-grooming [30]. Thus, the shift from a nonfocused response (body grooming) to a focused pain-related behaviour (licking the injected paw) after formalin injection, in anti-BEP pretreated rats reflects the antagonism of a physiological BEP modulatory role on the reactions to prolonged noxious input [31]. Formalin pain involves opioids since functional activity levels of several forebrain networks were increased in anti-BEP pre-treated animals even after shortlasting noxious stimulation in the absence of actual pain-related behaviour. This may be explained either by assuming a tonic inhibition of neural activity by BEP, or by BEP release even after a minor tissue injury. Opioid action (involving μ-opiate receptor) in medial thalamic and limbic structures, as well as in the locus coeruleus, is indeed likely to exert a more general effect on motivational and attention systems [32], and hence on the responsiveness of forebrain structures to a broad spectrum of stimuli in addition to a specific role in pain modulation. It has been suggested that the two phases of formalin pain are independent and are mediated by separate neural systems. In contrast to this most of the studies indicate that these two phases are interdependent when the events during the early phase influence the pain of the late phase [33, 34]. Formalin test, therefore, provides a means to check the integrity of the endogenous opioid status (EOS) and the analgesic system. Incidentally, opioids interact with MF too, thereby, presenting a unique natural state of complex interaction amongst opioids, MF and noxious stimuli. It was therefore, appropriate to select formalin model of pain for studying the effects of MF, which have been reported to mediate their effects through opioids.

Our results suggest that the exposure to magnetic field predominantly affect the late pain vis-à-vis the pain due to inflammation in group II rats. An increase in exposure sessions (group III) affects the initial pain too and thereby the processes underlying activation of nociceptors occurring during the initial phase of pain. As the processes in the initial phase of formalin pain have been identified to influence the processes of the late phase, it is also likely that the processes during the late phase when deviated from their base line repeatedly for a long period of time may influence the processes underlying the initial phase of formalin pain. Nonetheless, the process underlying late phase are more plastic and susceptible than those underlying initial phase.

The absence of effect in 15 days exposed rats could alternatively be due to the design of the study. The pain response was scheduled for test on the day after the exposure and therefore could be missed. There is a greater possibility of the exposure effects being reverted at the time of test that is about 18-20 h post-exposure. Nevertheless, the direction of response was same as in our 30 days exposure (group III) rats. However, when the number of sessions increased the recovery process was either absent or partial or incomplete thereby manifesting strong analgesia. There is sufficient evidence in the literature to believe that the mechanisms underlying temporal progression of MF exposure vary with time. The desensitisation effect of 5-HT auto-receptors is shown to be reversible after 1 h of acute exposure to 0.1-1.0 mT (εc close to 500 μT) [35] for 10 days and acute exposure for few minutes to hours leads to changes in pain responses, which are naloxone reversible.

The results of our experiment on phasic pain responses also indicate an analgesic response to MF exposure (17.9 μT) for groups of rats exposed for 15 days or more (groups II-V). The phasic pain tests, which revealed analgesia include latency of tail flick and threshold for tail flick and vocalization. In contrast to tonic pain a graded sensitivity of various responses with increase in sessions was not observed. The tests were conducted next day after receiving MF exposure as mentioned above. There was no statistically significant effect after lesser number of sessions (7 h × 8 days), whereas a total effect was observed when the number of sessions was increased to 15 (group II). We are reporting here an attenuated response to a variety of noxious stimuli, which is in line with several studies, while not supporting others [14, 15, 19, 20, 36].

A wide spectrum of responses ranging from no effect, analgesia to hyperalgesia is reported in literature. Our study design has an advantage of correlating temporal sequence of analgesia to various types of noxious stimuli, number and duration of MF having similar exposure conditions. The latter is another cause for discrepancy in the literature [20, 37]. It has been reported that the magnitude of inhibitory effects does not scale linearly with either the frequency or the amplitude of ELF-MF, whereas the static MF of the magnitude similar to ELF-MF affects the degree of inhibition linearly [20]. An inhibitory effect on opioid analgesia has been seen at amplitude of 40 μT, but not at 297 or 547 μT. Similarly, an inhibitory effect has been reported at a frequency of 30-35 Hz but not at 100 and 200 Hz. Therefore, ELF-MF of only specific combinations of amplitude and frequency exert inhibitory effects on opioid-induced analgesia. Our observations present a complete pattern of response to noxious stimuli in rats exposed to progressive duration but of similar MF conditions.

The reported literature is predominantly based on noxious thermal stimulus, which elaborates a motor response of tail representative of a withdrawal reflex mediated at spinal level. It is not indicative of pain, which has a wider definition. On the contrary, the vocalisation response involves the emotional component of pain in addition to the withdrawal, which is a better index of pain. To study the effect on pain threshold in the present study, the afferent fibres carrying pain information were directly stimulated circumventing the transduction process. An increase in the threshold of TF, SV and VA in the rats indicates that MF probably influences the processes beyond transduction, wherein calcium and potassium ions are amongst other important mediators. Several mechanisms are under investigation to explore the bio-interaction with MF including alterations in the levels of neural calcium and the stability of calcium binding on neuronal membranes [4, 8, 9]. The cellular detection site is suggested to be the Ca^{++}-calmodulin site in the neurological form of nitric oxide synthase—a site originally proposed by Lednev [38, 39, 40]. It predicts both increase and decrease in biological responses involving opioids [38]. The increased extracellular calcium levels have been reported to result in an increased influx of calcium during depolarization of enkephalinergic neurons, causing an increased release of enkephalin, which then causes analgesia [4]. Opioids have been shown to have both excitatory and inhibitory effect due to differential effects on Ca^{++} and K^+ channels [41, 42]. Low concentrations of opioids have excitatory effect leading to hyperalgesic actions and increased pain sensitivity [43], while at higher concentrations a predominant inhibitory effect leads to the induction of analgesia and decreased pain sensitivity.

Both an increase and decrease in pain are abolished by naloxone pre-treatment. The strong analgesic effect in tonic pain *per se* is opioid mediated since it was abolished by naloxone pre-treatment. The results are in line with several previous reports stating the opidergic-mediation of analgesic effects on responses to phasic noxious stimuli in acute/chronic MF exposed animals. This is the first report in the literature regarding involvement of opioids in MF induced graded effect on tonic pain.

The abovementioned phasic responses are mediated at the level of spinal cord, brain stem and limbic system, respectively, whereas the tonic pain includes periaqueductal grey matter, ventromedial hypothalamus (VMH) and also medial thalamus [25, 44]. Locus coeruleus, anterior pretectal nucleus, medial and lateral thalamus and nucleus accumbens are involved in nociceptive and antinociceptive mechanisms and receive BEP terminals. The results indicate that MF may have interacted with these sites in the neuraxis to influence both phasic and tonic pain. It is also likely that some higher area is afffected which in turn modulates these areas. Since, there is a generalized analgesia to various types of noxious stimuli it is likely that a neural site is involved which leads to a generalized response, bears a close and strong link with opioids, limbic brain and is also a pain modulation site. We hypothesize that one such site is VMH, which produces a change in pain response to several types of noxious stimuli in a similar direction when manipulated. Furthermore, hypothalamus is involved in adjustments to environmental stresses of heat, cold etc.; opioids are secreted from arcuate nucleus; opioid receptors are demonstrated in the neurons of VMH; modulate hormone secretion; and influence pain responses to stress and palatable food. It was, therefore, proposed to study stress responses and their modulation by palatable food in support of our proposed mechanism.

MF Modulation of Other Opioid Mediated Responses to Noxious Stimuli
The review of literature suggests that amongst the more dramatic effects of MF in both vertebrates and invertebrates are alterations in the actions of exogenous opiates and the activity of EOS. Since, opioid system is highly conserved during evolution it is reasonable to propose that MF affect the system reflecting in a broad range of endogenous and exogenous opiate mediated activities. Exposure to various types of electromagnetic stimuli has been shown to affect opiate-mediated analgesic, locomotor, reproductive and feeding behaviours [8, 16, 17, 45-53].

Palatable Food (Sucrose) Modulated Pain Behaviour
The results of our experiment 2 indicate that ingestion of sucrose increased both the TFL, threshold of TF and decreased pain rating in control rats. MF alone induced strong analgesia in all these tests but sucrose ingestion by them reduced the MF analgesia in all the other tests except for latency of TF. The data supports the role of sucrose ingestion as an antidote to MF vis-à-vis a substance restoring milieu interior.

Sucrose solution was available to the rats ad libitum in addition to the laboratory food pellets and tap water. They were not water deprived and therefore, they ingested it only because they preferred it over tap water. Acute sucrose ingestion *per se* leads to an immediate analgesia in rat or, human, infant and adult both. The analgesia is reported in spinally mediated reflex response (tail flick latency and threshold of tail flick) and tonic pain behaviour of rats. In infants and experimental pain in adult humans it is sufficient to relieve pain of heel lancing, circumcision, immunisation or venesection. In our rats sucrose feeding potentiated analgesia of MF in TFL only. It is possible that there is a cross tolerance to sucrose. In view of a dissociation between the latency and threshold of tail flick by sucrose ingestion in chronic MF exposed rats it is probable that the interaction is multifactorial and complex. The analgesia of sucrose ingestion involves a specific mechanism, which is probably partially separate from that of the MF.

The analgesia was inconsistent in the thresholds of SV and VA post-sucrose ingestion by control rats. This reflects the sparing of the mechanisms operating at the brain stem and limbic levels by the processes involved post-sucrose ingestion. Nonetheless, there is sufficient literature regarding the information of orally ingested palatable food arriving at ventromedial hypothalamus, leading to β-endorphin mediated analgesia [54, 55]. The effects are mediated by glucoreceptor neurons of the VMH [55]. Sucrose fed analgesia is also naloxone reversible [56, 57]. Since both the responses are opioid mediated, sucrose ingestion in MF group of rats pre- and post-exposure for even 15 days restores normalcy by cancelling the MF bio-interaction.

Stress Induced Pain Modulation

There is robust evidence in the literature regarding the involvement of opioids in the mediation of stress-induced analgesia. Therefore, it was pertinent to compare the responses to the repeated multiple stresses of chronic and intermittent pain of different kinds and restraint. Each of these has been reported to produce stress and thereby analgesia [1, 23]. This stress-induced analgesia is also abolished in our control rats ingesting sucrose per orally ad libitum [64]. We studied such a sucrose fed stress-alleviating mechanism in MF exposed rats. The response is again opioid mediated. The responses of chronic MF exposed rats to the moderately severe chronic stress of restraint and several noxious stimuli produced hyperalgesia unlike the analgesia in our control rats.

In control rats, the abovementioned stressors (restraint, noxious stimuli) *per se* produced analgesia, while sucrose ingestion (ad libitum after 3 h) *per se* produced hyperalgesia [64]. Both the responses involve opioids. However, the former is due to opioid release and the latter due to its insufficient release. Nevertheless, the effect of neither the stress nor sucrose ingestion is manifested when the rat ingests sucrose during stress period. It is clear that sucrose-ingestion could protect the rat from stress and counteracts the neurochemical changes of stress. Then the question arises about its benefit to the individual. Needless to say ingestion of sucrose has calming, satiating effect and therefore, cancellation of stress should be of advantage to the individual.

On the other hand, MF rats exhibited hyperalgesia during the same chronic stress of repeated noxious stimuli and restraint. The hyperalgesic response is believed to be due to deficiency of opioids, which is possible due to the cross-tolerance. One of the characteristic effects of repeated administration of opiates is the development of tolerance [8, 58]. Exposure to a rotating magnetic field for thirty minutes before the daily morphine administration significantly reduces the development of tolerance. This further support our observation of hyperalgesia in MF exposed rats undergoing stress. Because all the factors including chronic MF interaction, stress and noxious stimuli *per se* in MF exposed rats interact with opioids, it is quite possible that noxious stimuli are unable to release sufficient quantum of opioid thereby revealing its deficiency as hyperalgesia.

Sucrose ingestion in our MF exposed rats prevented the development of stress-induced hyperalgesia. Since the MF, stress and sucrose ingestion ineract through opioids there could be complex mechanism involved in their interaction, which is difficult to comment at this juncture. Nevertheless, sucrose ingestion has prevented the development of effects of MF as well as stress. Probably, sucrose ingestion releases opioids and when MF exposure is received it cannot interact. This appears to be a plausible explanation for the absence of any MF influence in sucrose fed rats although it cannot explain satisfactorily the data obtained from group III rats. These rats received sucrose solution to drink only for 2 weeks during the MF exposure of 60 days. The hyperalgesia of stress was also attenuated in them. The results only indicate that probably there are long-term effects of sucrose ingestion. The results of our experiments suggest that sucrose ingestion helps the body to maintain normalcy against deviating factors studied.

It has been reported that several types of stress may cause the release of β-endorphin while others do not [59]. The report gives direct evidence that the cold water swim (CWS) induced antinociception is regulated by the release of endogenous β-endorphin that subsequently activates ε-opioid receptors at the supra spinal site [60]. Thus, the ε-opioid system including descending enkephalinergic pathways may play an important role in environmentally induced anti-nociception/analgesia. A study on the above-mentioned affect of sucrose ingestion in CWS, a non-opioid mediated stress in MF exposed rats may reveal interesting aspects of such an interaction, since there is a discrimination between the two categories of stressors; namely propranolol-sensitive (restraint stress) and insensitive (formalin stress) β-endorphin responses have been identified, their sources of β-endorphin in plasma are also different. It is secreted from predominantly the melanotrophs of the intermediate lobe and corticorophs of the anterior lobe of pituitary, respectively. Furthermore, it is suggested that peptides are secreted in a fixed ratio but may be subject to stress-related differences in postsecretional mechanisms. It is worth noting that proopiomelancortin-derived peptides do show marked differences in clearance, distribution volume and other kinetic parameters. Peptide secreted from the intermediate lobe is also subjected to similar variation. It would be interesting to study the post-secretional mechanisms of the opioids in our sucrose-fed MF rats undergoing stress. It is likely that sucrose ingestion alters the kinetics of the stress hormones/modulators thereby alleviates stress effects.

Complex interaction with other neurotransmitter system is also indicated by the results of our experiment on aggressive behaviour. Foot shock induced aggression was reduced in our MF exposed group III and IV rats. The actual fight behaviour was noted profusely in control rats whereas an escape response was seen as a rule to the same stimulus in the MF exposed rats.

Increased aggression means the propensity of an individual to react aggressively in many circumstances (aggression as a trait characteristic of an individual); on other hand, it may refer to actual performance of aggressive behaviour. A close relation between serotonin and aggression has long been recognised.

Recently, Van der Vegt and co-workers [61] have shown that performance of aggressive behaviour increase 5HT neuronal activity and preventing this activation inhibits expression of aggressive behaviour. ELF-MF have been shown to alter both, the turnover and receptor reactivity of mono aminergic system incuding dopamine (DA) and serotonin systems [35]. Moreover, EMF exposure (low level 1000 mG, DC) to male rats for 1 month increased the concentration of 5HT in hypothalamus and DA metabolite, 3 methoxy tyramine in corpus striatum which dissipate after four month exposure [62]. Further, rodents exposed to a weak intermittent (5 min on/5 min-off) EMF for one hour exhibited increased pineal concentration of serotonin and 5-HIAA (hydroxy indole acetic acid) suggesting increased 5-HT activity [63]. On the other hand, primates exposed to 60 Hz EMF for 20 days [62] cycle exhibited decreased HVAA (Homovanillic acid) in CSF suggesting decreased turnover of both, the dopamine and 5-HT. The serotonergic system is predominantly involved in elaboration of an adaptive response of CNS to an external or internal stimulus. Therefore, it is involved in numerous physiological functions. Recent studies have shown that $5HT_{1B}$ receptor interact with MF (*in vivo* assays) inducing structural changes of the protein that   result in functional desensitisation of receptors [35]. It implies a decrease in efficacy of the retrocontrol of 5HT on the 5HT release at neuron terminals, which in turn will lead to an increase of 5HT availability in the synaptic cleft. However, these effects including the reversibility of the effect have been demonstrated after acute 1 h exposure (0.1 to 1 mt, EC 50 close to 500 μT). No datum has been yet collected under chronic exposure. It is hypothesized that a low level exposure for longer duration may possibly hypersensitize $5HT_{1B}$ receptors or induce constant blockade of the receptor which may contribute towards the decreased aggression in our rats [35].

Role of 5HT on Pain

Both catcholamine and $5HT_{1B}$ receptor have been implicated in the endogenous antinociception $5HT_{1B}$ receptor are negatively coupled to adenyl cyclase and their activation enhance K^+ current, which contributes to their inhibitory influence upon neuronal excitability. 5HT receptors are found in dorsal horn (lamina I and IV) DRG, NRM, PAG and nucleus tractus solitarius. It may, therefore, inhibit impulses at the peripheral afferent terminal at these sites and contribute to the antinociceptive effect. However, MF interacts by desensitisation of $5HT_{1B}$ receptors specifically in hypothalamus, which is incidentally also involved in pain modulation and aggressive behaviour. It is likely that the chronic exposure to MF leads to effective decrease in 5HT, which may finally contribute towards hyperalgesia and decreased aggression.

We, therefore, hypothesize that there is an initial opioid mediated MF interaction, which affects pain, pain induced stress, palatability responses, but a chronic (repeated) interaction may then attenuate 5HT system after an initial increase. The MF may be interacting with VMH to influence its functions including feeding, aggression, learning and memory, pain, palatability modulated responses.

However, the possibility of involvement of other neurotransmitter than opioids cannot be ruled out specially due to the fact that serotonin, GABA catecholamines, acetylcholine are affected by acute/chronic MF exposure. This is also indicated by our experiments on noxious stimulus related aggression, learning, memory behaviour of MF exposed rats.

References

1. Amir, S. and Amit, Z. Endogenous opioid ligand may mediate stress induced changes in the affective properties of pain related behaviour in rats. *Life Sci.* 1978; **23**: 1143–1152.
2. Basbaum, A.I. and Fields, H.L. Endogenous pain control systems: brainstem spinal pathways and endorphin circuitry. *Annu. Rev. Neurosci.* 1984; **7**: 309–338.
3. Kavaliers, M., Ossenkopp, K.P., Prato, F.S. and Carsen, J.J.L. Opioid systems and the biological effects of magnetic fields. In: AH Frey, editor. On the nature of electromagnetic field interactions with biological systems. Austin: RG Landes Co., 1994; 181–190.
4. Lipp, J. Possible mechanisms of morphine analgesia. *Clin Neuropharmacol.* 1991; **14(2)**: 131–147.
5. Millan, M.J. Descending control of pain. *Prog. Neurobiol.* 2002; **66(6)**: 355–474.
6. Redmond, D.E. and Krystal, J.H. Multiple mechanisms of withdrawal from opioid drugs. *Anu. Rev. Neurosci.* 1984; **7**: 443–478.
7. Kavaliers, M. and Ossenkopp, K.P. Magnetic field inhibition of morphine-induced analgesia and behavioral activity in mice: evidence for involvement of calcium ions. *Brain Res.* 1986; **379(1)**: 30–38.
8. Kavaliers, M. and Ossenkopp, K.P. Exposure to rotating magnetic fields alters morphine-induced behavioral responses in two strains of mice. *Neuropharmacology* 1985; **24(4)**: 337–340.
9. Blackman, C.F., Benane, S.G., House, D.E. and Joines, W.T. Effects of ELF (1-120 Hz) and modulated (50 Hz) RF fields on the efflux of calcium ions from brain tissue in vitro. *Bioelectromagnetics.* 1985; **6(1)**: 1–11.

10. Kavaliers, M., Ossenkopp, K.P. and Hirst, M. Magnetic fields abolish the enhanced nocturnal analgesic response to morphine in mice. *Physiol. Behav.* 1984; **32(2)**: 261–264.

11. Lindstrom, E., Lindstrom, P., Berglund, A., Mild, K.H. and Lundgren, E. Intracellular calcium oscillations induced in a T-cell line by a weak 50 Hz magnetic field. *J. Cell. Physiol.* 1993; **15(2)**: 395–398.

12. Yurinskaya, M.M., Kuznetsov, V.I., Galeyev, A.L. and Kolomytkin, O.V. Reactions of the receptor system of the brain to the action of low-intensity microwaves. *Biophysics* 1996; **41**: 869–875.

13. Betancur, C., Dell Omo, G. and Alleva, E. Magnetic field effects on stress-induced analgesia in mice: modulation of light. *Neurosci. Lett* 1994; **182(2)**: 147–150.

14. Del Seppia, C., Ghione, S., Luschi, P. and Papi, F. Exposure to oscillating magnetic fields influences sensitivity to electrical stimuli. I : Experiments on pigeons. *Bioelectromagnetics* 1995; **16(5)**: 290–294.

15. Papi, F., Ghione, S., Rose, C., Del Seppia, C. and Luschi, P. Exposure to oscillating magnetic field influences sensitivity to electrical stimuli. II: Experiments on humans. *Bioelectromagnetics* 1995; **16(5)**: 295–300.

16. Mathur, R., Singh, A.K., Behari, J. and Nayar, U. 50 Hz moderate intensity electric field exposure affects tonic pain behaviour in rats. In: Asia-Pacific Microwave Conference Proceedings, Ed. Gupta, R.S. Solar Print Process Pvt. Ltd. New Delhi, India, pp. 56–58, 1996.

17. Mathur, R., Singh, A.K., Nayar, U. and Behari, J. Nociceptive behaviour of rats exposed to 50 Hz moderate intensity electric field during development. IETE Technical Review 1997, **14(3)**: 201–203.

18. Hung, L.M. Cellular mechanisms of excitatory and inhibitory action of opioids in the pharmacology of opioid peptides, Teseng, L.F. (ed). Hardwood Academic Publishers 1995, 133–149.

19. Kavaliers, M. and Ossenkopp, K.P. Calcium channel involvement in magnetic field inhibition of morphine-induced analgesia. *Naunyn Schmiedebergs Arch Pharmacol.* 1987; **336(3)**: 308–315.

20. Prato, F.S., Carson, J.J.L., Ossenkopp, K.P. and Kavaliers, M. Possible Mechanisms by which extremely low frequency magnetic fields affect opioid function. *FASEB J.* 1995; **9**: 807–814.

21. Fan, S.F., Shen, K.F. and crain, S.M. Opioids at low concentration decrease openings of K^+ channels in sensory ganglion neurons. *Brain Res.* 1991; **558(1)**: 166–170.

22. Kirschvink, J.L. Uniform magnetic fields and double-wrapped coil systems: improved techniques for the design of bioelectromagnetic experiments. *Bioelectromagnetics.* 1992; **13(5)**: 401–411.

23. Alreja, M., Mutalik, P., Nayar, U. and Manchanda, S.K. The formalin test: a tonic pain model in the primate. *Pain* 1984; **20(1)**: 97–105.

24. Jain, S., Mathur, R., Sharma, R. and Nayar, U. Recovery from lesion-associated learning deficits by fetal amygdala transplants. *Neural Plasticity* 2002; **9**: 53–63.

25. Porro, C.A., Cavazzuti, M., Baraldi, P., Giuliani, D., Panerai, A.E. and Corazza, R. CNS pattern of metabolic activity during tonic pain: evidence for modulation by β-endorphin. *European Journal of Neuroscience* 1999; **11**: 874–888.

26. Dhawan, L. Nociceptive behavioural responses in rats exposed to magnetic field: role of opioid. Thesis submitted to AIIMS (1998).

27. Narasaiah, M. The role of limbic system in pain modulation: A behavioural and electrophysiological study in rats. Thesis submitted to AIIMS (1996).

28. Zangen, A., Herzberg, U., Vogel, Z. and Yadid, G. Nociceptive stimulus induces release of endogenous beta-endorphin in the rat brain. *Neuroscience.* 1998; **85(3)**: 659–662.

29. Loh, H.H., Tseng, L.F., Wei, E. and Li, C.H. Beta-endorphin is a potent analgesic agent. *Proce. Natl. Acad. Sci. USA* 1976; **73(8)**: 2895–2898.

30. Gispen, W.H., Wiegant, V.M., Bradbury, A.F., Hulme, E.C., Smyth, D.G., Snell, C.R. and de Wied, D. Induction of excessive grooming in the rat by fragments of lipotropin. *Nature* 1976; **264(5588)**: 794–795.

31. Porro, C.A., Tassinairi, G., Facchinetti, F., Panerai, A.E. and Carli, G. Central beta-endorphin system involvement in the reaction to acute tonic pain. *Exp. Brain Res.* 1991; **83(3)**; 549–554.

32. Yeung, J.C., Yaksh, T.L. and Rudy, T.A. Effect on the nociceptive threshold and EEG activity in the rat of morphine injected into the medial thalamus and the periaqueductal gray. *Neuropharmacology* 1978; **17(7)**: 525–532.

33. Vaccarino, A.L. and Melzack, R. Temporal processes of formalin pain: differential role of the cingulum bundle, fornix pathway and medial bulboreticular formation. *Pain* 1992; **49**: 257–271.

34. Dubuisson, D. and Dennis, S.G. The formalin test: a quantitative study of the analgesia effects of morphine, meperidine and brain stem stimulation in rats and cats. *Pain* 1977; **4**: 161–174.

35. Olivier, M., Grimaldi, B., Bailly, J.M., Kochanek, M., Deschamps, F., Lambrozo, J. and Fillon, G. Magnetic field desensitizes 5-HT$_{IB}$ receptors in brain: Pharmacological and functional studies. *Brain Research* 2000; **858**: 143–150.

36. Prato, F.S., Kavaliers, M. and Thomas, A.W. Extremely low frequency magnetic fields can increase or decrease analgesia in the land snail depending on field and light conditions. *Bioelectromagnetics* 2000; **21(4)**: 287–301.

37. Behari, J. and Mathur, R. Exposure effects of static magnetic fields on some physiological parameters of developing rats. *Indian Jour. of Experimental Biology* 1997; **35**: 894–897.

38. Lednev V.V. Possible mechanism for the influence of weak magnetic fields on biological systems. *Bioelectromagnetics.* 1991; **12(2)**: 71–75.

39. Kavaliers, M., Choleris, E., Prato, F.S. and Ossenkopp, K. Evidence for the involvement of nitric oxide and nitric oxide synthase in the modulation of opioid-induced antinociception and the inhibitory effects of exposure to 60 Hz magnetic fields in the land snail. *Brain Res.* 1998; **809(1)**: 50–57.

40. Kavaliers, M. and Prato, F.S Light-dependent effects of magnetic fields on nitric oxide activation in the land snail. *Neuroreport.* 1999; **10(9)**; 1863–1867.

41. Shen, K.F. and Crain, S.M. Dual opioid modulation of the action potential duration of mouse dorsal root ganglion neurons in culture. *Brain Res.* 1989; **491(2)**: 227–242.

42. Crain, S.M. and Shen, K.F. Opioids can evoke direct receptor-mediated excitatory effects on sensory neurons. *Trends Pharmacol Sci.* 1990; **11(2)**: 77–81.

43. Crain, S.M. and Shen, K.F. Ultra-low concentrations of naloxone selectively antagonize excitatory effects of morphine on sensory neurons, thereby increasing its antinociceptive potency and attenuating tolerance/dependence during chronic cotreatment. *Poc. Natl. Acad. Sci. USA* 1995; **92(23)**: 10540–10544.

44. Guilbaud, G., Peschanski, M. and Besson, J.M. Brain areas involved in nociception and pain. In: Melzack, R. and Wall, P. (eds.). Textbook of Pain, Churchill Livingstone, Edinburh, 1994, pp. 113–128.

45. Behari, J. and Mathur, R. Health hazards of electropollution—A Review, *Ann. Natl. Acad. Med. Sci. (India)* 1989; **25(3)**: 223–224.

46. Behari, J. and Mathur, R. Bioeffects of two different intensities of 50 Hz electric field in adult rats. In: Current Trends in Life Sciences, Vol. 17. Perspectives in Ageing Research. Eds. R. Singh and G.S. Singhal. Today's and Tomorrow's Publ. India, 1990, pp. 167–170.

47. Behari, J., Mathur, R. and Sharma, K.N. Behavioural ontogeny in rats exposed to extremely low frequency electric field. In: Nonlinear and Environmental Electromagnetics. Ed. H Kikuchi, Elsevier Pub., Amsterdam, 253–259, 1985.

48. Behari, J., Mathur, R., Sharma, K.N. and Datta, J.M. Biological effects on rats of chronic exposure to 50 Hz fields of moderate intensity. *Jour. of Bioelectricity* 1986, **5**(2): 335–342.

49. Mathur, R., Behari, J. and Sharma, K.N. Effect of chronic stress (electromagnetic field) on developing and adult rats. In: Brain and Psychophysiology of Stress. Eds. Sharma, K.N., Selevamurthy, W. and Bhattacharya, N., ICMR Pub., India, 1988, 213–220.

50. Singh, N., Rudra, N., Bansal, P., Mathur, R., Behari, J. and Nayar, U. Poly ADP ribosylation as a possible mechanism of microwave biointeraction, *Indian Jour. Physiol. Pharmacol.* 1994, **38**; 181–184.

51. Singh, N., Mathur, R. and Behari, J. Electromagnetic fields and cancer. IETE Technical Review 1997, **14**(3): 149–151.

52. Singh, N., Mathur, R., Azmi, S., Dhawan, D. and Behari, J. Effect of 50 Hz ELF field on rats-Poly ADP Ribosylation as a possible mechanism of signal transduction in Asia-Pacific Microwave Conference Proceedings. Ed. Gupta, R.S., Solar Print Process Pvt. Ltd. New Delhi, India, 1996, pp. 164–166.

53. Jha, P., Mathur, R. and Behari, J. Effect of Microwave exposure on circulating levels of testosterone in male rats. In: Asia-Pacific Microwave Conference. Eds Gupta R.S., Solar Print Process Pvt. Ltd. New Delhi, India, 1996, pp. -273–275.

54. Dutta, R., Mukherjee, K. and Mathur, R. Effect of VMH lesion on sucrose fed analgesia in formalin pain. *Japn. Journal Physiology* 2001; **51**(1): 63–69.

55. Mukherjee, K., Mathur, R. Nayar, U. Ventromedial hypothalamic mediation of sucrose feeding induced pain modulation. *Pharmacol. Biochem. and Behav.* 2001; **68**: 43–48.

56. Blass, E.M., Fitzgerald, E. and Kehoep, P. Interaction between sucrose, pain and isolation distress. *Pharmacol. Biochem. Behav.* 1987, **26**: 483–489.

57. Blass, E.M. and Hoffmeyer, L.B. Sucrose as an analgesic newborn infants. *Paediatric* 1991, **87**, 215–218.

58. Smart, D. and Lambert, D.G. The stimulatory effects of opioids and their possible role in the development of tolerance. *Trends Pharmacol. Sci.* 1996; **17**(7): 264–269.

59. Berkenbosch, F., Vermes, I. and Tilders, F.J. The beta-adrenoceptor-blocking drug propranolol prevents secretion of immunoreactive beta-endorphin and alphamelanocyte-stimulating hormone in response to certain stress stimuli. *Endocrinology.* 1984; **115**(3): 1051–1059.

60. Mizoguchi, H., Narita, M., Kampine, J.P. and Tseng, L.F. [Met 5]enkephalin and delta2-opioid receptors in the spinal cord are involved in the cold water swimming-induced antinociception in the mouse. *Life Sci.* 1997; **61**(7): L81–86.

61. Bea, J., Vegt, V.D., Lieuwes, N., Esther, H.E.M. and Wall, V.D. Activation of serotonergic neurotransmission during the performance of aggressive behaviour in rats. *Natural Neuroscience* 2003; **117**(4): 667–674.

62. Chance, W.T., Grossman, C.J., Newrock, G., Bovin, G., Yerian, S., Schmitt, G. and Mendenhall, C. Effects of electromagnetic fields and gender on neuro-transmitters and aminoacids in rats. *Physiology and Behaviour* 1995; **58**(4): 743–748.

63. Lerehl, A., Nonaka, K.O., Stokkan, K.A. and Reiter, R.J. Marker rapid alteration in nocturnal pineal serotonin metabolism in mice and rats exposed to weak intermittent magnetic field. *Bio. Chem. Bio. Phys. Res. Commun.* 1990; **169**: 102–108.
64. Mukherjee, K., Mathur, R. and Nayar, U. Nociceptive response to chronic stress of restrain and noxious stimuli in sucrose fed rats. *Stress & Health* 2001; **17**: 297–305.

Pain Updated: Mechanisms and Effects
Edited by R. Mathur

18. Chronic/Recurring Common Headaches: An Analysis

M.V. Padma Srivastava

Department of Neurology, C.N. Centre, All India Institute of Medical Sciences,
New Delhi-110 029, India

Introduction

The management of neurological diseases touches virtually all practicing clinicians, whether in hospital or in general practice. While providers of care struggle to meet innumerable quantitative criteria concurring the processes of diagnosis and management, it is important not to lose sight of the important related issue, which is the substance and quality of the actual medical care provided. The medical profession must lead from the front in the setting of standards of care based on the traditional but cogent twin pillars of good clinical practice, and their managerial colleagues. This article deals with the current perspectives of common headaches.

Headache is the most common of all neurological symptoms. There is none who has not experienced 'headache' in lifetime. Morbidity due to headache tension headache are major problems. Tension headaches outnumber migraine by 5 : 1. The overall incidence of migraine is about 10% of the population with a pronounced variation related to age. There is a higher incidence in women aged 20-24 years in a defined population. The overall lifetime prevalence of classic migraine is 5%, with a female to male ratio of 2 : 1, whereas, the overall lifetime prevalence of common migraine is 8%, with a female to male ratio of 7 : 1. Women are more likely to have common than classic migraine. In both types the most conspicuous precipitating factors are stress and mental tension. A list of common headaches at different ages is given in Table 1.

In general practitioners' clinic (surgery or hospital) over 95% of patients have tension headache, migraine, or atypical headache without a structural lesion. For such patients, whose symptoms are strongly influenced by social, personal and family problems, several therapeutic modalities are needed. The armamentarium is however limited. The frustration of implacable patients is reflected in their search for 'alternative therapies'. Medical science assesses its tools by rigorous analysis and scientific trials. Practitioners of alternative medicine should not daunt medicine, since, with rare exceptions, they have

Table 1   Common headaches at different ages

Sr. No.	3-16 (years)	17-60 (years)	60+ (years)
1	Migraine	Migraine	Referred from neck
2	Tension	Tension	Cranial arteritis
3	Psychogenic or fatigue	Cluster post-traumatic	Paget's disease of the skull
4	Post-traumatic	Cranial and dural tumors	Glaucoma, cranial and dural tumors
5	Occasional tumors	Cerebral tumors including abscess and subdural haematoma	Cerebral tumors including abscess and subdural haematoma
6	Tumors: Posterior fossa	Depression Referred from neck Paget's disease of skull	Rare cluster headache Paget's disease of skull Post-herpetic* and cranial neuralgias
	Intraventricular	Post-herpetic* and cranial neuralgias	Post-traumatic continuing tension headache Continuing migraine

*Uncommon presentation at this age.

so far failed to subject their unbounded claims of therapeutic triumphs to scientific scrutiny. When they do so and when their methods produce validated benefit, physicians should welcome and use them. Some of the most common recurring headaches are discussed.

Migraine
Various types of migraine are as follows:

(a) *Classic migraine*: Classic migraine is synonymous with aura which occurs in 20% of migraineurs. It is a paroxysmal disorder with headaches, often unilateral at the onset, associated with nausea, anorexia and after vomiting; it is preceded or accompanied by visual, sensory motor and mood disturbances and it is often familial.

(b) *Common migraine*: This is synonymous with migraine without aura. It occurs in 75% of headache patients. The term refers to similar paroxysmal headache without the aura. Both types of attack may occur at various times in the same patient. It is common for migraineurs to have tension headaches between their migraines; these should be identified to prevent misdirected treatment. Daily headache are never migrainous.

(c) *Migraine variants*: These are hemiplegic, basilar and opthalmoplegic, migraine sine cephalgia etc. It occurs in less than 5% of headache patients, usually requiring a neurologists appraisal and sometimes brain imaging.

Natural Course and Management
Migraine attack begins in childhood before the age of 10 years. These attacks may be overlooked if the child is unable to describe them. Sometimes, patient

can simply appear pale, ill, limp and inert; complaining of poorly localized abdominal pain. Headache is usually present, vomiting is common and there may even be fever, so that the suspicion of appendicitis or mesenteric adenitis often arises. The 80% of migraineurs have their first attack before the age of 30 years and the diagnosis should therefore be viewed with suspension if the age at onset is after 40. Attacks tend to lessen after the age of 50 years although, increased frequency of attacks at the menopause is common. Remission occurs in 70% of pregnancies. Exacerbation or complicated migraine with infarction may result from estrogen containing contraceptive.

Migraine attack lasts in adults for about 24 to 48 h but in children this lasts only for 2 to 6 h. In the latter, the headaches may disappear completely, attacks presenting with teichopsiae and no headache (migraine sine cephalgia). The apparent onset of migraine in the elderly implies atherosclerotic, thromboembolic diseases. Food idiosyncrasies, food allergies, red urines, specific dietary amines and omission of food are occasional precipitants. Emotional stress and fatigue, travel, sleeplessness are also important aggravating factors. A list of common precipitants is given in Table 2.

Table 2   Common precipitants of Migraine attack

1.	Fatigue, overwork, travel
2.	Relaxation after stress: holiday and Saturday morning headache
3.	Bright lights, disco
4.	Sleep excess or shortage: Sunday morning headache
5.	Missing meals
6.	Rare dietary sensitivity
7.	Alcohol, red wines
8.	Menstruation
9.	Exercise: vascular headaches such as footballer's migraine, coital cephalgia

Migraine is caused primarily by a neural (cerebral) mechanism with a fluctuating threshold, which determines the timing and pattern of attacks. A neural trigger activates the trigemino-vascular reflex, releasing vasogenic amines from blood vessel walls accompanied by their painful, pulsatile distension. The cerebral mechanisms respond to mood, emotions, tiredness, relaxation, hormonal changes, bright lights and noise. Its threshold is susceptible to hypothalamic function, which in turn is modulated by seasonal patterns, biological clock and hormonal factors. Personality and variations of mood and behaviour also influence the pattern of attacks, remissions and treatment.

Treatment
The treatment aims at controlling the symptoms and prevention or reduction of attacks. Many prophylactic drugs act by central serotonin (5 HT_2) antagonism, whereas control of an attack relies on construction of cranial vessels mediated by alpha adrenergic or 5 HT_1 receptors.

Analgesics Simple analgesics or non-steroidal anti-inflammatory agents must supplement risk, dark and quiet environment.

Ergotamine: Ergotamine (or dihydroergotamine) is an effective remedy for acute attacks in about 50% of cases. When overused, it can lead to habituation with ergotamine-dependent headache, similar to chronic analgesic-dependent headaches, which minimize migraine.

Sumatriptan: Sumatriptan is a specific and selective agonist of $5\,HT_1$ receptors on cranial blood vessels that causes vasoconstriction. The subcutaneous preparation (6 mg) gives relief of headache in 77% patients at 60 min and in 83% at 120 min with corresponding reduction in nausea, vomiting and photophobia. It is also effective in cluster headache with relief of symptoms at 15 min in 74% compared with 26% of those given placebo. Oral medication (100 mg) provides relief in about 70% of attacks within 2 hours. Sumatriptan is an effective, safe and prompt remedy, suppressing all the symptoms not headache alone. It works in 70% of sufferers, along with not in every patient.

Prophylaxis: Prophylaxis should only be considered if attacks occur more often than twice each month. Non-pharmacological techniques are successful in certain subjects. Prophylactic treatment aims to reduce the frequency. They should be given for 3 to 6 months and then reassessed. In patients with stress, amitriptyline in the night should be used. Beta-blockers without intrinsic sympathomimetic activity (propranol) reduce the frequency in about 60% of cases. It is most effective in the tense or hypertensive subjects with autonomic overdrive. Serotonin inhibitors are valuable in 60-70% of patients. Cyproheptadine and pizotifen may be tried. Calcium channel blockers such as flunarizine and verapamil have been established as useful prophylactic drugs. The newer prophylactic agents are valporate, divalprotic acid and lamotrigine.

Tension Headache

Tension headache is the most common of human complaints, constituting 70% of referrals to a headache clinic. Current systems classify the most common recurring headache as migraine or tension type. These two headache patterns are different expression of the same pathophysiological process having overlapping symptomatic presentations. Moreover, the same therapy has been shown to be effective for both types of headache patients. An alternative continuum classification model has been suggested, as there is an undoubled overlap between common migraine and tension headache.

In chronic tension headache (chronic daily headache), pain is felt diffusely all over the head, often located on the vertex, or forehead. Primary tension headache is psychogenic; its mechanisms are not fully understood. It is commonly bilateral, but may be unilateral. Patients characteristically complain of pressure, a feeling of tightness, or a heavy weight pressing on the crown. 'A tight band like a skull cap' is a common description. The symptoms may also seem to derive from inside the cranium: 'as if my head is bursting' or 'about to explode'. A 'creeping sensation (formication)' may be felt under the scalp, or a sense of sharp knives or burning hot needles drive in, may be related. Tension headache occurs daily and becomes worse in the evenings. Visuals disturbance, photophobia and vomiting seldom occur. Symptoms may continue for years without evident deterioration of general health. Symptoms are worse when the patient is tired or under pressure. Many sufferers are emotional and anxious with fears of brain tumors, or 'clot in the brain'. Treatment is most effective when the history is short. To cure such headaches after many years is a daunting and often unsuccessful task. Sensitive patients with fragile personalities may be unable to cope with life's stresses. They use 'headache' to escape from their responsibilities, which they cannot cope up with. Sedatives, tranquilizers and tension-relieving drugs are of limited value unless the psychological issues are adequately handled.

Patients often misuse analgesics, which aggravates the situation. However, with persuasion, the misuse can be reversed with dramatic benefit. Latent depression presenting as tension headache is easily overlooked. Early morning insomnia, negativism, guilt are suggestive of co-existing depression. The headache is worse in the morning (resembling that of raised pressure). Full doses of antidepressants are warranted. The prognosis for depression is often good.

Cluster Headache
The synonyms for cluster headache are Horton's syndrome and migrainous neuralgia. It predominantly affects males and begins at any age (often 20 to 50 years). It is manifested as daily bouts of unilateral headache of great severity lasting 30-120 min. The brevity, severity, lack of aura and vomiting occur daily in clusters. It may last for 4-16 weeks, which clearly differentiates it from migraine. It characteristically strikes at night; an hour or so after sleep and may recur during the day, often at the same time (alarm-clock headache). In many cases, the ipsilateral eye becomes red and bloodshot, watering profusely. The nostril may be blocked or run. Remissions are complete but the clusters recur every year or two.

Cervicogenic Headache
Head pain referred from cervical spondylosis is very common. It occurs on one or both sides of the neck and radiates to occiput, temple or frontal regions. It may be worse in the morning; lasts whole day and is aggravated by neck movement and tension. Vague and intermittent symptoms of tinnitus, dizziness and visual disturbances are sometimes attributed to compression of the vertebral arteries, although, it needs to be proved. Pain arises from the posterior zygapophyseal joints and related ligaments as a result of oesteophytes with irritation of the C_2 root or greater occipital nerves.

References

1. Classification and diagnostic criteria for headache disorders, cranial neuralgias and fascial pain. Headache Classification Committee of the International Headache Society. *Cephalagia* 1988; **8** (suppl. 7): 19–45.
2. Solomon S., Lipton R.B. Criteria for the diagnosis of migraine in clinical practice. *Headache* 1991; **31**: 384–387.
3. Davis P.A., Holm J.E., Myers T.C., Suda K.T. Stress, headache and physiological disregulation: a time-series analysis of stress in the laboratory. *Headache* 1998; **38(2)**: 116–21.
4. Pearce J.M. Sumatriptan : efficacy and contribution to migraine mechanisms. *J. Neurol. Neurosurg. Psychiatry* 1992; **55**: 1103–1106.
5. Saxena P.R., Den-Boer M.O. Pharmacology of antimigraine drugs. *J. Neurol.* 1991; **238** (suppl) S28–S35.
6. Kunkel RS. Muscle contraction (tension) headache. *Clin J Pain* 1989; **5**: 39–44.
7. Stang P.E., Yanagihara T., Swanson J.W., Beard C.M., O'Fallon W.M., Guess H.A., Melton L.J. Incidence of migraine headache: A population based study in Olmsted Country, Minnesota. *Neurology* 1992; **42**: 1657–1662.
8. Rasmussen B.K., Olesen J. Migraine with aura and migraine without aura: an epidemiological study. *Cephalagia* 1992; **12**: 221–228.
9. Lance J.W. A concept of migraine and the search for the ideal headache drugs. *Headache* 1990; **30** (1 suppl.) 17–23.
10. Kundrow L. Diagnosis and treatment of cluster headache. *Med. Clin. North. Am.* 1991; **75**: 579–594.

Pain Updated: Mechanisms and Effects
Edited by R. Mathur

19. Yoga as Relaxation Therapy for the Management of Headache

R.L. Bijlani

Department of Physiology, All India Institute of Medical Sciences,
New Delhi-110 029, India

Abstract: Since mental stress is a major causative factor for the majority of headaches, measures which relax the mind are helpful in treatment. In order to understand how yoga relaxes the mind, it is important to understand what yoga is. According to Sri Aurobindo, yoga is a process of working towards self-perfection with the ultimate aim of achieving union with the Divine. Improvement is the first step towards perfection, and the process should involve all aspects of the being—physical, emotional and intellectual. The core of the transformation is the yogic attitude, the first casualty of which is the separative ego. A seeker along the path of yoga starts developing the vision of basic unity behind the multiplicity of creation. From this vision follow the reduction, and eventual elimination, of desires, likes and dislikes, and clinging to life—the basic causes of stress according to Patanjali. In short, yoga gives the person a new way of looking at people, events and circumstances. Consequently, the person acquires inner calm and peace which are independent of external circumstances. However, besides this global change, among yogic practices there are specific techniques such as *shavasana* and meditation which are particularly relaxing. Swami Vivekananda Kendra at Bangalore has improvised some variations on these classical techniques, which they term quick relaxation, instant relaxation and deep relaxation techniques. While these techniques are helpful, it is important to keep in mind that a short time spent on these techniques, no matter how relaxing, cannot compensate for day-long turmoil. These techniques should be used only as facilitators of peace. The meditative poise of meditation should diffuse into the rest of the day for true relaxation.

Introduction

Headache is most commonly a physical manifestation of underlying mental stress; hence the term tension headache. Mental stress frequently leads to sustained contraction, or spasm, of head and neck muscles. Muscle spasm is a major contributor to tension headaches. Hence, measures which relax the mind are helpful in relieving both the muscle spasm and the headache. Although yoga is primarily a spiritual discipline rather than a relaxation technique, it does relax the mind. In order to understand how yoga relaxes the mind, it is important to look at what yoga is.

What is Yoga?

According to Sri Aurobindo, yoga is a process of working towards self-perfection with the ultimte aim of union with the Divine [1]. Improvement is the first step towards perfection, and the process should involve all aspects of the being—physical, emotional and intellectual. Since there is always room for improvement, and since yoga involves improvement in all aspects of life, yoga is a life-long process demanding commitment for 24 h a day, and yet the journey is unlikely to finish in a life-time. A long journey proceeds faster if we use a car than if we walk. Similarly, in yoga, techniques such as *asanas* and meditation can accelerate the progress. But techniques, which may take only a few hours a day are mere catalysts; the practice of yoga goes on throughout the day. Techniques are the visible part of yoga; the rest of yoga involves an inner transformation. The core of the transformation is the yogic attitude. The first casualty of the yogic attitude is the separative ego. A seeker along the path of yoga starts developing a vision of basic unity behind the multiplicity of creation. The basis of unity is the Spirit of the Creator, which is present in an unmanifest form in all creation. The Spirit represents the ultimate Reality which is behind the manifestation as well as working of the universe. Awareness of a common thread that runs through all creation helps the person rise above his little self, and look at people, events and circumstances from a broader perspective.

How Does Yoga Relieve Stress?

Ignorance (*avidya*) about the deeper unmanifest Reality of existence that pervades and runs the manifest universe is the basic cause of stress, and from this follow the other causes of stress enumerated by Patanjali, viz. ego (*asmita*), likes and dislikes (*ragadvesa*), and clinging to life (*abhinivesa*) [2]. Let us see how these sources of stress are eliminated by the yogic attitude. Ego is an expression of the wall that divides us from the rest of the universe. Awareness of the common Spirit that pervades the universe brings home to us the realization that the Spirit that unites us with the rest of the universe is more real than the dividing wall. Blurring of the boundary that separates us from others gives us a charitable outlook towards the people around us and an easier acceptance of events that may not be entirely to our liking. Once we accept a Reality higher than the manifest reality, we also indirectly acknowledge its supreme wisdom. Therefore grudging acceptance of events and circumstances gets replaced by cheerful accceptance of the will of the higher force that runs the universe. Thus the likes and dislikes that normally plague our minds get subdued. The broader perspective of the world around us also makes us aware that we are not indispensable, and therefore our continued existence as an individual is not a matter of much importance. This takes care of the last source of stress, viz. clinging to life. In short, yoga gives the person a new way of looking at people, events and circumstances. Consequently, the person acquires inner calm and peace which are independent of external circumstances.

Specific Techniques for Relaxation

While the change in attitude to life is more important than any relaxation technique, techniques do have a place in management of a crisis precipitated by prolonged unmitigated stress. All yogic postures (*asanas*) relax the mind to some extent because of the slow, gentle and graceful movements involved, the awareness with which *asanas* are supposed to be done, and the soothing atmosphere in which *asanas* are usually done. But there is also a specific *asana*, *shavasana* (the corpse pose), which is specially designed for relaxation.

Shavasana

Shavasana involves more than lying down in a well-defined comfortable posture. Muscles retain considerable tone even after lying down, as can be shown by the electromyographic (EMG) activity. Further, a conscious effort to relax the muscles can make the muscles completely flaccid, as can be shown by EMG silence. In *shavasana*, the person is encouraged to make such an effort. To facilitate the process, parts of the body from the feet upwards are relaxed successively, one at a time, before asking the person to relax the whole body. Relaxation is further facilitated by slow and deep abdominal breathing, and the peaceful atmosphere in which the exercise is conducted. *Shavasana* is frequently coupled with imagery and autosuggestion. The overall result is profound physical and mental relaxation, and relief of the spasm of the head and neck muscles which may be particularly marked in patients having headache.

Swami Vivekananda Kendra, Bangalore, has devised three variations of the classic *shavasana*. One of these, more or less like the classical *shavasana* described above, is called deep relaxation technique (DRT), and takes about 20 min. A variation, which involves progressive voluntary tightening of muscles followed by total relaxation takes 2 to 3 min, and is called Instant Relaxation Technique (IRT). IRT can be practised even in a chair in the office a few times a day, particularly when under unusually high pressure of stress. Another variation, which involves simultaneous voluntary relaxation of all parts of the body in the lying down posture takes 3 to 4 min, and is called quick relaxation technique (QRT) [3].

Meditation

Meditation is the yogic technique that is likely to be the first one to be mentioned while talking about relaxation through yoga. The classical technique of yogic meditation is based on the yoga sutras of Patanjali [4]. After preliminary moral purification (*yama* and *niyama*), the process of meditation involves assuming an appropriate posture (*asana*), slow and deep breathing with awareness (*pranayama*), sensory withdrawal (*pratyahara*), concentration (*dharana*), and developing the theme of concentration (*dhyana*). The goal of meditation is superconsciousness (*samadhi*) [5]. Although there are several techniques of meditation, they have a few basic features in common, which have been deduced and summarized by Herbert Benson as follows:

(a) quiet surroundings, (b) comfortable posture, (c) a mental device and (d) a passive attitude [6].

Although meditation is a very relaxing practice, and provides some relief from stress even if practised in isolation exclusively for mental relaxation, two reservations may be pointed out. First, unless the attitude to life becomes more positive, twenty minutes of meditation will not be able to compensate for day-long tension and turmoil. Second, meditative techniques in disciplines such as yoga were not devised for stress relief with a view to managing headaches. Their primary purpose was to silence the surface activity of the mind so that the seeker could get an unhindered experience of the spiritual basis of existence. Stress relief, or rather an experience of profound bliss, was only a pleasant side effect.

Does Yoga Help Relieve Headache?

We have so far discussed why yoga may be expected to be helpful in management of headache. Headache/migraine was found to be one of the seven top conditions thought to benefit the most from complementary and alternative therapies, including yoga, in a questionnaire-based survey [7]. But only well-conducted trials can confirm or reject these expectations and general impressions There are far more studies substantiating the stress-reducing effect of yoga, meditation and similar relaxation therapies than those addressed to headache *per se*. An 8-week meditation-based stress reduction program led to a significant reduction in anxiety and depression scores; the improvement was sustained during the 3-month follow up [8]. In a study of 1148 patients, a 10-week behavioral medicine intervention based on the relaxation response was found to improve psychological as well as physical symptoms significantly; the improvement was more marked in the high-somatizing group [9]. In a controlled, randomized prospective study, two group behavioural interventions involving relaxation response, awareness training and cognitive restructuring were significantly more effective than control treatment involving only information about stress management and its relationship to illness in reducing the symptom score of patients having a variety of psychosomatic complaints, including headache [10]. In a group of 51 patients having chronic pain, including headache, a 10-week stress reduction program based on mindfulness meditation led to a reduction of pain rating index by 33% or more in 65% of the patients [11]. In a group of 121 patients having headache or pain in the back, neck or face, a 4-week package which included behavioural group therapy, self-monitoring and biofeedback or relaxation training, led to a significant reduction in need for medication and improvement in verbal/non-verbal pain behaviour, physical functioning and employment status; the improvement was maintained at the 12-month follow-up [12]. In a case-report from Taiwan, mindfulness meditation was found effective by the patient himself in controlling his severe headaches associated with activities requiring concentration [13]. In a comparison of non-steroidal anti-inflammatory drugs (NSAID) and yoga, it was found that the spasm of muscles of the head and neck region, as judged by electromyography (EMG), was relieved more effectively by yoga than NSAID, although the patients in the yoga group were more severely affected than those in the NSAID group [14]. In an extensive review, Barrows and Jacobs have concluded that headache is one of the conditions for which there is moderate evidence that mind-body medicine techniques are helpful [15].

Conclusion

Thus the limited studies that are available, all suggest a role for yoga in the treatment of headache. There are several mechanisms by which it might work. First, it relieves stress by providing an alternative optimistic way of looking at life. Thus the situation remaining the same, the person does not bother about it any more because his cognitive appraisal of situation has now changed. This strategy is also used by modern psychology; but yoga, first, relies on it much more, and secondly, in yoga there is a firm philosophical foundation for the optimistic outlook. That is why Sri Aurobindo called yoga nothing but practical psychology [16]. There may be other more tangible mechanisms also behind the pain relief provided by yoga. Meditation possibly releases corticotropin releasing hormone (CRH), which in turn releases beta-endorphin [17], of which one of the effects is pain relief. Relying on the endogenous pharmacy is preferable to prescription drugs because, as Deepak Chopra says, only the endogenous chemicals are associated with the 'know-how' which leads to release of just the right amount of the chemical at just the right place accompanied by a simultaneous increase in the receptivity to the drug where its action is most needed [18]. Although endorphins are a more fascinating and convincing mechanism, cognitive reappraisal should be considered more important because no matter which therapy, including yoga, is used, some headaches will refuse to go away. In that situation, only the willing and cheerful surrender embodied in yoga will help the person remain happy in spite of the headache. Thus the headache may persist, but that is not reason enough for the suffering also to persist. Absence of suffering is what yoga guarantees, and there can be nothing better any system of medicine can offer.

References

1. Sri Aurobindo. The Synthesis of Yoga. Pondicherry: Sri Aurobindo Ashram, 4th Edition, 1970, p. 2.
2. Patanjali's Yoga Sutras, II: 3.
3. Nagendra H.R., Nagarathna R. New Perspectives in Stress Management. Bangalore: Vivekananda Kendra Yoga Prakashana, 4th edition, 1997, p. 58.
4. Patanjali's Yoga Sutras, II: 46-55, III: 1-3.
5. Pandit M.P. Dhyana. Pondicherry: Dipti Publications, 3rd Edition, 1972.

6. Benson H. The Relaxation Response. New York: Avon Books, 1975, pp. 159–161.

7. Long L, Huntley A., Ernst E. Which complementary and alternative therapies benefit which conditions? A survey of the opininons of 223 professional organizations. *Complement Ther Med.* 2001; **9**: 178–185.

8. Kabat-Zinn J., Massion A.O., Kristeller J., Peterson L.G., Fletcher K.E., Pbert L., Lenderking W.R., Santorelli S.F. Effectiveness of a meditation-based stress reduction program in the treatment of anxiety disorders. *Am J Psychiatry* 1992; **149**: 936–943.

9. Nakao M., Myers P., Fricchione G., Zuttermeister P.C., Barsky A.J., Benson H. Somatization and symptom reduction through a behavioral medicine intervention in a mind/body medicine clinic. *Behav. med.* 2001; **26**: 169–176.

10. Hellman C.J., Budd M., Borysenko J., McClelland D.C., Benson H. A study of the effectiveness of two group behavioral medicine interventions for patients with psychosomatic complaints. *Behav. Med.* 1990; **16**: 165–173.

11. Kabat-Zinn J. An outpatient program in behavioral medicine for chronic pain patients based on the practice of mindfulness meditation: theoretical considerations and preliminary results. *Gen. Hosp. Psychiatry.* 1982; **4**: 33–47.

12. Cinciripini P.M., Floreen A. An evaluation of a behavioral program for chronic pain. *J. Behav. Med.* 1982; **5**: 375–389.

13. Sun T.F., Kuo C.C., Chiu N.M. Mindfulness meditation in the control of severe headache. *Chang Gung Med. J.* 2002; **25**: 538–541.

14. Bhatia R. Assessment of endogenous opioid system in control and chronic pain subjects. M.D. (Physiology) thesis, All India Institute of Medical Sciences, New Delhi, 2002.

15. Barrows K.A., Jacobs B.P. Mind-body medicine: An introduction and review of the literature. *Med. Clin. North Am* 2002; **86**: 11–31.

16. Sri Aurobindo. *The Synthesis of Yoga.* Pondicherry: Sri Aurobindo Ashram, 4th Edition, 1970, p. 39.

17. Harte J.L., Eifert G.H., Smith R. The effects of running and meditation on beta-endorphin, corticotropin-releasing hormone and cortisol in plasma, and on mood. *Biol. Psychol.* 1995; **40**: 251–265.

18. Chopra D. Quantum Healing: Exploring the frontiers of mind/body medicine. New York: Bantam Books, 1989, p. 41.

20. Status of Central Opioidergic System and Muscle Spasm in Chronic Tension Type Headache: Perspective Role in Management

R. Bhatia[1], N. Gupta[2], M. Tripathi[3], G.P. Dureja[4],
R.L. Bijlani[1] and R. Mathur[1]

Department of [1]Physiology, [2]Endocrinology, [3]Neurology and [4]Anesthesiology,
All India Institute of Medical Sciences, New Delhi-110029, India

Introduction

Chronic tension type headache (TTH) embraces a number of commonly used terms like tension headache, muscle contraction headache, psychomyogenic headache, stress headache, ordinary headache and psychogenic headache [1]. It affects 14% of adult population once or more per week and 3% are affected almost daily [2]. The pathophysiology of tension type headache remains to be determined. A few electromyographic (EMG) studies suggest muscle spasm as the primary pathology underlying chronic TTH [3], whereas, other studies report no link between muscle spasm and the symptoms of chronic TTH [4]. Nevertheless, the most consistent abnormality in the EMG of chronic TTH patients is a reduction or abolition of second exteroceptive suppression period (ES_2) during the voluntary contraction of temporalis muscle [5], which indicates the involvement of central serotonergic and probably opioidergic mechanism in pathogenesis of chronic TTH. Besides, mental stress and tension are the most frequent precipitants of this type of headache [6]. Despite serious efforts of the researchers a clear understanding of underlying pathophysiology and, therefore, a specific treatment is not available. Moreover, noxious stimuli per se activate endogenous analgesic system significantly involving the opioidergic system [7, 8]; about the status of which we are totally ignorant in chronic TTH patients. This article aims to determine the status of the muscle spasm and opioidergic pain control mechanism in chronic TTH. The status of the former was adjudged by recording EMG of pericranial muscle (temporalis) at rest, while the latter by naloxone challenge test (NCT). Further, it was attempted to study the effectiveness of mental relaxation and yoga in relieving the headache in chronic TTH patients.

Subjects and Methods

Chronic tension type headache patients were selected from Pain and Neurology Clinics of All India Institute of Medical Sciences. The subjects ranged from 18-50 years in age with a history of headache for more than 15 days a month or 180 days a year for at least 2 years (Table 1). Patients with a history of prescription of muscle relaxants, hormones, morphino-mimetics drugs; practice of yoga; drug addiction or abnormal menstrual history were excluded from the study. A written informed consent of the patients was obtained as a prerequisite to the study. The patients were then divided into three groups on the basis of the intervention undertaken. To determine the role of pericranial muscle spasm, the EMG of temporalis muscle was recorded during rest, pre- and post-life style management course (yoga group, $n = 6$) or neuro muscular relaxant, botulinum toxin injection (BOTOX group, $n = 3$). The third group of patients ($n=6$) comprised of simple pharmacological mediation by non-steroidal anti-inflammatory drugs (NSAID group) whereas the fourth group of healthy volunteers ($n = 6$) was selected to serve as controls. Their endogenous opioid system was assessed by neuroendocrine method (naloxone challenge test) while the muscle spasm was confirmed by recording the EMG of pericranial muscle temporalis, bilaterally. Both the tests were performed before and after one month of respective interventions namely NSAIDs, BOTOX injection or life style management course.

Table 1   Pain duration of the patients in different study groups

S. No.	Pain duration (years)		
	Yoga group	NSAID group	BOTOX group*
S1	6	3	5
S2	8	2	4
S3	15	6	2
S4	8	2	–
S5	10	6	–
S6	11	2	–

*Only three patients in BOTOX group completed the study. The patients who preferred to undergo life style management course had a longer duration of chronic TTH.

Naloxone Challenge Test

Principle: The naloxone challenge test is based on the principle of withdrawal of the tonic inhibition exerted by opioids on hypothalamic luteinizing hormone releasing hormone (LH-RH) neurons. The reversal of this inhibition through a receptor antagonist such as naloxone is accompanied by discharge of LH-RH neurons, which induces a release of LH in plasma [9, 17].

The study was approved by the Institutional Ethical Committee for studies in human and was conducted in compliance with its regulation, policies and principles. The subjects signed the informed consent. The study was conducted in the morning after an overnight fast and bed rest for a mean of 8 hours. The blood samples were collected under all aseptic precautions from a heparinised canula introduced in the antecubital vein. The blood samples (numbers 3 of 2 ml each) were withdrawn at an interval of 15 min (basal). Naloxone (Samarth Pharma Pvt. Ltd., Mumbai, India) was administered by a rapid intravenous injection (0.1 mg/ml/kg bw within 4 min) and blood samples (numbers 7) were collected after naloxone injection similarly (post-naloxone). The blood samples were centrifuged at 2000 rpm for 20 min. The serum was separated. It was stored at −20°C till LH levels were estimated in these samples by utilising IRMA kits (Medicorp., Canada). The female subjects were instructed to report for NCT on day 17-22 of their menstrual cycle. Immunoradiometric assay was done for estimation of LH concentrations. Intra-assay variation was <5% and the inter assay variation was also <5%.

Electromyography
In order to assess the role of muscle spasm in chronic TTH, EMG of muscle temporalis was recorded using two Ag/AgCl disc electrodes, placed bilaterally to record the bipolar EMG of each muscle. One electrode was placed 10 mm lateral to the external angle of the orbit and second directly above the first. The EMG was recorded using Biopac Student Lab (BSL, V3.6.2) system, (Biopac System Inc., 42 Aero Camino Santa Barbara, CA93117). It is computerized equipment having a software programme and MP30 hardware unit. It has four channels and a smart sensor, attached to Channel-3 for all the recordings. EMG of the muscle. temporalis was recorded for 1 min duration for each side while the subject was instructed to remain in a complete state of rest.

Injection of botulinum toxin: Botulinum toxin type A (BOTOX-A) is one of seven neurotoxin serotypes produced during the fermentation process by the bacteria clostridium botulinum. The neurotoxin molecule is a 15,0000 Dalton di-chain peptide consisting of heavy chain linked by a disulfide bond to a light chain. It is believed to act selectively on peripheral cholinergic nerve endings and blocks the release of acetylcholine from presynaptic cholinergic nerve endings, without affecting the neuronal conduction or acetylcholine synthesis or storage. Once injected, the type A neurotoxin molecule binds to the motor nerve terminal through high affinity receptor selectivity. After binding, the botulinum toxin is internalized, the light chain of neurotoxin molecule is released into the cytoplasm of the nerve terminal and then acts to block vesicle fusion in the nerve membrane, thereby preventing the release of acetylcholine into the neuromuscular junction. Evidence indicates that chemical denervation of neuromuscular junction by this toxin results in expansion of end plate region and growth stimulation of collateral axonal sprouts. Eventually a nerve sprout is thought to establish a new neuromuscular junction with muscle activity gradually returning over a period of approximately 3 months. Therefore, repeat injections may be required for described clinical effect.

The intramuscular injections are given at the local sites of muscle tenderness, which can be identified by manual palpation [10]. Botulinum toxin A (BOTOX 50-60U) was divided into 10-12 doses and injected using a fine needle into multiple sites in temporalis muscle. The injection sites were selected by the physician according to the intensity of pain felt by patient.

Life style management course: The subjects were registered at Integral Health Clinic in the Department of Physiology, AIIMS for 2 weeks. Each session extended from 08:30 to 11:30 h. Integral Health Clinic aims at inculcating the yogic attitude in daily life of the patients in order to improve their quality of life, besides weaning them from heavy medication. The life style management course consists of lectures on yoga, meditation, fundamentals of nutrition along with personalized advice on diet and physical activity. Moreover, there are practical sessions when the experts teach various 'asanas', meditation and other relaxation techniques and patients practice under their supervision. The patients were also advised to continue this regimen for at least one month (period of observation).

Data Analysis

The total EMG record of 1 min was analysed bin (10 sec) wise for comparison of EMG amplitude during rest, before and after the intervention. Three alternate bins of 10 sec each were considered. Friedman test did not reveal significant difference amongst the three bins therefore; the mean of these bins was used for rest of the statistical analysis. The average leutinizing hormone levels at each time period was also compared between the groups using Kruskal Wallis test. In case of significant results, multiple comparison test was carried out to identify the pairs of groups having significantly different results. The comparison between first and second visit of the same group of patients was done by Wilcoxon Signed Rank test in all the groups. The data was considered significant at 5% level of significance ($p < 0.05$).

Results

The chronic TTH patients were 18-46 years of age while male to female ratio was nearly 1 : 1. The blood pressure of all the patients was in the normal range (systolic, 100-130 mmHg and diastolic 70-90 mmHg). The duration of pain ranged from 2 to 10 years (Table 1). The duration of each episode of pain was 4-6 h with a frequency of 2-3 episodes per day. Most of the patients complained of a band like pain throughout the head.

EMG During Rest

In control subjects at rest the mean amplitude of muscle temporalis were

12.91 ± 5.51 μV and 13.48 ± 8.72 μV of left and right side, respectively (Fig. 1, Table 2). In pre-NSAID group the EMG amplitude of left and right muscle temporalis were 26.18 ± 21.11 μV and 28.84 ± 14.7 μV, respectively; whereas in pre-BOTOX group it was 48.44 ± 42.58 μV and 49.25 ± 46.71 μV, respectively and in pre-yoga group it was 54.54 ± 36.99 μV ($p = 0.015$) and 49.95 ± 25.76 μV, respectively (Fig. 1, Table 2). The EMG amplitude in pre-yoga group was significantly higher as compared to the controls ($p = 0.33$).

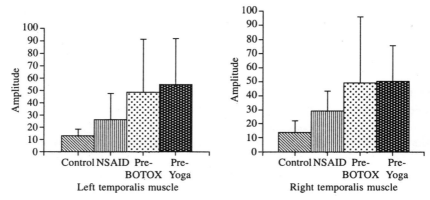

Fig. 1.   EMG amplitude (μV) of temporalis muscle at rest in the study groups

Table 2   EMG amplitude (μV) of temporalis muscle before and after various interventions

| Group | EMG amplitude* (μV) | | | | p-value |
| | Left muscle temporalis | | Right muscle temporalis | | |
	Before intervention	After intervention	Before intervention	After intervention	
NSAID	26.18±21.11	11.75±1.13	28.84±14.7	15.02±4.93	0.04
BOTOX	48.44±42.58	9.05±1.41	49.25±46.71	9.62±3.31	1.10
Yoga	54.54±36.99	29.18±21.00	49.95±25.76	26.63±25.78	0.02

*EMG amplitude of left and right muscle temporalis in control volunteers was 12.91 ± 5.51 and 13.48 ± 8.72 μV, respectively. $p < 0.05$ is significant.

One Month Post-intervention

In NSAID group the EMG amplitude of muscle temporalis after intervention (NSAIDs therapy) were 11.57 ± 1.13 μV ($p = 0.04$) and 15.02 ± 4.93 μV ($p = 0.04$) for left and right side, respectively, suggesting an improvement in the status of muscle spasm by oral NSAID therapy (Fig. 2, Table 2). There was a decrease in EMG amplitude after the intervention in BOTOX group also (9.05 ± 1.41 μV and 9.62 ± 3.31 μV for left and right side, respectively). The EMG amplitude was significantly lower as compared to the controls

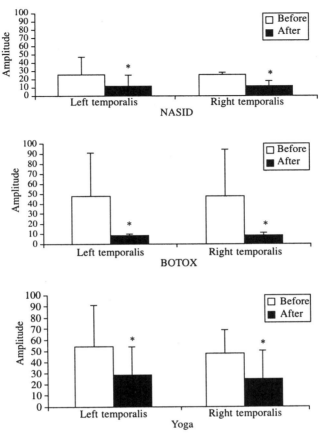

Fig. 2. Effect of different treatment modalities namely NSAID medication, BOTOX injection and life style management course on EMG amplitude of temporalis muscle at rest.

indicating markedly flaccid muscles too. It was observed that EMG activity during rest for left and right muscle temporalis was 29.18 ± 21.00 μV and 26.63 ± 25.78 μV, respectively. These values were comparable to controls as well as when compared to their first visit. The values for left ($p = 0.028$) and right ($p = 0.028$) muscle temporalis were significantly higher as compared to their first visit (Fig. 1, Table 2).

Naloxone Challenge Test

Controls: The basal LH levels ranged from 2.8 ± 1.3 to 3.5 ± 1.7 U/L. After 30 min of naloxone injection the LH levels started increasing gradually attaining a maximum at 60 min (5.68 ± 2.19 U/L), and then gradually declining to reach the pre-naloxone level 135 min from the start of study (Fig. 3).

NSAID group: In this group the basal LH levels ranged from 3.1 ± 2.7 to

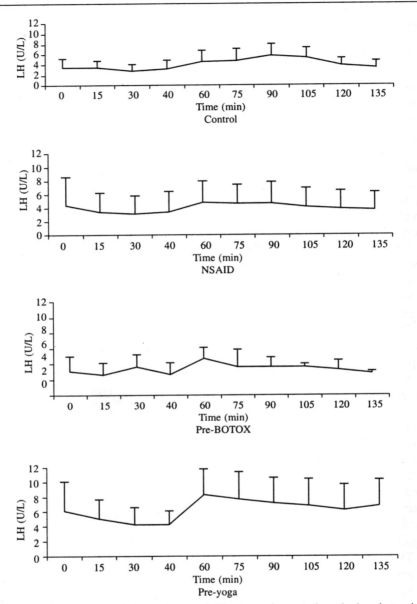

Fig. 3. The LH pattern during naloxone challenge test in controls and chronic tension type headache patients.

4.4 ± U/L, which were comparable to the control group of subjects. The LH levels started increasing post-naloxone 30 min and a peak was attained (4.48 ± 2.22U/L) at 60 min post-naloxone after which the levels started gradually declining.

Pre-BOTOX group: Basal LH levels ranged from 2.6 ± 1.6 to 3.6 ± 1.7 U/L. The levels started increasing at 30 min and attained a peak at 60 min (4.7 ± 1.4 U/L). This was followed by a sharp fall in the levels at 45 min post-naloxone.

Pre-yoga Group: Basal LH levels ranged from 4.2 ± 2.4 to 6.1 ± 4.0 U/L. After naloxone challenge, the LH levels increased to $8.18 + 3.6$U/L. The levels decreased 45 min post-naloxone, which did not return to baseline until the period of observation.

One Month Post-intervention
The comparison between the two visits of same group of patients was done by Wilcoxon Signed Rank Test. It revealed that after yoga the pattern of LH levels attained a peak at the same time, i.e. 30 min (6.8 ± 2.0 U/L) after naloxone but the rise in LH levels was gradual followed by a gradual decline to 5.6 ± 1.8 U/L (90 min) (Fig. 4) which was comparable to the pattern obtained in controls suggesting a beneficial role of life style management course. Similarly, the pattern of LH rise and fall was comparable to controls in NSAID group also but the BOTOX group did not show much improvement in the pattern of LH levels after treatment.

The intensity of headache perceived by the patients was subjectively assessed on visual analogue scale before and after intervention (Table 3). VAS also supported a significant improvement after NSAID therapy, BOTOX injection or life style management course although the improvement was more in patients undertaking life style management course ($p = 0.027$).

Discussion
The results of present study indicate that in chronic tension type headache patients, there exists an over activity of muscle temporalis at rest as compared to the controls. After undertaking respective interventions, namely, analgesic medication, muscle relaxant (BOTOX injections) or life style management course, it was observed that the muscle activity of muscle temporalis at rest declined in all the headache patients. The decline was comparatively more significant in life style management course group.

The chronic pain extends for a long period of time, represents low levels of underlying pathology, which often fails to explain the presence and extent of pain [11]. Besides, this chronic pain states have a great impact on affective state of an individual leading to emotional distress and at times physical disability too [11]. Despite significant advances in medicine, the treatment of chronic pain remains a difficult task because pain continues even in the absence of an obvious pathology. Persistent pain leads to a cascade of events, which are directed towards drawing the individual's attention and protection simultaneous with some other responses necessary for self-propagation. This includes an all out effort on the part of the body, which ranges from neural, biochemical, behavioral to an emotional adjustment to pain. Part of this

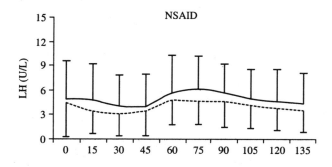

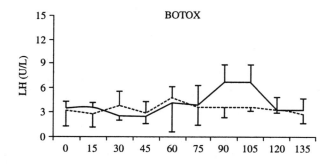

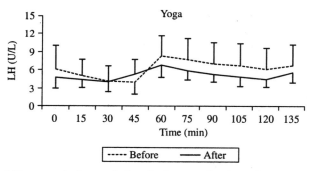

Fig. 4.   LH pattern before and after the intervention in various study groups.

Table 3.   Visual analogue scale (VAS) score before and after various interventions

	Visual analogue scale score		
Group	Before intervention	After intervention	*p*-value
NSAID	7.40 ± 1.50	3.67 ± 1.97	0.026
BOTOX	8.67 ± 1.50	2.67 ± 2.08	1.109
Yoga	7.00 ± 2.10	2.00 ± 1.26	0.027

p < 0.05 is significant.

adjustment is activation of endogenous opioid system in order to reduce the pain which has three major neural components namely periaqueductal gray (PAG) in mid brain, several nuclei of rostroventral medulla (RVM) and the spinal dorsal horn [12]. The stimulation of peripheral nociceptors send afferent input (A-delta fibers for fast pain and C fibers for slow pain) to dorsal horn of spinal cord (lamina II). The spinothalamic tract conveys the information to PAG, reticular formation, thalamus, hypothalamus and arcuate nucleus where opioid receptors are present in abundance [13].

Aberration of endogenous opioid system characterizes a number of chronic pain states, e.g. migraine, cluster headache, slipped disc and syndrome X [9]. There are some reports indicating the involvement of EOS in headache patients too. CSF opioid levels have been assessed in cluster headache patients [14] and it has been reported that in 72% of cluster attacks a concomitant increase in plasma beta endorphin levels was observed [15]. Buratti [16] estimated beta endorphin levels in circulating mononuclear lymphocytes. However, these methods may not reflect the true central opioid tone besides their feasibility in all the patients. Therefore, evaluation of central opiate activity was assessed by utilizing a neuroendocrine approach, i.e naloxone challenge test. The naloxone challenge test is based on the principle of withdrawal of the tonic inhibition exerted by opioids on hypothalamic lutenizing hormone releasing hormone (LH-RH) neurons. The reversal of this inhibition through a receptor antagonist such as naloxone is accompanied by discharge of LH-RH neurons, which induces a release of LH in plasma [17]. The test involves an intravenous injection of opioid antagonist, naloxone and assessing the response in terms of serum LH levels. In common migraine (CM), migraine with interparoxysmal headache (MIH), classical migraine and chronic cluster headache patients, plasma LH levels were estimated after naloxone challenge. The response to naloxone challenge was lacking in two-thirds of MIH and half of CM patients [17]. Another group of investigators studied the correlation between hyperalgesic state with the opioid status in syndrome X and angina patients utilizing this test [9]. They also reported a low LH release after naloxone administration in syndrome X patients suggesting an aberration in endogenous opioid system contributing significantly towards the symptoms as headache or chest pain vis-à-vis hyperalgesic states.

However, no such studies have been reported for chronic tension type headache, although an aberration in central pain control mechanisms has been suggested by the suppression or absence of the second exteroceptive suppression period (ES2) of temporalis muscle [5]. The ES2 is the inhibition of voluntary EMG activity of temporalis muscle on electrical stimulation of trigeminal nerve through a multisynaptic reflex mechanism suggesting a central dysfunction. The disturbance is believed to be in the limbic control of brain stem centers (PAG, Raphe magnus and lateral reticular nucleus). Incidentally, these areas are involved in pain control [18]. On the other hand, the overactivity of pericranial and cervical muscles have been implicated suggesting a role of peripheral mechanism in chronic tension type headache [19]. In our study also there is an overactivity of temporalis muscle at rest indicating a peripheral mechanism for chronic TTH, which is in line with the previous reports [6]. Besides, the naloxone challenge test also revealed an aberration in the opioid tone as reflected by the abnormal LH pattern in our patients as compared to the healthy volunteers indicating a significant contribution of endogenous opioids in chronic TTH either in etiology or persistence of headache or both. Therefore, it was pertinent to select life style management course, vis-à-vis yogic way of life and meditation, which could target both the aspects, viz. pathophysiology of TTH and the chronic pain syndrome. The former includes the peripheral muscle spasm; the central opioid status, while the latter includes the emotional and anxiety aspects of chronic TTH patients.

Yoga and transcendental meditation have been used as a combined approach towards mental and physical well being for a long time. Garfinkel et al [20] treated patients of osteoarthritis of hand by yoga-based intervention. Mental relaxation has shown positive results in patients suffering from chronic backache, chest pain, pain of carcinoma and bullet wounds [21]. Cinciripini and Floreen [22] reported beneficial effect of behavioural programme for management of chronic pain in back, head, neck and face region. Our study also highlights the beneficial effect of the change in life style in chronic tension type headache management. The patients were given three types of treatment modalities, viz. oral NSAID, local injection of botulinum toxin and the third group attended life style management course. The muscle spasm of pericranial muscle (temporalis muscle) decreased while the opiate status was corrected and became comparable to controls after the life style management course. The subjective assessment of pain done by visual analogue scale further reflected a decrease in the scores, suggesting the general well being of these patients after life style management course.

Despite successful cure by such a traditional approach a question is often posed that whether the changes in pain behavior correlate with changes in nociception. However, a careful look at the pain behavior includes several components of pain such as physiological sensations, affective changes and visible manifestation of discomfort or physical impairment. These components are linked to each other although they may be dissociated. Therefore, the perception of noxious stimulus can be modulated at several steps in the neuraxis, while being processed for motor, autonomic or emotional aspects of it. Yoga may be attenuating these responses specifically more so at the limbic brain processing. This is in line with the previous study where Schepelmann et al. [18] compared ES2 of fibromyalgia syndrome, and chronic TTH patients and controls. The duration of ES2 in fibromyalgia patients was comparable to controls whereas that of chronic TTH was significantly shortened. But ES2 changes are not correlated with headache intensity, EMG levels, and pain threshold. They point towards a CNS dysfunction, probably a disturbance of limbic control of these brain stem centers (e.g. PAG, raphe magnus and lateral reticular nucleus) which control the excitability of medullary ES2 inhibitory interneurons via serotonergic and presumably opioidergic mechanisms. The pathology of chronic TTH is unsettled and increase in muscle activity is sometimes demonstrable in EMG [3, 23, 24]. Therefore, it is valid to use mental relaxation techniques to relieve chronic headache because it corrects various aberrant aspects of chronic TTH.

References

1. Olesen J., Bach F.W., Langemark M. and Secher N.H. Plasma and cerebrospinal fluid beta endorphin in chronic tension type headache. *Pain* 1992; **51** (2): 163–168.
2. Rasmussen B.K., Jensen R., Schroll M. and Olesen J. Epidemiology of headache in a general population a prevalence study. *J. Clin. Epidemiol.* 1991; **44**: 1147–1157.
3. Pfaffenrath V. and Isler H. Evaluation of the nosology of chronic tension type headache. *Cephalalgia* 1993; **13** (Suppl 12): 60–62.
4. Simons D.G. and Mense S. Understanding and measurement of muscle tone as related to clinical muscle pain. *Pain* 1998; **75**: 1–17.
5. Schoenen J., Gerard P., De Pasqua V. and Sianard-Gainko J. EMG activity in pericranial muscles during postural variation and mental activity in healthy volunteers and patients with chronic tension type headache. *Headache* 1991; **31**: 324–4.
6. Jensen R. Mechanism of spontaneous tension type headaches and analysis of tenderness, pain threshold and EMG. *Pain* 1996; **64**: 251–256.
7. Milan J.M. Descending control of pain. *Progress in Neurobiology* 2002; **66**: 355–474.
8. Narita M. and Tseng F. Evidence of the existence of the β-endorphin sensitive 'ε-opioid receptor' in the brain : the mechanism of ε-mediated antinociception. *Jpn. J. Pharmacol.* 1998; **76**: 233–253.
9. Fransesco F., Luciano A., Marco P., Pierluig C., Giulia B., Gluseppina M. and Antonio V. Role of endogenous opiate systems in patients with syndrome X. *Am. Heart J.* 1998; **136**: 1003–1009.
10. Smuts J.A., Baker M.K. and Smuts H.M. Botulinum toxin type A as a prophylactic treatment in chronic tension-type headache. *Cephalalgia* 1999; **19**: 454.
11. Bonica J. with collabortion of Loeser J.D., Chapman C.J. and Fordyce W.E. The management of pain. Philadelphia. Lipincott Williams and Wilkins, Third edition, 2001.
12. Basbaum A.L., Fields A.L. and Fields H.L. Endogenous pain control mechanisms: review and hypothesis. *Ann. Neurol.* 1978; **4**: 451–62.
13. Tsou K., Jang C.S. Studies on the site of analgesic action of morphine by intracerebral microinjection. *Sci. Sin.* 1964; **13**: 1099.
14. Hardebo J.E., Ekman M., Eriksson M., Holgersson S. and Ryberg B. CSF opioid levels in cluster headache. In: Clifford Rose (ed.) Migraine, Kargel, Basel, 1985: 79–85.
15. Franceschini R., Leandri M., Gianelli M.V., Cataldi A., Bruno E., Rolandi E. and Barreca T. Evaluation of beta-endorphin secretion in patients suffering from episodic cluster headache. *Headache* 1996; **36**: 603–607.

16. Buratti T. Decreased levels of β-endorphin in circulating mononucleus leucocytes from patients with acute myocardial infarction. *Cardiology* 1998; **90**: 43–47.

17. Facchinetti F., Martignoni E., Gallai V., Mucieli G., Petraglia F., Nappi G. and Genazzani A.R. Neuroendocrine evaluation of central opiate activity in primary headache disorders. *Pain* 1988; **34**: 29–33.

18. Schepelmann K., Dannhausen M., Kotter I., Schabet M. and Dichans J. Exteroceptive suppression of temporalis muscle activity in patients with fibromyalgia, tension-type headache, and normal controls. *Electroencephalogr. Clin. Neurophysiol.* 1988; **107**: 196–199.

19. Jensen R. Pathophysiological mechanisms of tension type headache: a review of epidemiological and experimental studies. *Cephalalgia* 1999; **19**: 602–621.

20. Garfinkel H., Schumacher R. Jr., Husain A., Levy M. and Reshetar R. Evaluation of a yoga based regimen for treatment of osteoarthritis of the hands. *Journal of Rheumatology* 1994; **21**: 2341–2343.

21. French A.P. and Tupin J.P. Therapeutic application of a simple relaxation method. *Am. J. Psychotherapy*, 1990: 282–287.

22. Cinciripini P.M. and Floreen A. An evaluation of a behavioral program for chronic pain. *Journal of Behavioral Medicine* 1982; **5(3)**: 375–389.

23. Merskey H., Bogduk N. Classification of chronic pain, Descriptions of chronic pain syndromes and definitions of pain terms, 2nd ed. Seattle WA, IASP Press 1994.

24. Silberstein S., Mathew N., Saper J. and Jenkins S. For BOTOX® Migraine clinical research group. *Headache* 2000; **40**: 445–450.

Pain Updated: Mechanisms and Effects
Edited by R. Mathur

21. Cognitive Behavioural Therapy in Management of Headache

Manju Mehta

Professor of Clinical Psychology, Department of Psychiatry,
All India Institute of Medical Sciences, New Delhi-110029, India

Abstract: The 8 to 10% children and adolescent attending psychiatric clinics in general hospital report with complaints of headache. The common cause of headache is stress, tension, anxiety, depression, reinforcement of illness behaviour and imitation of pain behaviour as it is present in other family members also. Family environment plays a very important role in genesis of pain behaviour. Comprehensive assessment can help in finding factors that maintain pain behaviour. Cognitive behavioural methods like reinforcement of non-pain behaviour, distraction, imagery, problem solving, learning of positive coping skills and social skills are helpful in managing headache. Family members should be included as co-therapist in the management.

Introduction

There is a high incidence of tension type headache and migraine in children and adolescents attending child psychiatry clinic, specially in a general hospital. Prevalence of headache is reported to be 11% in girls and 4% in boys aged 12 to 16 years [1]. During a year, in the Child Psychiatric Clinic at AIIMS, approximately 8 to 10% cases are of headache [2]. This condition not only poses a challenge to the treating physician but also to the family members. The family members become apprehensive about the seriousness of the problem, as the child continues to suffer from headache.

Recurrent headache causes suffering and disability in a person. It interferes with the academics as well as the extra curricular activities of the child. The frequency, intensity and duration of headache are affected by several factors. The psychological and environmental factors contribute to the causation of headache. Some studies have also shown the relationship between the depression in mother and the headache in the child [3, 4]. Besides, the diverse environmental factors like weather conditions, sound and light exposure; exertion, family circumstances, mental stress and academic stress also contribute to headache [5].

Emotional distress has been identified not only as a fundamental component of pain but also as a cause of pain and as a concurrent problem attracting the attention of diagnosticians during assessment of pain disorders [6]. Persisting emotional distress can trigger new pain or reinstate old pain in the absence of pathological organic states. Emotional stress may be associated with increased pain by precipitating activity in biological systems that are also responsive to noxious stimulation. Anxiety, depression, anger and other emotions may provoke substantial autonomic, visceral and somatic activity. Tension headaches have been assumed to be the result of sustained contractions of the muscles of the face, scalp and neck in the absence of permanent structural changes, usually as a reaction to life stress.

Therefore, it is important to understand the nature, causes, assessment methods and management of the headache to reduce the treatment cost in terms of minimizing the number of investigations, decreasing the reinforcement to illness behaviour in the child and reducing distress in parents.

Assessment

Effective management of pain in children depends on comprehensive assessment made on the following guidelines:

1. *Self report of pain—Experience and perception*: The child's report about his experience of pain is taken in detail, with regard to his perception, the meaning, time of occurrence of pain; relieving factors and the degree of distress it causes. Visual analog scales can be used to assess intensity of pain.

2. *Headache diary*: Child is asked to maintain a headache diary in which he records frequency and severity of pain every day. He is also asked to write about the things he liked most and so also hated the most during the day. This provides a good clue about the disturbing factors.

3. *Behavioural observation of the child's pain*: This includes assessment of pain behaviour with the help of parents. Parents are given Antecedent, Behaviour, Consequence (ABC) chart for recording of pain behaviour and factors contributing to pain. Besides this, information on child's activities, play behaviour, social skills and school attendance is also recorded. All the activities which are affected by pain are noted.

4. *Medical screening*: All relevant investigations should be ordered to rule out any organic cause of headache.

5. *Cognitive functioning*: Cognitive developmental level can be assessed on any standardized test. Generally there is a discrepancy in the expectation and achievement level in scholastic performance. School adjustment of the child should be assessed.

6. *Psychosocial factors*: Psychosocial factors also play an important role in the variability of perceived pain. Family members having similar type of pain, psychosocial adjustment of the child, family environment and stresses are instrumental in the perception and reporting of pain [7–9]. Table 1 shows psychosocial factors that influence headache.

7. *Baseline recording*: Baseline record of the frequency, severity and duration of pain should be done. Parents are asked to record these aspects of

the pain behaviour for 6 days before starting the treatment. Baseline information is very useful for several reasons, for example,

(a) it serves to ensure parent's compliance with instructions and their willingness to keep records.
(b) it helps in the selection of treatment procedures.
(c) most of the parents think that the pain was due to organic causes but after one-week record on ABC charts they could understand the psychosocial aspect of the pain.
(d) the effects of treatment can be compared with baseline.

8. *Ongoing assessment*: Parents are asked to continuously record the frequency, severity and duration of pain as it helps in monitoring the effects of intervention. Besides, the parents become more confident about improvement in their child.

9. *Assessment of family*: Parents and other family members should be assessed for anxiety, coping ability, stresses, pain behaviour and their expectation from the child. Both objective and subjective methods can be used.

Table 1   Psychosocial factors in headache

1.	Anxiety level specially related to academic tasks
2.	Attention seeking behaviour
3.	Pain in other family members
4.	Parental anxiety and overprotection for the child
5.	Parental discord
6.	Poor coping skills
7.	School-stress
8.	Recent change of school
9.	Temperament, sensitive, easily upset over trivial matter

Methods of Intervention

In the management of headache cognitive behaviour techniques are very effective. Table 2 summarizes various techniques used in pain management.

Table 2   Techniques of pain management

Behavioural	Cognitive
Parental counseling	Relaxation therapy
Behavioural contracting	Attention and distraction
Time out from reinforcement	Guided imagery
Modeling	Coping skills training
Social skill training	Problem solving
	Information

Behavioural Intervention

These techniques alter pain through the modification of overt action.

1. *Parental counseling.* The belief of a child and parents dictate the method utilized to relieve pain during the episode of headache besides shaping their broader efforts to resolve the cause of headache. Parent's untoward anxiety and apprehension usually increases the child's pain, distress and disability. Thus the behavioural observations help in understanding the parents of the sick child, which in itself is one of the important causes of headache. Moreover, it also increases treatment compliance. Behavioural techniques used in pain management are mainly based on operant conditioning.

2. *Behavioural contracting.* A contract is made with the child in which whenever he is not complaining of the pain and manages his pain by himself he gets a reward. While, complaint of pain, display of illness behaviour like lying down on the bed, sleeping, not doing any thing is subjected to response cost, no reward and negative marking [10].

3. *Time out from reinforcement.* Parents are asked to use time out from reinforcement whenever the child reports pain. Pain free periods are rewarded by giving more attention to the child. Attention seeking can be reduced.

4. *Modeling.* Parents and older sibs are asked to tolerate pain whenever they experience it so that they set an example for the younger sick child in the family. Their interaction with the child and family environment is necessary to be modified.

5. *Social skill training.* Children who are perceived to be deficient in social skills, namely, inability to make friends, mix with other children, express their feelings, are given social skill training. Generally the child restricts its activity whenever he suffers from pain. Therefore, the child should be encouraged to engage himself in a wide variety of activities ranging from mild to moderate stressor tasks. It helps to build confidence in the child.

The goal of the operant conditioning approach is to decrease pain behaviour and replace it with well behaviour. In my experience ABC charts recorded by the parents to determine cause and affect relationship are of significant help. After analyzing these, the parents could be easily convinced of the psychological nature of the problem in their child. Manipulation of social environmental contingencies and verbal reinforcement are very powerful methods of intervention in the management of headache in children.

Cognitive Strategies

These techniques influence pain through the medium of thoughts or cognition. Cognitive techniques used are:

1. *Relaxation training.* Anxiety and tension are often the underlying causes of headache. Relaxation training is useful in reducing anxiety. Patients are taught the sequential tensing and relaxation of large muscle groups and deep breathing to achieve total body relaxation. They are instructed to practice

daily. Anxious and sensitive children improve by relaxation exercises as it conditions their autonomic nervous system.

2. *Attention and distraction.* Distracting attention from pain to other activities helps in reducing pain. Children are asked to divert their attention on some interesting task of their choice whenever they suffer from pain. They may opt for listening to music or watching television, taking a break from their academic activity, or sit in the balcony of their house to enjoy nature.

3. *Guided imagery.* Children are trained to imagine pleasant scenes which they have experienced in the past wherever they experience an episode of headache. The scenes should be from nature like watching waves on the sea beach, or sunset or looking at fresh flowers.

4. *Coping skills training.* Most of the children with headache have poor coping skills. They tend to use more often the negative ways of coping than positive methods. Better coping methods to deal with problems are taught to these children through role play, modeling and group discussions.

5. *Problem solving.* Headache is often associated with academic tasks. Detailed assessment reveals that such children have a faulty method of studying. Therefore, they are trained in simple problem solving, studying in small units and remaining relaxed at the time of the study.

Cognitive such as distraction and significance of the pain for the individual and emotional variables like anxiety influence pain. The cognitive techniques reduce the anxiety level of the child. Both, the reduction in the anxiety level and the problem solving technique, improve their performance at school. The punch line is that the ability of the child to manage stressful events has to be increased in order to avoid anxiety and negative mood.

Parents as Co-therapists

The cognitive behavioural treatment requires about 10 to 15 sessions. Its practice at home is very essential. Thus parents should be actively involved in the treatment. Besides, they have to take the responsibility of correcting their own behaviour, in terms of decreasing overprotection of the child, reinforcement of pain behaviour and increasing focus on pain free behaviour. They also need to supervise relaxation exercises and other cognitive exercises. In my experience, I have found that the parents can be successful co-therapists if only they are highly motivated; able to accept the psychological nature of the problem; ignore illness behaviour; postpone the demands of the child; remain consistent in delivering rewards and punishments and have therapeutic compliance. While, the parents were unsuccessful as co-therapist when they themselves had poor coping skills, high anxiety level, low frustration tolerance and over emphasized their pain and disability.

A combination of behavioural and cognitive techniques can effectively control pain. For each child a set of specific techniques can be selected from the above list according to the contributing factors. The implementation of therapy depends upon providing a feedback of cause and contributing factors to the child and parents. Rationale for treatment should be provided to motivate both the parents and child to accept the treatment. The frequency and intensity of pain gradually decreases as the child's adaptability to stress improves. The parents are then asked to let the child resume its previous activity level, namely, going to school, participation in play and household activities.

Drugs should not be arbitrarily given because they would only support the family's concept of pain, in addition to the dependence of the child on drugs. At times, when pain is acute the drugs can be used as placebo. Later on, it should be followed by behavioural methods. For the success of the intervention, parents' cooperation and their understanding of the problem is essential.

References

1. Varni, J.W., Dietrich, S.L. Behavioural pediatrics towards a reconceptionalization, *Behavioural Medicine Update*, 1981; **3**: 5–7.
2. Mehta, M. Headache in children. In :. Sharma K.N., Nayar U., Bhattacharya N. (eds). Current trends in pain research and therapy. Vol. II, Stimulus produced analgesia. Prachi Prakashan, Delhi, 1986, 115–119.
3. Zuckerman, B., Stevenson, J. and Bailey, V. Stomach and headache in community sample of preschool children. *Paediatrics* 1987; **79**: 677–689.
4. Mortiner, M.J., Kay, J., Grown, A. and Good, P.A. Does a history of maternal migraine or depression predisposes children to headache and stomachache? *Headache* 1992; **32**: 353–355.
5. Mehta, M. Cognitive behavioural intervention in abdominal pain. In: Sharma K.N., Nayar U., Bhattacharya N. (eds). Current Trends in Pain Research and Therapy. Vol. IV, Chronic pain reactions, mechanisms and modes of therapy. 1989; 169–173.
6. Feurestein, M. and Skjei, E. Mastering pain. Bantam Books, Inc. New York, 1979.
7. Dutta S. and Mehta, M. Stress in children with recurrent abdominal pain: A clinical study. *Ind. Jr. Paed.* 1997; **64**: 555–561.
8. Khurshid, A.K. Temperament, stressful life events and family psychopathology in children with recurrent abdominal pain. M.D. Thesis submitted at AIIMS; 1997.
9. Sethi, S.S. Role of selected family characteristics in children with functional somatic complaints. M.D. Thesis submitted at AIIMS, 1995.
10. Fordyce, W.E., Fowler, R.S., Lehman, I.R., Delatem, B.I. and Triesshmann, R.B. Operant conditioning in the treatment of chronic pain. *Arch. Physic. Med. Rehab*, 1973; **54**: 399–408.

22. Endogenous Opioids Status in Idiopathic Trigeminal Neuralgia Patients: Effect of Cervical Sympathetic Blockade

J. Rengarajan[1], G.P. Dureja[1], T.S. Jayalakshmi[1],
N. Gupta[2] and R. Mathur[3]

Departments of [1]Anesthesiology and Intensive Care, [2]Endocrinology and [3]Physiology,
All India Institute of Medical Sciences, New Delhi-110 029, India

Introduction

Trigeminal neuralgia is a severe, lightening like pain in the trigeminal nerve territory that can be triggered by touch, cold wind, strong whiff of air etc. [1]. The pathophysiology of trigeminal neuralgia has been much debated, the pain being ascribed variously to hyperactivity or abnormal discharges arising from Gasserian ganglion, nerve compression, nerve regeneration, sympathetically maintained and immune mediated pain [2-4]. In sympathetic maintained pain, nociceptors are thought to develop an alpha-adrenergic sensitivity probably as the result of expression of alpha-adrenergic receptors at their terminals. It has been reported that the initial trauma to the peripheral nervous system activates nociceptors and produces a sprouting of alpha-adrenergic receptors on the nociceptors [5].

Besides, trigeminal neuralgia is a chronic pain state wherein the endogenous analgesic system is likely to have a significant contribution. However, no reports are available about the status of endogenous opioidergic system in either the pathophysiology or progression of it. In several chronic pain/ hyperalgesic states including headache (common migraine, migraine with interparoxysmal headache, classical migraine and chronic cluster headache) and syndrome X, the symptoms have been attributed to an abnormality in the beta-endorphin response [6, 7]. Assessment of the endogenous opioid system on the basis of both CSF and plasma beta-endorphin levels is reported to have a limited value and is more conveniently now estimated in the circulating mononuclear leucocytes [8]. The procedure is very expensive and tedious, therefore cannot be used as a scanning test. Recently, a simple alternative approach to assess central endogenous opioid system activity by measuring plasma leutinizing hormone in response to intravenous naloxone administration (naloxone challenge test) has been reported. It has been utilized to evaluate the beta-endorphin levels indirectly vis-à-vis opioid status in the above-mentioned chronic pain states [6, 7]. It is pertinent that pain should be assessed objectively while searching for a stable measure in the management of trigeminal neuralgia. No study has so far compared the efficacy of Stellate ganglion block in trigeminal neuralgia. This study was designed to evaluate the role of sympathetic component (Stellate ganglion block) in trigeminal neuralgia by utilising clinical, electrophysiological and biochemical methods.

Materials and Methods

Stellate ganglion was blocked in 10 patients of trigeminal neuralgia (of either division), diagnosed on the basis of criteria suggested by International Headache Society (IX). The patients were selected from the pain clinic of the department of Anesthesiology and Intensive Care at AIIMS, New Delhi. The study was conducted in strict compliance with the rules and regulations of the Institutional Ethics Committee for studies on humans, after its approval.

Patients were explained and introduced to the concept of visual analogue scale (VAS) and noxious electrical stimulus after obtaining informed consent. A baseline VAS in response to noxious electrical stimulus were recorded and the fasting blood samples were taken for the estimation of endogenous opioids. A total of 10 samples were collected at every 15 min interval of which the first 3 samples constituted the basal samples. After the third sample 4 mg naloxone was injected intravenously slowly and 7 more samples were collected at 15 min interval, stored at $-20°$ C for assay of leutinizing hormone level by immuno-radiometric method (details are described elsewhere in this monograph).

Pain response by VAS

The detailed method is described elsewhere in this monograph. Briefly, the stimulating electrodes (Ag-AgCl cup electrodes) were applied on the skin over the retromalleolar aspect of the foot. The subject was first acquainted with an electrical stimulus (current strengths varying from 1 to 5 mA). The subject was asked to rate his sensation on a VAS after explaining to him the same. The sural nerve was stimulated with a train of 5, 1 msec pulses at intervals of 1 msec and incremental current strength (1, 3, 5, 7 and 9 mA) at intervals of 5 min. The current was gradually increased from 1 mA in steps of 2 mA and the maximum ceiling limit was 11 mA. However, if the subjective report of pain reached 10 on VAS, further electrical stimulation was not given.

Each time the subject was asked to rate his pain on the VAS.

Gasserian Ganglion Block

The patient was placed in supine position with cervical spine in extended position. Medial edge of sternocleidomastoid muscle was then displaced laterally with 2 fingers and the tissues overlying the transverse process of C_6

(Chassaignac's tubercle) were compressed. The pulsations of carotid artery were then identified under palpating fingers. The skin medial to the carotid pulsations was prepared with antiseptic solution and a 22 gauge $1\frac{1}{2}$ inch needle was advanced until contact was made with the transverse process of C_6. After bony contact was made needle was withdrawn approximately 2 mm to bring needle tip out of the body of longus colli muscle. Bupivacaine (10 ml solution of 0.25%) was carefully injected after negative aspiration. Patients were observed for 1 hour. One injection per day was given for five days (total 5 injections).

Results

Duration and Frequency of Pain
Duration of the disease varied from 2 to 10 years (mean 3.56 years) (Fig. 1). They had approximately 6.67 painful episodes/hour with each episode lasting for 13 sec. After a mean of 3.44 ±1.130 Stellate ganglion blocks the patients experienced pain relief. The pain relief was effective for 2.44 ± 2.97 months after the Stellate ganglion block. Prior to block the mean VAS score was 8 ± 1.014, after 24 h of block 77% of patients showed significant reduction in pain (mean score 4.11 ± 2.522) (Fig. 2). After 1 month the mean VAS score was 4.22 ± 2.438 while after 2 months it was 4.56 ± 2.603. This was statistically significant in comparison to pre-block VAS score. The number of patients who had pain relief gradually decreased at 6 months.

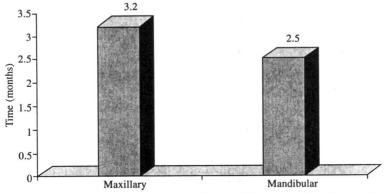

Fig. 1. Duration (months) of relief in pain after the Stellate ganglion block trigeminal neuralgia patients of either division.

Patients had 6.67 episodes of pain/hour which immediately decreased to 2.44 episodes/h after 24 h following cervical sympathetic blockade. The decrease in painful episodes at the end of 24 h, 1 month, 3 months were statistically significant ($p < 0.05$). All the patients (100%) presented with trigger zone allodynia; 77% of patients were relieved of allodynia after 1 month and 66% at the end of 2 months, which were statistically significant.

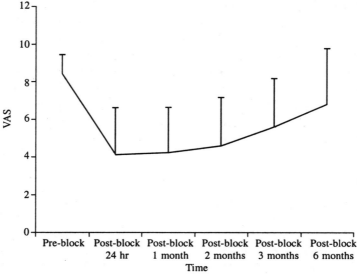

Fig. 2. Pain response on VAS (mean ± SD) at various time periods in trigeminal neuralgia patients. An immediate significant relief in pain was noted, which continued for 2 months post-block.

After 6 months 77% of the improved patients showed recurrence of pain and trigger point allodynia.

Effect of Increasing Current Strength on Pain Response

Pain perceived by the patient was reported utilizing VAS whose rating was recorded with each increment in the current strength from 1 to 11 mA in a stepwise manner (2 mA increments). In patients prior to block the pain score (VAS) at 1 mA was 1.44. At the end of 24 h after the block, the pain scores were 2.67 and at the end of 2 months it was 1.7. The comparison of pre-block pain scores with scores after the block showed no statistical significance among them (Table 1).

Table 1 Comparison of pain with stimulation (mean VAS) at different current intensities

Current (mA)	Pre-block	Post-24 h	Post-2 months
1	1.44±1.878	2.67±3.24	1.7±1.994
3	4±2.598	3.56±3.283	3.67±2.906
5	6.22±1.986	6.22±2.906	5.9±3.284
7	7.56±1.333	8.78±1.394	7.94±1.108
9	8.67±1.118	9±1	9.22±2.706
11	9.54±3.567	9.33±0.5	9.56±0.527

p-value insignificant between pre- and post-24 h, pre- and post-2 month, post-24 h and post-2 months.

Current Intensities for Threshold Pain

Current intensity at which the initial pain response was reported is considered as the threshold of pain. The mean threshold current intensity prior to the block was 4.11 mA. The threshold current intensity for pain increased to 5.89 mA 24 h post-block, which was statistically significant. The pain threshold decreased to 5.44 at the end of 2 months. When compared with pre-block threshold current intensity the difference was statistically significant ($p = 0.05$).

Effect of Chronic Pain on Endogenous Opioid Status

Indirect estimate of endogenous opioids through lutenizing hormone (LH) level estimation was done after giving naloxone (Fig. 3, Table 2). First three values (0 min, 15 min, 30 min) were basal levels while next 7 (45, 60, 75, 90, 105, 120 and 135) were post naloxone values. LH level prior to the block was compared with those at 2 months after the block (at each point of time).

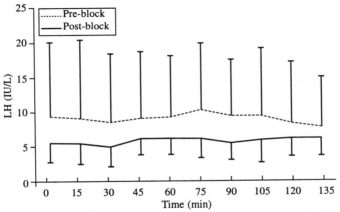

Fig. 3. LH concentration before and 2 months post-Stellate ganglion block in two patient groups.

Table 2   Change of endogenous opioids level at different time periods

Time (min)	Pre-block	Post-block IU/L	Rate of rise
0	9.39 ± 10.78	5.51 ± 2.67	6.58 ± 60.65
15	9.15 ± 11.40	5.46 ± 2.98	−27.41 ± 100.00
30	8.62 ± 9.88	4.99 ± 2.89	−15.16 ± 92.50
45	9.15 ± 9.68	6.16 ± 2.37	−48.90 ± 119.80
60	9.34 ± 8.86	6.19 ± 2.38	−21.69 ± 86.70
75	10.37 ± 9.66	6.15 ± 2.79	−3.40 ± 75.41
90	9.50 ± 8.17	5.54 ± 2.42	9.36 ± 56.65
105	9.50 ± 9.78	5.94 ± 3.23	−11.09 ± 92.84
120	8.49 ± 8.86	6.19 ± 2.59	−48.58 ± 117.78
135	7.86 ± 7.37	6.24 ± 2.56	−55.46 ± 134.00

There was a decrease in the LH levels both basal as well as post-naloxone values after the 2 months of ganglion block in comparison with pre-block. The values did not attain statistical significance probably because of the larger standard deviation in the pre-block condition of the patient.

Rate of Change of Endogenous Opioids
The rate of change of endogenous opioids at different points of time was computed

$$\frac{\text{(Post-value)} - \text{(Pre-value)}}{\text{Pre-value}}$$

Rate of rise of endogenous opioids between pre- and post-block at different time intervals was statistically insignificant probably because of the small sample size although, the pre-block values were greater than the post-block values (Fig. 4, Table 2).

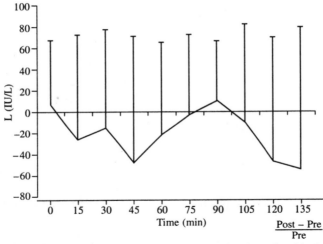

Fig. 4. Difference in LH levels of pre- and post-Stellate ganglion block conditions.

Discussion
Trigeminal neuralgia is one of the most painful human afflictions. It is characterized by recurrences and remissions, and successive recurrences may incapacitate the patient. Due to the intensity of the pain, even the fear of an impending attack may prevent activity. Unfortunately, over the time, the pain of trigeminal neuralgia usually becomes more severe and more frequent, requiring higher dosage and more continuous use of medications. As a result, many patients whose pain was initially well controlled with medication have to increase the drug dosages to nearly toxic levels in order to control their pain.

Role of Sympathetic Nerves in Trigeminal Neuralgia
The main objective of this study was to explore the role of cervical sympathetic blockade in the treatment of trigeminal neuralgia. This study establishes the sympathetic component in trigeminal neuralgia. The pathophysiological mechanisms proposed for neuropathic pain were central neuronal sensitization, central sensitization related damage to nervous system inhibitory functions, and abnormal interactions between the somatic and sympathetic nervous systems [8]. The fact that sympathetic fibers also communicate with the trigeminal nervous system at the level of Gasserian ganglion supports our hypothesis [9]. The results indicate that 77% patients had significant pain relief after the cervical sympathetic blockade. This effect persisted till 3 months in 44% of patients. The number of pain episodes had also significantly decreased following the intervention and persisted till 3 months. The hallmark of neuropathic pain is chronic allodynia and hyperalgesia. All our patients had trigger point allodynia and 77% of patients had relief from it at the end of 1 month after cervical sympathetic blockade. According to Bonica [10] and others [2, 11] if a patient reports good pain relief after a sympathetic block the patient can be said to have sympathetic mediated pain. Based on the aforementioned facts, pathophysiology of trigeminal neuralgia can be considered similar to other sympathetic mediated pain such as complex regional pain syndrome and it is amenable to treatment with sympathetic blocks.

Pain Relief in Trigeminal Neuralgia by Stellate Ganglion Block
In this study the duration of pain relief following cervical sympathetic blockade was approximately 2.44 ± 2.97 months in 66 % of patients which is comparable to the report of Max et al. [14] involving peripheral nerve block procedures. The effective pain relief claimed in their study was for 2 months in 74% of the patients.

In a study by Oturai et al. [13] involving peripheral nerve blocks for 45 patients trigeminal neuralgia, pain recurred in 50% of patients within a month. Eye problems and dysaesthesia were reported in 5-8% of patients. Serious complications such as cutaneous necrosis, bony sequestrum, diplopia, facial nerve palsy and loss of vision were reported in other studies [14, 15]. Several published series suggest a high level of initial success (87-98%) with microvascular decompression, experiencing immediate pain relief. Even in experienced hands, a mortality rate of 0.2 to 1% was described [16]. Complications reported by Max et al. [14] following alcohol injection were crawling sensations in 48%, burning discomfort in 33% and complete numbness in 3.7% of patients. A significant advantage of Stellate ganglion block in our patients was achievement of adequate pain relief without any complications such as cutaneous necrosis, facial nerve palsy, corneal anaesthesia or sensory loss.

However, some of the unpleasant side effects of Stellate ganglion blockade result from Horner's syndrome (ptosis, miosis and nasal congestion). Common complications result from diffusion of local anesthetic into the nearby nerves resulting in recurrent laryngeal nerve involvement. This is indicated by the complaints of the patient of hoarseness of voice, feeling of lump in the throat and sometimes subjective shortness of breath. The diffusion of local anesthetic may block phrenic nerve causing temporary paralysis of the diaphragm and can lead to respiratory embarrassment specifically in patients where respiratory reserve is already severely compromised. Partial brachial plexus block can also occur. The two most feared complications are intraspinal injection and intravascular injection of local anesthetic. Respiratory embarrassment and need for mechanical ventilation can result from injection into intrathecal space. Intravascular injection most often involves the vertebral artery and can cause unconsciousness, respiratory paralysis, seizures and sometimes severe arterial hypotension. In our study, no patient encountered any of these dreadful complications.

Response to Novel Noxious Stimulus

In the present study, a novel noxious stimulus (electrical stimulus) was required to be assessed by the patients in the background of chronic severe neuralgic pain. The phenomenon of altered perception of a novel stimulus in the background of severe almost continuous pain is reported in both animal and human studies [17, 18]. The novel experimental stimulus is highly reproducibly quantifiable unlike the chronic pain and, therefore, it is the assessment of novel stimulus per se obviously determined by the central neural state in the background of the chronic pain. The response to experimental vis-à-vis novel pain in a patient of chronic pain is now being utilized to assess chronic pain indirectly [19, 20, 21]. There is an altered threshold and suprathreshold response, a decrement in pain tolerance as well as in the ability to discriminate between sensations. Chronic pain itself, as per its definition induces stress and altered neurochemical profile thereby providing a different neurochemical milieu for processing fresh noxious stimuli [22, 23]. A number of recent studies have assessed the influence of baseline or induced mood on subjective and psychological responses to experimental stimulation. Baseline [24] and induced [25] anxiety have been shown to increase pain ratings to thermal or pressure pain ratings, while an experimentally induced depressive mood (induced by presentation of text with depressing themes) decreased tolerance to cold press or pain [26]. Pain memory processes have been investigated using experimental painful stimulation [27]. These studies provide experimental examples of how the experience of chronic pain can exert subtle influence on cognitive processes and mood besides the response to noxious stimulus. Pain itself can also impair cognitive and psychomotor performance [28].

Our results strongly support this contention. There was an increase in the threshold current for the pain associated with stimulation in our patients. Comparison of threshold amplitude with VAS at the end of 24 h and 2 months after the block revealed statistically significant decrease in the pain rating at 1 mA and 3 mA current strength, even though the difference at higher current intensities was not statistically significant. In chronic pain patients it is also reported that discriminating noxious stimuli from non-noxious stimuli is lost at higher intensity of stimulation [17].

Role of Endogenous Opioids

Endogenous opioids play an important role in pain control both at the spinal level and at the supraspinal level involving descending pathways [29]. It has been postulated that in sympathetic mediated pain, normal increase in endogenous opioids in regional sympathetic ganglia to prevent excessive autonomic activity, is lost [10]. Since the estimation of endogenous opioids and its correlation with pain relief is the main problem in various studies; beta endorphin in plasma, CSF [30], and circulating mononuclear leucocytes have been estimated in several chronic pain conditions [6, 7, 31]. CSF opioids estimation is an invasive technique and has a poor patient compliance, particularly for longitudinal studies. These procedures are expensive, tedious, and therefore cannot be used as a scanning test. Hence, we utilised leutinizing hormone levels following naloxone challenge to indirectly estimate the endogenous opioid system based on the study of Facchinetti et al. [6].

Our results revealed a decrease in LH levels of 5.808 IU/L post-sympathetic block compared to laboratory normal value of 13-20 IU/L. When compared with the pre-block values this decrease in the LH levels post-sympathetic block was not statistically significant, probably because of smaller sample size. Another interesting finding was that the LH surge following naloxone injection was not seen in the trigeminal neuralgia patients both pre- and post-block.

One explanation for this in chronic pain states could be the derangement in central opioidergic axis due to tonic inhibition which leads to an either impaired secretion or altered receptors status or both. Alternative explanation is that there is imbalance in the activity of several limbic and non-limbic areas involved in modulating pain due to the severe pain of trigeminal neuralgia itself. This may affect the opioid secretion. In our study, we have not directly measured the concentration of opioids, but the concentration of leutinizing hormone. The opioids are inhibited by the anti-opioid, naloxone, which in turn withdraws a tonic inhibition on the LH-RH neurons. Thereby involving a change in the excitability of the neurons. It is also likely that the neuronal excitability has altered due to the neuronal processes involved in severe chronic pain conditions or due to a concurrent change in the local neurochemical profile. It is difficult to comment on these aspects in human studies. It is hypothesized that there is tonic derangement of endogenous opioids secretion either at the level of higher cortical centers or at the level of periaqueductal gray. There is also a possibility of derangement of feedback loop of endogenous opioids system (EOS). Depending on the mechanism of disarray involved, patients may present with either an increase or decrease in endogenous opioids level that may or may not coincide with the degree of analgesia achieved. However, larger sample size and more sophisticated tests (NMR, PET) may provide a clear picture. There was no statistical difference in this study between premenopausal and postmenopausal women as well as males and females in terms of LH levels.

The data suggest that repeated cervical sympathetic blockade (Stellate ganglion blocks) with 0.25% Bupivacaine 10 ml, provides effective pain relief in majority of patients with trigeminal neuralgia. Cervical sympathetic blockade increases the pain threshold and therefore, probably breaks the vicious circle of neuropathic pain. The threshold current for pain perception can be used to assess the effectiveness of pain relief following the cervical sympathetic blockade in trigeminal neuralgia patients. Cervical sympathetic blockade results in supraspinal and/or spinal mediated analgesia. No life threatening complications or morbidity was seen following cervical sympathetic blockade in our study. It is a minimally invasive technique compared to other techniques. The results provided by estimation of leutinizing hormone in lieu of endogenous opioid per se for pain relief in trigeminal neuralgia by cervical sympathetic blockade although was not statistically significant exhibited a characteristic different pattern. Patients acceptance for the procedure was excellent.

To conclude, the pain of trigeminal neuralgia is sympathetically mediated and repeated cervical sympathetic blockade provides effective pain relief. However, studies with larger number of patients and longer duration of follow-up are needed to validate our findings.

References

1. Anonymous classification and diagnostic criteria for headache disorders, cranial neuralgias and facial pain. Headache Classification Committee of the International Headache Society. *Cephalalgia* 1988; **8**: 1–96.
2. Wall Patrick K.D. Textbook of pain (3rd ed), Churchill Livingstone, Harcourt Publishers Limited, p. 691.
3. Browsher D. Pain as a neurological emergency. Neurological Emergencies in Medical Practice, 1988: pp. 118–136.
4. Central pain complicating information following subarachnoid haemorrhage. *Br. J. Neurosurgery* 1989; **3**: 435–442.
5. Campbell R., Parks K.W. and Dodds R.N. Chronic facial pain associated with endodontic neuropathy, *Oral Surg Oral Med Oral Pathol.* 1990; **69**: 287–290.
6. Facchinetti F., Martignoni E., Gallai V., Mucieli G., Petraglia F., Nappi G., and Genazzani A.R. Neuroendocrine evaluation of central opiate activity in primary headache disorders. *Pain* 1988; **34**: 29–33.
7. Fransesco F., Luciano A., Marco P., Pierluig C., Giulia B., Gluseppina M, and Antonio V. Role of endogenous opiate systems in patients with syndrome X. *Am. Heart J.* 1998; **136**: 1003–1009.
8. Mori T., Terai T. and Hatano M. et al. Stellate ganglion blocks improved loss of

visual acuity caused by Retro bulbar optic neuritis after herpes zoster. *Anesthesia Analgesia* 1997; **85**: 870–871.

9. Stanton-Hicks M., Prithvi Raj P. and Racz G.B. Use of Regional Anesthetics in the Diagnosing Reflex Sympathetic Dystrophy and Sympathetically Maintained Pain. Editors Janig W., Stanton-Hicks M. Reflex Sympathetic Dystrophy: a reappraisal. IASP Press, Seattle 1996; 217– 23.

10. Bonica's Management of Pain 3rd Ed, Editor Johan D. Loeser J.D. Chapman C.J., Fordyce W.E., Stephan H.B. and Dennis C.T., Lippincott Williams and Wilkins, Philadelphia, 2001; p 390 .

11. Lichtor T. and Mullan J.F. A 10-year follow-up review of percutaneous microcompression of the trigeminal ganglion. *J. Neurosurg.* 1990; **72**: 49–54.

12. Guieu R., Blin O., Pouget J. and Serratrice G. Analgesic effect of Indomethacin showed using the nociceptive flexion reflex in humans. *Annals of Rheumatic Diseases* 1992; **51**: 391–393.

13. Oturai A.B., Jensen K. Erikson -J. and Marsden F. Neurosurgery for trigeminal neuralgia: Comparison of alcohol block, neurectomy and radiofrequency coagulation. *Clin. J. Pain* 1996; **2**: 311–1 .

14. Max M.P. et al. Trigeminal neuralgia. A revision of six hundred and eightynine cases with a follow-up study on sixtyfive percent of the group. *J. Neurosurg* 1952; **9**: 367–71.

15. Fardy M.J. and Patton D.W. Complications associated with peripheral alcohol injections in the management of trigeminal neuralgia. *Br Oral Maxillofac Surg.* 1994; **32**: 387–91.

16. Barker F.G., Jannette P.J., Bissonette D.J., Larkins M.Y. and Jho H.D. The long-term outcome of microvascular decompression for trigeminal neuralgia. *N. Eng. J. Med.* 1996; **334**: 1077–83.

17. Sood S. Brain evoked potential correlates in chronic pain. Ph.D. thesis submitted to AIIMS, 2000.

18. Fordyce W.E. A learning in pain. In: RA Sternbach (Ed). Psychology of pain, Raven Press, New York 1976; **49**: 22.

19. Gracely R.H. Psychophysical assessment of human pain. In: Bonica JJ, Liebeskind J.C., Able-Fessard DG (eds.). Adances in pain research and therapy 1979; Raven Press, New York.

20. Price D.D., Rafii A., Watkins L.R. and Buckingham B. A psychophysical analysis of acupuncture analgesia. *Pain* 1984; **19**: 24–42.

21. Gibson S.J., La Vasseur S.A. and Helme R.D. Cerebral even related responses induced by CO_2 laser stimulation in subjects suffering from cervico-brachial syndrome. *Pain* 1991; **47**: 173–182.

22. Leppler J.G., Greenberg H.J. The P3 potential and its clinical usefulness in the objective classification of demands. *Cortex* 1984; **20**: 427–433.

23. Gamsa A. Is emotional disturbance a precipitator or a consequence of chronic pain? Elsevier, *Pain* 1990; **42**: 183–195.

24. Gaughan A.M. and Gracely R.H. A somatisation model of repressed negative emotions: defensiveness increase affective rating of thermal pain sensations. Society of Behavioral Medicine Abstracts, 1989.

25. Cornwall A. and Donderi D.C. The effect of experimentally induced anxiety on the experience of pressure pain. *Pain* 1988; **35**: 105–113.

26. Zelman D.C., Howland E.W., Nicholas S.N. and Cleeland C.S. The effects of induced mood on laboratory pain. *Pain* 1991; **46**: 105–11.

27. Seltzer S.F. and Yarczower M. Selecting encoding and retrieval of affective words during exposure to aversive stimulation. *Pain* 1991; **47**: 47–51.

28. Lorenz J. and Bromm B. Event-related potential correlates of interference between cognitive performance and tonic experimental pain. *Psychophysiol.* 1997; **34**: 436–445.

29. Elias M., Chakerian M., Repeated Stellate ganglion block using a catheter for pediatric Herpes zoster opthalmicus. *Anesthesiology* 1994; **80**: 950–952.

30. Hardebo J.C., Ekman M., Eriksson M., Holgersson S. and Ryberg B. CSF opioid levels in cluster headache. In: Clifford Rose (ed) Migraine, Kargel Basel 1985; 79–85.

31. Buratti T. Decreased levels of β-endorphine in circulating mononuclear leucocytes from patients with acute myocardial infarction. *Cardiology*, 1998; **90**: 43–47.

23. Cyclooxygenases: As Novel Drug Target(s) in CNS Related Disorders

S.K. Kulkarni, Ashish Dhir and Pattipati S. Naidu

Pharmacology Division, University Institute of Pharmaceutical Sciences,
Panjab University, Chandigarh-160 014, India

Introduction

Approximately 17 million Americans take non-steroidal anti-inflammatory drugs daily for the treatment of pain and inflammation. These drugs are non-selective inhibitors of cyclooxygenase (COX) enzyme. Cyclooxygenase is a key enzyme that converts arachidonic acid derived from membrane phospholipids to prostaglandins, which have important signaling, and housekeeping functions [1]. Three isoforms of cyclooxygenase enzyme have been identified and they are found to be present almost in all tissues including the brain. It is generally accepted that, in intact brain, neurons are the predominant cell group expressing cyclooxygenase-2 (COX-2) [2]. Expression of COX in brain resulted in its involvement in various CNS related disorders such as neuroinflammatory and neurodegenerative disorders, e.g. as in Alzheimer's, Parkinson's, Amyotrophic lateral sclerosis, epilepsy, memory, AIDS-induced dementia, stroke, and other diseases including depression, mania, pain, fever etc. In all these disorders, COX-2 isoform enzyme has been reported to be expressed and the role of cyclooxygenase-1 (COX-1) in various neurological diseases has been therefore overlooked. Moreover, COX-2 inhibitors are reported to be beneficial in some of the abovementioned CNS disorders.

Pathway of Arachidonic Acid Release and Metabolism

Arachidonic acid is the most important precursor of the eicosanoids. It is a 20 carbon chain fatty acid. For eicosanoid synthesis to occur, arachidonic acid must first be released or mobilized from membrane phospholipids by one or more lipase of the phospholipase A_2 type. At least three phospholipase types mediate arachidonic acid release from membrane phospholipids. They are cardiac PLA_2 ($CPLA_2$), cytosolic PLA_2 and secretory PLA_2. Following mobilization from membrane phospholipids, four different routes, i.e. Lipoxygenase(s), Epoxygenase(s), Cyclooxygenase(s) and Free radical(s) [3] oxidize arachidonic acid. After its release from the membrane phospholipids, arachidonic acid is acted upon by cyclooxygenase isoenzyme and form prostaglandins. The two isoforms are COX-1 and COX-2. If acted upon by COX-1 it leads to the formation of constitutive prostaglandins and if acted upon by COX-2 isoenzyme it leads to formation of regulated prostaglandins that have both pathophysiological and adaptive roles in the body system (Fig.1) [6]. Protective PG's, which preserve the integrity of the stomach lining and maintain normal renal functions in a compromised kidney, are synthesized by COX-1. In addition COX-1 is also present in platelets that lead to thromboxane A_2 production, causing aggregation of platelets to prevent inappropriate bleeding [4]. COX-2 on the other hand can be induced by inflammatory stimuli and by cytokines in migratory and other cells, suggesting that the anti-inflammatory action of NSAIDs are due to the inhibition of COX-2, whereas the unwanted side effects such as damage to the stomach lining and toxic effects on the kidney are due to the inhibition of the constitutive enzyme COX-1, respectively [5].

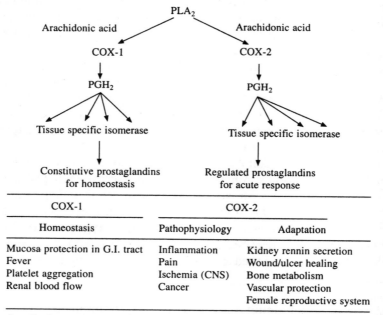

Fig. 1. Cyclooxygenase pathway and the functions of cyclooxygenase isozymes.

Location of Cyclooxygenases in Brain

Prostaglandins are unevenly distributed throughout the brain and specific PG's are more abundant in some species than others. In 1991, Tsuborkuro et al [7] were the first to localize COX-1 to neurons and glial cells in monkey brain. In 1993, Yamagata et al [8] first described the basal COX-2 expression in rat brain.

Cyclooxygenase is expressed in the neuron and the glial cells of the brain. Indeed, brain is one of the few tissues that contains detectable levels of

COX-2 mRNA under normal conditions. Highest level of COX expression was observed in olfactory bulbs, followed by midbrain and hypothalamus, with the lowest levels in hippocampus [9]. COX-1 was mostly expressed in the dorsolateral tegmentum, the dentate gyrus, the superior colliculus, distinct hypothalamic regions, the raphe nuclei and the nucleus of the solitary tract [10]. COX-2 mRNA was localized by Yamagata et al using COX-2 specific antiserum. COX-2 immunoreactivity was found in subcortical nuclei, including the paraventricular and median preoptic nuclei of the hypothalamus, the dorsal raphe nuclei, the lamina terminalis etc. [11]. COX-2 expression was abundantly expressed in neonatal microvasculature and cortex, but decreased in older animals.

Glial cells such as microglia, astrocytes and oligodendrocytes also express cyclooxygenases. Different studies indicate its expression in microglia. COX-2 is induced in cultured microglia by lipopolysaccharide (LPS) [12]. COX-1 immunoreactive glial cells are observed in human, monkey and rat brain using different antibodies. COX-1 immunoreactivity in astrocytes has not been observed in vivo [13]. These cyclooxygenases in glial cells get over-expressed during the inflammatory process in brain and NSAID's can prevent the inflammation.

In general, cyclooxygenase-1 is present in:

(a) cortical layer 2 of frontal, temporal, parietal, occipital lobe.
(b) hypothalamus.
(c) all regions of hippocampus [14].

Extensive COX-1-ir was found throughout cholinergic neurons of human basal forebrain [15].

Cyclooxygenase-2 is present in:

(a) pyramidal cells of hippocampus.
(b) dentate gyrus.
(c) piriform cortex.
(d) layer 2 and 3 of neocortex.

Neocortical regions and subcortical structures include amygdala, striatum, thalamus, hypothalamus [11]. Neuronal cell bodies, i.e. in proximal and distal dendrites and dendritic spines. Majority of cyclooxygenases are excitatory and glutamatergic neurons and it is generally accepted that in intact brain, neurons are the predominant cell group expressing COX-2 in all species examined and COX-2 is majorly present in all parts of brain [16].

Cyclooxygenases in Various CNS Related Disorders

Neuroinflammatory and Neurodegenerative Disorders
Oxidative stress in the brain is produced by the generation of free radicals like reactive radicals of oxygen such as superoxide anion, hydroxyl radical

and peroxy radical, reactive non-radicals of oxygen such as hydrogen peroxide and singlet oxygen and also includes radicals of C, N and S [18]. These free radicals cause damage to neurons and involved in various neurodegenerative disorders such as Alzheimer's disease, Parkinson's disease, HIV induced dementia and Amyotrophic lateral sclerosis [19].

Involvement of the cyclooxygenase enzyme in neurodegeneration and neuroinflammation is shown in Fig. 2 [17].

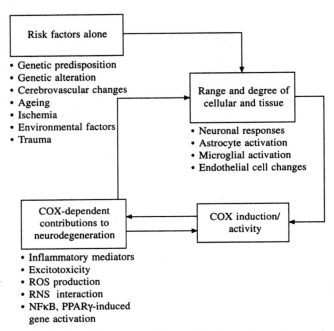

Fig. 2.   Involvement of cyclooxygenase in neuroinflammation and neurodegeneration.

Cyclooxygenase and Alzheimer's Disease

Alzheimer's disease is the most common form of dementia in the ageing population, affecting more than four million people in the USA alone. The disease generally persists with memory impairment, and as it progresses over 5-10 year period it affects most of the cortical functions, consistent with pathological changes. These changes include neuronal and synaptic loss, the presence of intracellular cytoskeletal tangles and extracellular accumulation of amyloid beta peptides as "plaques".

NSAIDs delay the onset and slow the progression of Alzheimer's diseases. Jenkinson's et al. [20] reported that AD was less prevalent in patients with rheumatoid arthritis than in general population and it was suggested that the negative association of rheumatoid arthritis and AD might be due to the significant use of anti-inflammatory agents in these patients [21]. In addition to neurofibrillary tangles and amyloid beta deposition, there is a marked inflammatory reaction in AD patients characterized by glial activation and endogenous expression of the pro-inflammatory cytokines, complement components and acute phase reaction proteins [22, 23]. Thus NSAIDs may act to slow or prevent AD by inhibiting ongoing inflammatory processes in Alzheimer's brain. In one study, PGD_2 levels were found to be significantly higher in AD brain relative to control and it was speculated that neuronal cyclooxygenase activity was increased in Alzheimer's disease [24]. There was an increase in COX-2 mRNA (25%) levels in frontal cortex of nine AD patients [25]. The COX-2 immunostaining of tangle bearing neurons of AD and Down's syndrome patients was reported by Oka and Takashima [26]. The National Institute of Ageing (NIA) in 2000 launched a clinical trial to determine whether treatment with certain NSAIDs will slow cognitive and clinical decline in people with AD. The study evaluates two NSAIDs namely rofecoxib and naproxen a selective COX-2 inhibitor and a non-specific COX inhibitor, respectively. This was the first clinical trial.

Cyclooxygenase and Parkinsonism

Parkinson's disease is a common neurodegenerative disorder whose clinical manifestations include resting tremor, slowness of movement, rigidity and postural instability. Proinflammatory cytokines, IL-10, TNF-α and IFN-α, induce CD-23 expression in glial cells which triggers iNOS expression and NO release. NO may amplify the production of cytokines within the glial cells but also diffuse to neighboring dopaminergic neurons. It is debated that whether infiltrated T lymphocytes could be the cellular source of IFN-γ in patients of Parkinson's disease brains. NO produced by activated glial cells can react with superoxide (O^{2-}) to form peroxynitrite ($ONOO^-$), which can damage proteins and other cell constituents. NO also may contribute to oxidative stress by releasing iron from ferritin [16].

Several studies have been carried out on the basis of the role of COX in Parkinson's disease. In one study, 6-hydroxydopamine lesioned rats (model for Parkinson's disease), the level of TNF-α, was found to be enhanced both in striatum and substantia nigra. It has been demonstrated that targeted deletions of the COX-2 gene in mouse confers some protection against MPTP induced dopaminergic cell death [27]. A higher dose of amino salicylic acid (ASA) (100 mg/kg) and meloxicam (50 mg/kg) showed an almost complete protection against MPTP induced cell loss. It normalizes the compensatory increase of dopamine turnover and alters the MPTP induced decrease in locomotor activity [28].

Cyclooxygenase in HIV-induced Dementia and Other CNS Infections

Dementia is an important complication of HIV infection. Pathological hallmark of AIDS dementia include neuronal loss and cytokine dysregulation. In CNS, macrophage and microglia are infectively infected with HIV [29]. Prostaglandins were elevated in the brain of subjects with HIV associated dementia [30]. Intracerebroventricular injection of HIV recombinant protein gp-120 COX-2 immunoreactivity in cortical neurons while indomethacin reduced apoptic neuronal death induced by gp-120 in neocortex [31]. COX-2 is also unregulated in other CNS infections. For example, increased levels of cyclooxygenase-2 were observed in cortical neurons and glia of rats injected with Borna disease virus [32].

Cyclooxygenase and Amyotrophic Lateral Sclerosis

The pathogenesis of cell death in amyotrophic lateral sclerosis (ALS) may involve glutamate mediated excitotoxicity, oxidative damage and apoptosis [33]. Recent evidences provide important support for a pathogenic role of COX-2, an inducible enzyme that increases in brain after synaptic activity, seizures or ischemia and in the spinal cord after direct physical trauma to the cord [34]. COX-2 was found to be increased in spinal cord of transgenic ALS mice and there are increased levels of PGE_2. It causes the release of calcium ions in astrocytes, which is necessary and sufficient to cause glutamate release [35] leading to excitotoxicity. Celecoxib, a selective COX-2 inhibitor decreased PGE_2 formation and thereby showing beneficial effects. Another mechanism by which COX-2 inhibitors may be protective in ALS is by interruption of inflammatory process that causes the production of reactive oxygen species (ROS), free radicals, proinflammatory cytokines and other toxic molecules.

Cyclooxygenase and Memory

Cyclooxygenase-2 inhibitors have a role in memory. There is a role of COX-2 in cell signaling [14]. Some evidences, which indicate a potential role of COX in physiological mechanisms underlying memory formation, are as follows:

1. Cardiac phospholipase A_2 ($CPLA_2$) also produces intracellular platelet activating factor (PAF). PAF is a putative retrograde messenger in hippocampal long-term potentiation (LTP) [36] and PAF has a regulatory effect on COX-2 transcription [37] indicating a possible interaction between intracellular PAF function and prostaglandin pathway in memory.
2. The role of excitatory amino acid (NMDA) receptors in memory has been well documented and COX-2 is expressed in neurons as an immediate early gene [7] in an NMDA receptor dependent manner, in which COX causes the impairment of adrenergic, and glutamatergic neurotransmission.

Cyclooxygenase and Seizures

Epilepsy is a common neuropsychiatry disorder affecting about 0.5-1% of the world population. Clinical signs of epilepsy arise from the intermittent, excessively synchronized activity of the group of neurons. Different neurotransmitters and neuro-modulators are known to play a role in epilepsy. At least four important neurotransmitters namely GABA, glutamate, dopamine and acetylcholine are reported to play a key role in the normal functioning of limbic system, the area that play an important role in the onset of seizure activity. The neuromodulation by prostaglandins and their possible role in epileptogenesis has recently [38] been studied. Cyclooxygenase-2 expression is markedly and transiently up regulated in neurons in response to excitatory stimuli such as seizures and kainic acid as compared to COX-1 expression [36]. Selective COX-2 inhibitors reduce the onset of convulsions in pentylenetetrazol (PTZ)-induced seizure model suggesting the role of COX-2 in epilepsy.

In another model of lithium chloride and tacrine (5 mg/kg i.p.) induced status epilepticus seizures. There was also an expression of COX-2 enzyme protein particularly in dorsal hippocampus and elevated brain PGE_2 levels. Similarly, following kainic acid treatment there was significant rise (upto seven folds) in contents of PGE_2, $PGF_2\alpha$, PGD_2 over normal brain contents [39].

Some recent studies have indicated that NSAIDs can exacerbate seizures and prostaglandins have protection against convulsions, while other suggested that COX inhibition may be beneficial in some seizures paradigms. Therefore, it is controversial whether prostaglandins and COX-2 are epileptogenic or anti-epileptogenic.

Cyclooxygenase and Multiple Sclerosis

A limited number of studies investigating the pathogenesis of multiple sclerosis suggests the induction of iNOS and NO and oxygen free radicals by macrophages and microglia may be important in disease progression [40]. There is abundant accumulation of nitrotyrosine in active multiple sclerosis plaques as well as in lesions of acute experimental autoimmune encephalitis, a model for multiple sclerosis [41]. However, the extent to which these effects involve COX associated pathway is not yet clear.

Cyclooxygenase and Focal Ischemia

COX isoenzyme has also a role in focal ischemia. Inhibiting iNOS activity attenuated PGE_2 expression in brain even in the presence of abundant COX-2 expression. Cells like macrophages and neutrophils are capable of producing superoxide anion and nitric oxide during inflammatory process. It damages metabolic enzymes. Nitric oxide radical also reacts with oxygen radicals to form powerful and toxic oxidant, i.e. peroxynitrite free radical [16, 42]. Peroxynitrite free radical can act as peroxide source of oxidizing equivalents required to activate the peroxidase activity of COX and initiate COX turnover. Net effect of this is enhanced COX turnover include the production of pro-inflammatory associated PGE_2 [43].

Cyclooxygenase and Drug Addiction

Chronic ethanol treatment (4 days) produces a pattern of COX-2 induction that was generally similar to that induced by excitatory amino acids. Chronic ethanol treatment causes COX-2 expression in limbic cortex, cingulate medial prefrontal cortex and perirhinal cortex (150% increase), isocortex (150% increase in deeper layers) amygdala (70% increase). It is possible that induction of COX-2 in these limbic cortical regions during chronic ethanol treatment contributes to progressive nature of ethanol dependence and alcoholism [44]. Withdrawal from chronic ethanol treatment elicits a host of behavioral and neurological changes, including hyperactivity, anxiety, tremors and seizures [45]. These effects are due to over-activation of glutamate and under-activation of GABA neurotransmission [46]. There is 200% increase over control in COX-2 immunostaining found in infralimbic region of the medial prefrontal cortex and perirhinal cortex during withdrawal [43].

Cyclooxygenase and Schizophrenia

Schizophrenia is a devastating psychiatric disorder affecting about 1% of the population worldwide. Horrobin [47], speculated that in schizophrenia, there could be a failure of normal synthesis of prostaglandin in brain and drugs like aspirin increased the schizophrenia symptoms. In another study Watt [48] reported an increase in PGE levels in CSF of schizophrenics. There may be defect in 1 series prostaglandins with normal or near normal production of the 2 series leading to an imbalance between the two groups of compound. Further studies are needed to probe the role of cyclooxygenases and their metabolites in schizophrenia.

Cyclooxygenase and mania

Although very little is known about the role of COX enzyme in mania, Rapoport and Bosetti [49] hypothesized that lithium, an antimanic drug, acted by targeting parts of the arachidonic acid cascade which may be functionally hyperactive in mania. Thus, selective COX-2 inhibitors like celecoxib and rofecoxib could be used as an add on therapy with lithium, as lithium itself reduced COX-2 level in brain and the concentration of prostaglandin E_2. When lithium concentration reaches 0.7 nm in brain after administration of lithium chloride for four weeks, it results in the reduction of arachidonic acid turnover by 75%. COX-2 inhibitors also have a role in depression [50] and may be used in bipolar disorders.

Cyclooxygenase and Spreading Depression

Spreading depression (SD) is a wave of sustained depolarization challenging the energy metabolism of the cell without causing irreversible damage. Spreading depression is a wave of ionic transients involving release of K^+ and uptake of Ca^{2+}, Na^+ and Cl^- and it is most likely initiated and propagated by massive presynaptic release of glutamate and activation of N-methyl-D-aspartate receptors subsequent to local brain injury including focal brain ischemia [51]. It was described as a transient negative interstitial direct current potential that spreads from the site of initiation at a rate of 2-5 mm/min followed immediately by a prolonged disappearance of spontaneous electrocortical activity. When SD triggers a massive Ca^{2+} influx, which in energy compromised neurons is enough to initiate cell death cascade. Koistinaho and Chan [52] reported that SD directly induced COX-2 expression in focal brain ischemia by stimulating the NMDA receptor and activating phospholipase A_2. Only a few postmortem studies, however, reported COX-2 expressions in human brain ischemia [53]. Cyclooxygenase-2 gene expression increased by 1.6 fold in the SD group as detected using a DNA microarray.

Cyclooxygenase and CNS Tumors
It has been observed that there is increased COX-2 expression in many types of cancer [54]. Levels of arachidonic acid and PGE_2 were significantly higher in gliomas and meningiomas than in control brain tissue [55]. Prostaglandins synthesis may favor tumor growth by any mechanism that includes increased angiogenesis, increased proliferation and decreased tumor cell apoptosis [55].

COX-1 expressing microglia/macrophages were commonly found within tumor parenchyma and in areas of tumor infiltration and COX-2 positive cells were observed in surrounding areas of necrosis [56].

Cyclooxygenases and Pyrexia
Fever is one of the symptoms associated with infectious disease and inflammation. Enhanced production of PGE_2 in the brain has been associated with pyrexia [57].

LPS administration increases PGE_2 levels. in the brain in parallel with concomitant increase in body temperature [58]. There is strong evidence for a direct relationship between LPS induced expression of COX-2 in the brain and LPS induced fever. Further the idea that COX-2 rather than COX-1 is involved in fever is supported by recent evidences showing that LPS induced fever is impaired in COX-2 deficient but not in COX-1 deficient mice [59].

Conclusions
Cyclooxygenase and its products are extensively involved in neuroinflammation and neurodegenerative states. There is still much to be learnt about the roles of prostaglandins and cyclooxygenases in the CNS. These molecules exert an immediate effect and can also exacerbate secondary, long-lasting cascades of event that lead to significant pathology. The mechanisms by which COX and its products exert their damaging effects have yet to be fully defined. COX can also contribute to the free radical production and oxidative stress in a variety of ways. Although, COX-2 appears to participate in a variety of CNS disorders, the potential contribution of COX-1 should not be ignored. Sorting out clinically relevant roles for the therapeutic intervention and

understanding mechanisms by which COX isoforms contribute to CNS disease processes remain important areas for future research investigation.

References

1. Griffin MR. Epidemiology of nonsteroidal anti-inflammatory drug associated gastrointestinal injury. *Am J Med* 1998; **104**: 23S-29S, Discussion 41S-42S.
2. Lipsky P. Cyclooxygenase-2 specificity and its clinical implication. *The American Journal of Medicine* 1999; **106**: 51S-57S.
3. Foegl ML and Ramwell PW. In : Basic and clinical Pharmacology, 8th edition, Edited by BG Katzung (McGraw-Hill) 2001; 311.
4. Funk CD, Funk LB, Kennedy ME, Pong AS and Fitzgeroid GA, Human Platelet/ Erythroleukemia Cell Prostaglandin G/H Synthase: cDNA cloning expression and gene chromosomal assignment. *FASEB J* 1991; **5**: 2304–2312.
5. Vane JR, Michell JA, Appleton I, Tomlison A, Bishop BD, Croxtall J and Willoughby DA. Inducible isoforms of cyclooxygenase and nitric oxide synthase in inflammation. *Proc Natl Acad Sci USA* 1994; **91**: 2046–2050.
6. Kulkarni SK, Jain NK and Singh A. Cyclooxygenase isoenzyme and newer therapeutic potential for selective COX-2 inhibitor. *Methods and Findings in Experimental and Clinical Pharmacology* 2000; **22**: 291–298.
7. Tsuborkura S, Watanabe Y, Ehara H, Imamura K, Sugimoto O, Kagamiyama H, Yamamoto S and Hayaishi. Localisation of prostaglandin endoperoxide synthase in neurons and glia in monkey brain. *Brain Res* 1991; **543**: 15.
8. Yamagata K, Andreasson KI, Kaufmann WE, Barnes C A and Worley PF. Expression of a mitogen inducible cyclooxygenase in brain neurons: regulation by synaptic activity and glucocorticoids. *Neuron* 1993; **11**: 371–386.
9. Kawasaki M, Yoshihara Y, Yamaji M and Watanabe Y. Expression of prostaglandin endoperoxide synthase in rat brain. *Brain Res Mol Brain Res* 1993; **19**: 39–46.
10. Norton JL, Adamsom SL, Bocking AD and Han VK. Prostaglandin-H synthase-1 (PGHS-1) gene is expressed in specific neurons of the brain of the late gestation ovine fetus. *Brain Res Dev Brain Res* 1996; **95**: 79–96.
11. Breder CD, Dewitt D, Kraig RP. Characterization of inducible cyclooxygenase in rat brain. *J Comp Neurol* 1995; **355**: 296–315.
12. Minghetti L, Polazzi E, Nicoline A, Cerminon C and Levi G. Up-regulation of cyclooxygenase-2 expression in cultured microglia by prostaglandin E_2 cyclic AMP and non-steroidal anti-inflammatory drugs. *Euro J Neurosci* 1997; **9**: 934–940.
13. O'Banion MK, Miller JC, Chang JW, Kaplan MD and Coleman PD. Interleukin-1 beta induces prostaglandin G/H synthase-2 (Cyclooxygenase-2) in primary murine astrocyte culture. *J Neurochem* 1996; **66**: 2532–2540.
14. Breder CD, Smith WL, Raz A, Masferrer J, Seibert K, Needlemen P and Saper CB. Distribution and characterization of cyclooxygenase immunoreactivity in the ovine brain. *J Comp Neurol* 1992; **322**: 409–438.
15. Yermakova A and O'Banion MK. Cyclooxygenase-1 immunoreactivity in human nucleus basalis cholinergic neurons. *Soc Neurosci Abstr* 2002; **24**: 1994.
16. Kaufman WE, Worley PF, Pegg J, Bremer PJ and Isakson P. COX-2 a synaptically induced enzyme is expressed by excitatory neurons at postsynaptic sites in rat cerebral cortex. *Proc Natl Acad Sci USA* 1996, **93**: 2317–2321.
17. Maida ME and O'Banion MK. The cyclooxygenase in neuroinflammation

and neurodegeneration: Emerging perspectives. *Inflammatory Events in Neurodegeneration* 2001: 189.

18. Thomas JA. Oxidative stress and oxidant defense. In modern nutrition in health and disease. Published by Williams and Wilkins, Baltimore, 1998; 751–760.

19. Strong R, Mattammal MB and Andron AC. Free radicals, the aging brain and age related neurodegenerative disorders. In: Free radicals in aging (YUBP ed), CRC Press, Bocarton 1993; pp. 223–246.

20. Jenkinson ML, Bliss MR, Brain AT and Scott DL. Rheumatoid arthritis and Senile dementia of the Alzheimer's type. *Br J Rheumatol* 1989; **28**: 86–88.

21. McGeer P L, McGeer E, Rogers J and Sibly J. Anti-inflammatory drugs and Alzheimer's disease, *Lancet* 1990; **335**: 1037.

22. McGeer PL and McGeer EG. The inflammation response system of the brain: implications for the therapy of Alzheimer and other neurodegenerative diseases. *Brain Res Rev* 1995; **21**: 195–218.

23. Rogers J and O'Brarr S. Inflammatory mediators in Alzheimer's disease. In: Molecular Mechanism of Dementia Edited by Wasco W and Tnazi RE, Humana Press Inc., Totowa NJ, 1997; 177.

24. Iwamoto N, Kobayashi K and Kosaka K. The formation of prostaglandins in the postmortem cerebral cortex of Alzheimer's type dementia patients. *J Neurol* 1989; **236**: 80–84.

25. Pasinetti GM and Aisen PS. Cyclooxgenase-2 expression is increased in frontal cortex of Alzheimer's disease brain. *Neuroscience* 1998; **87**: 319–324.

26. Oka A and Takashima S. Induction of cyclooxygenase-2 in brains of patients with Down's syndrome and dementia of the Alzheimer's type specific localization in affected neurons and axons. *Neuroreport* 1997; **8**: 1161–1164.

27. Teismann P, Jackson-Lewis V, Vila M and Przedborski S. Cyclooxgenase-2 deficient mice are resistant to MPTP (Abstract). *Soc Neurosci Abstr* 2001; **688**: 2.

28. Teismann P, Schwaninger M, Weih F, Ferger B. Nuclear factor-kappaB activation is not involved in a MPTP model of Parkinson's disease. *Neuroreport* 2001; **12**: 1049–1053.

29. Petito CK, Adkins B, Tracey K, Roberts B, Torres-Munoz J, McCarthy M and Czeisler C. Chronic systemic administration of tumor necrosis factor alpha and HIV gp120: effects on adult rodent brain and blood-brain barrier, *J Neurovirol* 1999; **5**: 314–318.

30. Griffin DE, Wesselingh SL and McArthur JC. Elevated central nervous system prostaglandin in human immunodeficiency virus associated dementia. *Ann Neurol* 1994; 35:592–597.

31. Bagetta G, Corasaniti MT, Paoletti AM, Berliocchi L, Nistico R, Giammarioli AM, Malorni W and Finazzi-Agro A. HIV-1, gp120-induced apoptosis in the rat neocortex involves enhanced expression of cyclooxygenase-2(COX-2). *Biochem Biophys Res Comm* 1998; **244**: 819–824.

32. Röhrenbeck AM, Bette M, Hooper DC, Nyberg F, Eiden LE, Dietzschold B and Weihe E. Upregulation of COX-2 and CGRP expression in resident cells of the Borna disease virus-infected brain is dependent upon inflammation. *Neurobiol Dis* 1999; **6**: 15–34.

33. Drachman DB, Frank K, Dykes-Hoberg M, Teismann P, Almer G, Pizedborski S and Rothstein JD. Cyclooxygenase-2 inhibition protects motor neurons and prolong survival in a transgenic mouse model of ALS. *Ann Neurol* 2002; **52**: 771–778.

34. Resnick DK, Graham SH, Dixon CE and Marion DW. Role of cyclooxygenase-2 in acute spinal cord injury. *J Neurotrauma* 1998; **15**: 1005–1013.

35. Bezzi P, Carmignoto G, Pasti L, Vesce S, Rossi D, Rizzini BL, Pozzan T and Volterra A. Prostaglandins stimulate calcium-dependent glutamate release in astrocytes, *Nature* 1998; **391**: 281–285.

36. Clark GD, Happel LT, Zorumski CF and Bazan NZ. The role of platelet activating factor in the release of excitotoxic neurotransmitters. *J Lipid Mediators and Cell Signaling* 1994; **10**: 95.

37. Bazan NG, Fletcher BS, Herschman HR and Mukherjee PK. Platelet-activating factor and retinoic acid synergistically activate the inducible prostaglandin synthase gene. *Proc Natl Acad Sci* 1994; **91**: 5252–5256.

38. Takemiya T, Suzuki K, Sugiura H, Yasuda S, Yamagata K, Kawakami Y and Maru E. Inducible brain COX-2 facilitates the recurrence of hippocampal seizures in mouse rapid kindling. *Prostaglandins and Other Lipid Mediators* 2003; **71**: 205–216.

39. Ciceri P, Zhang Y, Shaffer AF, Leahy KM, Woerner MB, Smih WG, Seibert K, Isakson PC. Pharmacology of celecoxib in rat brain after kainate administration. *J Pharmacol Exp Ther* 2002; **302**: 846–852.

40. Vander Veen RC, Hinton DR, Incardonna F and Hofman FM. Extensive peroxynitrite activity during progressive stages of CNS inflammation. *J Neuroimmunol* 1997; **77**: 1–7.

41. Cross AH, San M, Stern MK, Keeling RM, Salvemini D and Misko TP. A catalyst of peroxynitrite decomposition inhibits murine experimental autoimmune encephalomyelitis. *J Neuroimmunol* 2000; **107**: 21–28.

42. Gross SS and Wolin MS. Nitric oxide pathophysiological mechanism. *Ann Rev Physiol* 1995; **57**: 737–769.

43. Padmaja S, Squadrito GL and Pryor WA. Inactivation of glutathione peroxidase by peroxynitrite. *Arch Biochem Biophys* 1998; **349(1)**: 1–6.

44. Knapp DJ and Crews FT. Induction of cyclooxygenase-2 in brain during acute and chronic ethanol treatment and ethanol withdrawal. *Alcoholism: Clinical and Experimental Research* 1999; **23**: 633–643.

45. Pohorecky LA, Cagan M, Brick J and Jaffe SL. The startle response in rats: effect of ethanol. *Pharmacol Biochem Behav* 1976; **4**: 311–316.

46. Frye GD, McTown TJ and Breese GR. Characterization of susceptibility to audiogenic seizures in ethanol dependent rats after microinjection of gamma-aminobutyric acid (GABA) agonists into the inferior colliculus substantia nigra or medial septum. *J Pharmacol Exp Ther* 1983; **227**: 663–670.

47. Horrobin D. Prostaglandins and schizophrenia. *The Lancet* 1980; **1(8170)**: 706–707.

48. Watt D. Prostaglandin and Schizophrenia. *The Lancet* 1979; **1(8117)**: 668–669.

49. Rapoport SI and Bosetti F. Do lithium and anticonvulsants target the brain arachidonic acid cascade in bipolar disorder. *Arch Gen Psychiatry* 2002; **59**: 592–596.

50. Leonard BE and Song C. Changes in the immune system in rodent model of depression. *International Journal of Neuropsychopharmacology* 2002; **5**: 345–356.

51. Kraig RP and Nicholson C. Extracellular ionic variation during spreading depression. *Neuroscience* 1978; **3**: 1045–1059.

52. Koistinaho J and Chan PH. Spreading depression-induced cyclooxygenase-2 expression in the cortex. *Neurochem Res* 2000; **25**: 645–651.

53. Iadecola C, Froster C, Nogawa S, Clark HB and Ross ME. Cyclooxygenase-2 immunoreactivity in the human brain following cerebral ischemia. *Acta Neuropathol* (Berl) 1999; **98**: 9–14.

54. Williams CS, Mann M and Dubois RN. The role of cycloxygenase in inflammation cancer, and development. *Oncogene* 1999; **18**: 7908–7916.

55. Kokoglu E, Tuter Y, Snadikci KS, Yazici Z, Ulakoglu EZ, Sonmez H and Ozyurt E. Prostaglandin E_2 levels in human brain tumor tissue and arachidonic acid levels in the plasma membrane of human brain tumors. *Cancer Lett* 1998; **132**: 17–21.

56. Deininger MH and Schluesener HJ. CP-10 a chemotactic peptide, is expressed in lesions of experimental autoimmune encephalomyelitis uveitis and in C6 gliomas. *J Neuroimmunol* 1999; **93(1–2)**: 156–163.

57. Stitt JT. Prostaglandin E as the mediator of the febrile response. *Yale J Biol Med* 1986; **59**: 137–149.

58. Sirko S, Bishas I and Coceani F. Prostaglandin formation in the hypothalamus in vivo: effect of pyrogens. *Am J Physiol* 1989; **256**: R616–R624.

59. Lis Wang Y, Matsumura K, Ballou LR, Morham SG and Blatteis CM. The febrile response to lipopolysaccharide is blocked in cyclooxygenase-2(-*l*-) but not in cyclooxygenase-1(-*l*-) mice. *Brain Res* 1999; **825**: 89-94.

24. Antinociceptive Effect of Cyclooxygenase and Lipooxygenases (COX/5-LOX) Inhibitors

Mahendra Bishnoi, Anil Kumar,
C.S. Patil and S.K. Kulkarni

University Institute of Pharmaceutical Science, Panjab University,
Chandigarh-160014, India

Abstract: NSAIDs are well known to produce antinociceptive effect via the inhibition of the cyclooxygenase enzyme. However, lipooxygenases pathway is also involved in nociceptive process. In the present study, effect of dual inhibition of cyclooxygenase and lipooxygenase pathways were assessed in chemonociceptive model of pain. Naproxen (5-20 mg/kg, p.o.), nimesulide (1-4 mg/kg, p.o.), rofecoxib (1-4 mg/kg, p.o.) and AKBA (50-200 mg/kg, p.o.) [a 5-LOX inhibitor] produced a dose dependent and significant antinociceptive effect in acetic acid-induced chemonociception in mice. Co-administration of subeffective dose of naproxen (5 mg/kg p.o.), nimesulide (1 mg/kg p.o.) and rofecoxib (1 mg/kg p.o.) with AKBA (100 mg/kg p.o.) produced a significant antinociceptive effect as compared to *per se*. However, the effect of nimesulide (a preferential COX-2 inhibitor) with AKBA was more pronounced as compared to other combinations with AKBA. The present study provides an evidence for beneficial effect dual inhibitors (COX/LOX).

Introduction

Oxidized arachidonic acid (AA) derivatives, collectively termed as eicosanoids (prostaglandins and leukotrienes) are now well established to play a key role in sensitization of nociceptors and nociceptive processing [1]. Isoforms of COX (COX-1 and COX-2) enzymes are produced in inflammation and pain related conditions. Various theories have also been put forward to explain how the efficacy of cyclooxygenase increases with 5-lipooxygenase enzyme inhibitors [2-3].

Lipooxygenases products of arachidonic acid metabolism are generated by the sensory neurons and have been implicated directly in activating the capsaicin sensitive vanilloid receptors (VR-1) [4-6]. Besides this they also activate extracellular signal regulated kinase (ERK) through the pertussis toxin (PTX), sensitive G-protein (Gi/Go) and PKC dependent pathways [1, 7]. MK 886, a 5-LOX inhibitor blocked carrageenan induced knee joint incapacitation, a measure of tonic pain [8].

Based on possible activity of both cyclooxygenase and lipooxygenases metabolites, various theories have also been put forth to explain how the efficacy of cyclooxygenase was increased with 5-lipooxygenase enzyme inhibitors [2-3]. Therefore, in the present study various cyclooxygenase inhibitors such as naproxen, nimesulide, rofecoxib and AKBA, a specific LOX inhibitor (acetyl-11-keto-β-boswellic acid), have been tried to explore their synergism. AKBA is one of the four major pentacyclic tripterpenic acids (boswellic acids) present in the acidic extract of *Boswellia serrata* gum resin. 3.8% AKBA is present in the complete acidic extract. AKBA is a novel highly specific inhibitor of the 5-lipooxygenase, the key enzyme for starting the synthesis of all leukotrienes. It has been suggested that AKBA inhibit 5-LOX either by directly interacting with 5-LOX or interacting with the 5-lipooxygenase activating protein (FLAP).

Materials and Methods

Animals: Laka mice (20-30 g) of either sex, bred in central animal house (CAH) of Panjab University, Chandigarh, maintained at 12 h light and dark cycle were used in the study. Animals were housed under standard lab conditions, with free access to food and water. All behavioral experiments were carried out between 0900 and 1700 h. The experimental protocols were approved by IAEC of the university.

Drugs, dose and treatment: The drugs used were naproxen (5, 10, 20 mg/kg), nimesulide (1, 2, 4 mg/kg), rofecoxib (1, 2, 4 mg/kg) and AKBA (50, 100, 200 mg/kg). All the drugs were dissolved into 0.5% CMC and administered per orally (p.o.) 45 min prior to the acetic acid (1%, i.p.) administration.

Acetic acid induced writhing assay [9]: Acetic acid solution (1%, 10 ml/kg i.p.) was used to produce writhing in mice. The number of wriths (constriction of abdomen, turning of trunk/twist, extension of hind legs) due to acetic acid was expressed as nociceptive response. Number of wriths per animal was counted during a 20 min session, beginning 3 min after the injection of acetic acid.

Statistical analysis: Results were expressed as mean ± SEM. The difference in response to test drugs and controls was determined by one-way ANOVA followed by Dunnets test. $P < 0.05$ was considered statistically significant.

Results

Antinociceptive Effects of Different COX and LOX Inhibitors

Naproxen (5, 10, 20 mg/kg), nimesulide (1, 2, 4 mg/kg), rofecoxib (1, 2, 4 mg/kg), AKBA (50, 100, 200 mg/kg) exerted a significant dose dependent antinociceptive effect (reduction in the number of wriths) against acetic acid induced chemonociception in mice (Figs. 1 and 2).

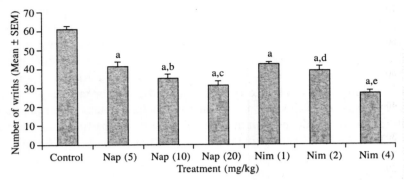

Fig. 1.   Dose response effect of naproxen and nimesulide in acetic acid induced writhing test. [a]$P < 0.05$ as compared to control, [b]$P < 0.05$ as compared to Nap (5), [c]$P < 0.05$ as compared to Nap (10), [d]$P < 0.05$ as compared to Nim (1), [e]$P < 0.05$ as compared to Nim (2).

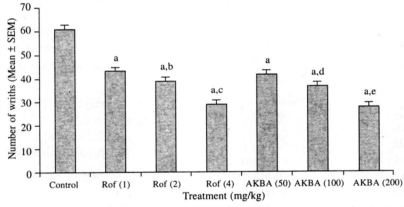

Fig. 2.   Dose response effect of rofecoxib and AKBA in acetic acid induced writhing test. [a]$P < 0.05$ as compared to control, [b]$P < 0.05$ as compared to Rof (1), [c]$P < 0.05$ as compared to Rof(2), [d]$P < 0.05$ as compared to AKBA (50), [e]$P < 0.05$ as compared to AKBA (100).

Modification of Antinociceptive Effect of Cyclooxygenase Inhibitor by AKBA

In combinational studies, the sub therapeutic doses of naproxen (5 mg/kg), nimesulide (1 mg/kg), rofecoxib (1 mg/kg) produced a significant anti-nociception when combined with AKBA (100 mg/kg) as compared to *per se.* The effect of combination of nimesulide (1 mg/kg) and AKBA was more pronounced than the combination of naproxen (5 mg/kg) and rofecoxib (1 mg/kg) with AKBA (100 mg/kg) (Fig. 3).

Discussion

The abdominal constriction response induced by acetic acid is a very sensitive procedure that enables the detection of antinociceptive properties of drug

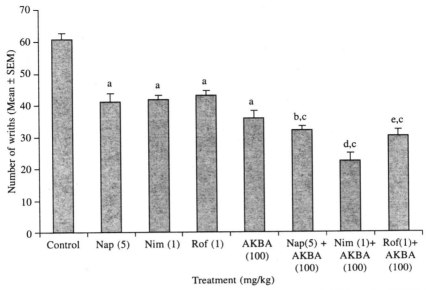

Fig. 3. Modification antinociceptive effect of cyclooxygenase inhibitors by AKBA in acetic acid induced writhing test. [a]$P < 0.05$ as compared to control, [b]$P < 0.05$ as compared to Nap (5), [c]$P < 0.05$ as compared to AKBA, [d]$P < 0.05$ as compared to Nim (1), [e]$P < 0.05$ as compared to Rof (1).

[9]. Role of cyclooxygenase and lipooxygenases system in nociception is now well documented [3, 10]. The cyclooxygenase and lipooxygenases pathways produce their respective metabolites (prostaglandins, leukotrienes and thromboxanes) that are involved in nociception process [11]. Therefore, dual inhibitions of cyclooxygenase and lipooxygenases pathways are now being tried in the management of pain. Therefore, present study was carried out with the aim to assess the antinociceptive property of dual inhibitors by blocking both pathways.

In the present experiment, naproxen, a selective cyclooxygenase (COX-1) inhibitor, nimesulide (preferential COX-2 inhibitor), rofecoxib (selective COX-2 inhibitor) and AKBA (nonspecific 5-LOX inhibitor) produced significantly dose-dependent antinociceptive effect. Further, when subeffective dose of naproxen (5 mg/kg p.o.), nimesulide (1 mg/kg p.o.) and rofecoxib (1 mg/kg p.o.) was administered along with AKBA (100 mg/kg p.o.), synergistically increased antinociceptive effect was produced which was found to be significant as compared to their *per se* effect. However, of all the drug combination, nimesulide and AKBA combination was found to produce maximum antinociceptive effect.

This suggests that conventional cyclooxygenase inhibitors can be used in reduced dose (subeffective) along with lipooxygenases inhibitor (AKBA). This will also help to reduce the dose of latter drugs that are known to produce various side effects such as gastrotoxicity.

References

1. Aley KO, Levine JD. Contribution of 5- and 12-lipooxygenase products to mechanical hyperalgesia induced by prostaglandin E_2 and epinephrine in the rat. *Exp Brain Res* 2003; **148**: 482–487.
2. Rioja I, Terencio C, Ubeda A, Molina P, Alcaraz MJ. A pyrroloquinazoline derivative with anti-inflammatory and analgesic activity by dual inhibition of cyclooxygenase-2 and 5-lipooxygenase. *European Journal of Pharmacology* 2002; **434**: 177–185.
3. Griswold DE, Marshall P, Martin L, Webb EF. Analgesic activity of SK&F 105809, a dual inhibitor of arachidonic acid metabolism. *Agents Actions Suppl.* 1991; **32**: 113–117.
4. Piomelli D. The ligand that came from within. *Trends Pharmacol Sci* 2001; **22**: 17–19.
5. Craib SJ, Ellington HC, Pertwee RG, Ross RA. A possible role of lipooxygenase in the activation of vanilloid receptors by anandamide in the guinea-pig bronchus. *Br J Pharmaco* 2001; **134**: 30–37.
6. Hwang SW, Cho H, Kwak J, Lee SY, Oh U. Direct activation of capsaicin receptors by products of lipooxygenases: endogenous capsaicin-like substances, *Proc Natl Acad Sci USA* 2000; **97**: 6155–6160.
7. Raso E, Tovari J, Toth K, Paku S, Trikha M, Honn KV, Timar J. Ectopic alpha2 beta3 integrin signaling involves 1, 2-lipooxygenase- and PKC-mediated serine phosphorylation events in melanoma cells. *Thromb Haemost* 2001; **85**: 1037–1042.
8. Tonussi CR, Ferreira SH. Tumour necrosis factor-alpha mediates carrageenin-induced knee-joint incapacitation and also triggers over nociception in previously inflamed rat knee-joints. *Pain* 1999; **82**: 81–87.
9. Jain NK, Singh A, Kulkarni SK. Analgesic, antiinflammatory and ulcerogenic activity of zinc naproxen complex in mice and rats. *Pharm Pharmacol Commun* 1999; **5**: 599–602.
10. Janusz JM, Young PA, Ridgeway JM, Scherz MW, Enzweiler L et al. New cyclooxygenase-2/5lipooxygenase inhibitors: 1,7-tert-butyl-2,3-dihydro-3,3-dimethylbenzofuran derivatives are gastrointestinal safe anti-inflammatory and analgesic agents: Discovery and variation of the 5-keto substituent. *J Med Chem.* 1998; **41**: 1112–1129
11. Cashman J, McAnulty G. Nonsteroidal anti-inflammatory drugs in perisurgical pain management: mechanisms of action and rationale for optimum use. *Drugs* 1995; **49(1)**: 51–70.

25. Herbal Remedies for Pain

Rajani Mathur[1] and S.K. Gupta[2]

[1]Department of Pharmacology, All India Institute of Medical Sciences,
New Delhi-110 029, India

[2]Delhi Institute of Pharmaceutical Sciences and Research, New Delhi-110 017, India

Abstract. The use of natural products, especially medicinal plants, for healthcare is increasing world-wide. These plant-derived drugs are sold freely at pharmacies and health stores without any professional advice. These herbs have pharmacological activity, adverse effects and even interactions with conventional drugs. We discuss here some of the species (*Cannabis salix, Capsicum, Azadirachta indica, Glycine max, Piper longum, Panax ginseng*) that hold promise as analgesic drugs and present their supporting evidence. One of the most important analgesic drug employed in clinical practice today continues to be the alkaloid morphine. Recently discovered antinociceptive substances include alkaloids, terpenoids and flavonoid. The development of new analgesics is important for understanding the complex pathways related to electrophysiological and molecular mechanisms associated with pain transmission. Plant-derived substances have, and will certainly continue to have, a relevant place in the process of drug discovery, particularly in the development of new analgesic drugs. Health care professionals can no longer ignore their widespread use. Clinicians should ask the patients about their use of herbs in a non-judgmental way, and should document the patient's use of these drugs. Finally, we must be more aware of the side effects and the potential drug interactions of these herbs, and advise our patients to avoid long term use of these drugs due to lack of information regarding the safety of these medicines.

Introduction

Pain therapies from natural sources date back thousands of years to the use of plant and animal extracts for a variety of painful conditions and injuries. Since 1875, the hydrolyzed product of bitter glycoside from the Willow bark (*Salix alba*) has been used to relieve pain and fever. Its product acetylsalicylic acid still finds favor as aspirin. Plant-derived analgesic compounds such as opium derivatives from *Papaver somniferum* and local anesthetics isolated from coca leaves are in use since late 1800s [1].

Owing to renewed interest in outsourcing novel drugs from plant source, many molecules have been identified as potential analgesics. Medical professionals working in the field of pain are aware that a sizeable percentage of their patients have tried herbal therapies for pain relief. Surveys in both the US and other industrialized nations suggest that it is pain related disorders, including headaches, back pain and arthritis that are most likely to drive people to use herbal remedies [2]. To alleviate suffering from unmitigated pain, patients often see alternative therapies such as nutritional supplements and herbal medicines. However, clinching data linking dietary components to analgesia are lacking. Since the establishment of National Center for Complementary and Alternative Medicine (NCCAM) at the National Institute of Health, in 1992, this area of research has seen active work being conducted and results obtained [2, 3]. Some of the plant derived molecules that are being pursued as potential analgesics are discussed here.

Cannabis sativa

Marijuana contains over 60 different types of cannabinoids, which are its medicinally active ingredients. Cannabinoids have the capacity for neuromodulation through direct, receptor-based mechanisms at many levels within the nervous system, providing therapeutic properties that may be applicable to the treatment of neurologic disorders. These include antioxidation, neuroprotection, analgesia, anti-inflammation, immunomodulation, modulation of glial cells, and tumor growth regulation [4].

Its synthetic congeners like ajulemic acid (AJA), also known as CT-3 and IP-751, are emerging as potential analgesic and anti-inflammatory candidates. In preclinical studies AJA has displayed many of the properties of non-steroidal anti-inflammatory drugs (NSAIDs). In initial short-term trials in healthy human subjects, as well as in patients with chronic neuropathic pain, it proved to be more effective than placebo as measured by the visual analog scale. Moreover, there was complete absence of psychotropic effects and dependency after withdrawal of the drug. Its mechanism of action has been tentatively explained as the activation of peroxisome proliferation activating receptor-γ (PPAR-γ) regulation of eicosanoid and cytokine production [5].

Azadirachta indica

Azadirachta indica (or neem) is an evergreen tree cultivated in all parts of India. Its parts like bark, leaves, branches, flowers, fruits, seeds have been reported to have pharmacological properties including analgesia. In experimental models of pain, A. indica has shown to act by both peripheral and central mechanisms in its antinociceptive effects [6].

Piper methysticum

Piper methysticum extract (kava kava) is a traditional herbal remedy and possesses numerous therapeutic properties for which it is included in various polyherbal formulations of Ayurvedic medicine. Traditionally, fruits, stem and even whole plant has been used for treatment of palsy, gout, rheumatism. P. methysticum extract containing kavalactones, kavain, dihydrokavain, methysticin, dihydromethysticin, yangonin, or desmethoxy-yangonin have been tested for their anxiolytic and analgesic property [7, 8].

Panax ginseng

Ginseng, the root of *Panax ginseng*, is a mild oriental folk medicine that is reported to relieve a variety of ailments. The main constituents include ginsenosides or ginseng saponin that are responsible for its pharmacological activity. The studies indicate that analgesic effects induced by ginsenosides are limited to an action at the spinal level. Ginsenosides induce differential or modality specific antinociception. They may inhibit the release of neurotransmitters involved in transmission of nociception from afferent presynaptic nerve terminal as opioids. They may also produce antinociception by blocking transmission of nociceptive information to secondary post-synaptic neurons at spinal cord following stimulation [9].

Linalool

Linalool is the naturally occurring enantiomer. This monoterpene is commonly found as a major volatile component in several aromatic plant species like *Salvia sclarea*, many of which are used in traditional medicine to cure a variety of acute and chronic ailments [10].

Linalool is a known competitive antagonist of N-methyl-D-aspartate (NMDA) receptors and this may be the mechanism underlying antinociception. Additionally, linalool also possesses weak *in vitro* anti-cholinesterase activity. Since muscarinic neurotransmission is involved in antinociception at the spinal level, this may also contribute towards antinociceptive activity of linalool. Antinociception exerted by linalool appears to depend both on opiodergic and cholinergic neurotransmission [10].

Glycine max

Soybean (*Glycine max*) and its products have been used as a primary source of protein in the diet of Asians. It contains proteins, oil, fiber and carbohydrate. Soy oil is unsaturated with high concentration of essential fatty acids like linoleic and α-linolenic acid and vitamin E. In addition isoflavones, saponins, phytic acid and trypsin inhibitors are also present. The isoflavones share structural similarity with mammalian estrogens. Primary isoflavanoids that are bioactive are genistein, daidzin, glycetin. These are effective antioxidants, free radical scavengers leading to antinociception [3].

Dietary soy proteins also significantly contribute towards antinociceptive activity associated with edema, thermal hyperalgesia and inflammation. Studies conducted in rodents have shown that pretreatment with soy-containing diet for 28 days prevented development of tactile and heat allodynia, but not mechanical hyperalgesia in the animals. This dietary effect was not correlated with calorie intake and weight gain or dietary concentration of fat and carbohydrates [11].

Capsicum frutescens

The efficacy and tolerance of a capsicum plaster in non-specific low back pain was investigated in a double-blind, randomized, placebo-controlled multicentre parallel group study. The superiority of the treatment of chronic non-specific low back pain with capsicum plaster compared to placebo was clinically relevant and highly statistically significant. No systemic side-effects were observed. The capsicum plaster offers a genuine alternative in the treatment of non-specific low back pain [12].

In other studies fixed combination herbal preparation having capsicum as one of the constituents, was used for the treatment of acute tonsillitis. More than half of the patients reported marked alleviation of the principal symptom, moderate or severe difficulty in swallowing, within the first 5 days of treatment. Comparable improvements occurred in other outcome measures, including earache, headache and fatigue. No adverse effects were reported [13].

In interesting animal studies oral administration of capsicum solution and low capsaicin (8-methyl-N-vanillyl-6-nonenamide) doses during gestation produced an increase in the latency of the thermonociceptive escape response of rat offspring [14]. Thus, there is increasing data indicating the therapeutic utility of capsicum.

Conclusion

These studies indicate the rising possibility of plant derived molecules in influencing aspects of pain. Further research will help determine if their use as mainline or adjunct therapy in conditions of acute and chronic pain. They may help to overcome the dose related side effects associated with long term use of conventional analgesics.

References

1. Reisner L. Biologic poisons for pain. *Curr Pain Headache Rep.* 2004; **8(6)**: 427–34.
2. Wendy BS. Research methodology: implications for CAM pain research. *Clin J Pain* 2004; **20**: 3–7.
3. Tall JM, Raja SN. Dietary constituents as novel therapies for pain. *Clin J Pain* 2004; **20**: 19–26.
4. Carter GT, Ugalde V. Medical marijuana: emerging applications for the management of neurologic disorders. *Phys Med Rehabil Clin N Am.* 2004; **15(4)**: 943–54.
5. Burstein SH, Karst M, Schneider U, Zurier RB. Ajulemic acid: A novel cannabinoid produces analgesia without a "high". *Life Sci.* 2004; **75(12)**: 1513–22.
6. Khanna N, Goswami M, Sen P, Ray A. Antinociceptive action of *Azadirachta indica* (neem) in mice: possible mechanism involved. *Indian J Exp Biol.* 1995; 848–850.
7. Smith KK, Dharmaratne HR, Feltenstein MW et al. Anxiolytic effects of kava extract and kavalactones in the chick social separation-stress paradigm. *Psychopharmacology* (Berl) 2001; **155**: 86–90.
8. Coimbra HS, Royo AV, de Souza VA et al. Analgesic and anti-inflammatory activities of (-)-o benzyl cubebin, a (-)-cubebin derivative, obtained by partial synthesis. *Boll Chim Farm.* 2004; **143(2)**: 65–9.

9. Yoon SR, Jin JN, Young HS et al. Ginsenosides induce differential antinociception and inhibit substance P induced nociceptive response in mice. *Life Sci.* 1998; **62**: 319–325.

10. Peana AT, Aquila PSD, Chessa ML et al. (–) linalool produces antinociception in two experimental models of pain. *Eur J Pharmacol* 2003; **460**: 37–41.

11. Shir Y, Sheth R, Campbell JN, Raja SN, Seltzer Z. Soy-containing diet suppresses chronic neuropathic sensory disorders in rats. *Anesth Analog.* 2001; **92(4)**: 1029–34.

12. Frerick H, Keitel W, Kuhn U, Schmidt S, Bredehorst A, Kuhlmann M. Topical treatment of chronic low back pain with a capsicum plaster *Pain.* 2003; **106(1-2)**: 59–64.

13. Rau E. Treatment of acute tosilitis with a fixed-combination herbal preparation. *Adv Ther* 2000; **17(4)**: 197–203.

14. Pellicer F, Picazo O, Leon-Olea M. Effect of red peppers (*Capsicum frutescens*) intake during gestation on thermonociceptive response of rat offspring. *Behav Brain Res.* 2001; **119(2)**: 179–83.

Pain Updated: Mechanisms and Effects
Edited by R. Mathur
Copyright © 2006 Anamaya Publishers, New Delhi, India

26. Relevance of Social Science Concepts to Health Systems: Eualgesic State Management

Nirupama Prakash

Humanistic Studies, Hospital and Health System Management,
Birla Institute of Technology and Science, Pilani-333031, India

Introduction

This article aims to explain the social organization of health system vis-à-vis eualgesic state through concepts related to social structure of society. After completing this module, we should be able to:

(a) explain the significance of relationship between health/eualgesia and society.
(b) distinguish between concepts of health/eualgesia and medicine.
(c) describe the social organization of health system.
(d) explain important social science concepts and apply its relationship to health care organizations and health systems.

Significance of Health/Eualgesia and Society

The society is the system of usage and procedures, of authority and mutual aid, of many groupings and divisions, of controls of human behaviors and liberties. It is the web of social relationship. This is how society has been defined. Society must be organized and in a well-organized society various processes such as political, social, health system management, economic and cultural are structured and each organ performs its duties efficiently. The social behavior of each member in the society is determined by the health and sensitivity to painful stimuli albeit in a pain free state. The concept of health has evolved and expanded including it to be not only a pain free state but also emotionally sound. In the early 1900s, health was defined biologically, thus restricting health to the absence of death, chronic diseases/chronic mild irritation or pain and/or physical disabilities. Recently, pain is defined as an "unpleasant sensory and emotional experience associated with actual or potential tissue damage or described in terms of such damage." In the decades since then, health has undergone a "de-biologization". In the more recent years, a more holistic, multisectoral approach to the determinants of health has political processes and sociocultural factors. Here, a variety of social, economic, political and cultural issues are seen as additional determinates of society's health [1].

It is a common notion to consider areas of health and medicine from a technical perspective. Take the example of AIDS. The general belief is that AIDS is a medical problem. Now, it is widely accepted that sociology has a great deal to say not only about the causes of disease but about their cures as well. It is beyond doubt that such patients are emotionally disturbed/pained and need tender care. There are numerous cases of people affected by AIDS being discriminated against in their places of work, in their homes, prisons, hospitals and wide variety of social contacts. Thus, respect for human right, tolerance and compassion is needed to make them pain free and emotionally stronger.

The Social Medicine

This has primarily been a European specialty. Pioneers sowed the seeds that medicine is a social science. However, the germ theory of disease and discoveries in microbiology checked the development of these ideas. Alfred Grothan revised the concept of social medicine in 1911 that stressed the importance of social factors in the etiology of disease, which was called *social pathology* [2]. Development in the field of social sciences like sociology, psychology and anthropology, rediscovered that man is not only a biological animal but also a social being. Disease has social causes, social consequences and social therapy. Social medicine is the study of man as a social being in his total environment. Its focus is on the health of the community as a whole. Social medicine stands on two pillars, namely, medicine and sociology. In broad sense, social medicine is an expression of the humanitarian tradition in medicine. It could be identified with care of patients, prevention of disease, administration of medical services or any area in the field of health and welfare. In the more restricted sense, social medicine is concerned with knowledge based in epidemiology and the study of medical care of society.

It is well know that laughter therapy works wonders for patients with cancer pain. This is a glaring example of social behavioral pattern, which has a positive impact on health care. Erdman [3] points out that humor is an important part of life. Care should be taken to ensure that humor persists even during the bleakest times for patients, families and medical personnel. Laughter eases the mind, diffuses tension among people and has positive physiologic effects on patients. Thirteenth century medical history depicts laughter as being used as an anesthetic for surgical procedures. It has also been known to be a treatment for colds and depression. While laughing, a person experiences an increase in heart rate, which in turn stimulates circulation. Laughter also release endorphins, which provide the body with natural pain relief. Laughing exercises the muscles used for breathing and movement. It is a common belief that laughing 100 times a day is equal to 10 min of rowing and that relaxation follows the stimulation produced by laughter, resulting in a cool-down period with decrease in heart rate, blood pressure and muscle tension.

In addition to its physiologic benefits, humor serves communicative, social-interactive and psychological functions. Doctors/nurses can assess the laughter needs of the patients and interject "humor breaks" into the nursing care plan. The bottom line is that the use of humor and a laughter with patients and families serves to improve the quality of their lives, it makes the hospital environment more enjoyable for everyone and also hastens the process of healing thereby reducing the pain and agony.

The question then arises as to how does the doctor determine which patients are likely candidates for humor therapy. Some people are not accustomed to humor in their lives; therefore, nurses and physicians often do not know the background of the patient. It may be helpful to identify the likely candidates for humor therapy on the basis of the following questionnaire:

1. Do you like to laugh?
2. Before you became ill, did you laugh a lot?
3. What makes you laugh? Give examples such as a comedy, jokes, cartoons etc.
4. When is the last time you had a good belly laugh?
5. With whom do you laugh? What is about that person that invites you to laugh?
6. Can you remember a painful experience that was soothed by humor?
7. In which area in your life you would like to add humor?

If the answer is 'No' to Question 1, then it may be helpful to try to determine the reasons (such as financial difficulties, cultural limitations and the nature of disease). A shared laugh between the patient and the nurse can bridge communication. Sharing humor leads to a caring personal response, which in turn helps to individualize patient care. A variation of social humor in health care known as *play therapy* has been used for years to encourage children to face difficult procedures or discussions [3].

Distinction Between Concepts of Health and Medicine

Health can be defined as a state of mind, physical and social well-being. It involves not merely the absence of pain/illness but a positive sense of soundness as well. This definition put forth by World Health Organization draws attention to the interplay of psychological, physiological and sociological factors in a holistic sense of being.

Medicine can be defined as an institutionalized system for the scientific diagnosis, treatment and prevention of disease, illness and other damage to the mind or the body. It is concerned with the physiological and psychological conditions that prevent a person from achieving a healthful state [4]. There is a dichotomy of medicine into two major branches, namely, curative medicine and public health or preventive medicine. With advances in medical and bio-medical sciences, acute infectious diseases could be controlled. However, modern diseases such as cancer, diabetes mellitus, cardiovascular, mental illness and accidents come into prominence in industrialized countries. These diseases could not be treated or explained on the basis of germ theory of disease.

One can list various factors or causes in the etiology of diseases, namely, social, economic, genetic, environmental and psychological, although each of these factors are equally important. Most of these factors are linked to man's lifestyle and behavior.

The primary objectives of the curative medicine are the alleviation of disease from the patient rather than from the masses. It employs various modalities to accomplish this objective, such as diagnostic techniques and the treatment. Around middle of 20th century, a profound revolution was brought in allopathic medicine, which has been defined as treatment of disease by the use of a drug, which produces a reaction that itself neutralizes the disease, by the introduction of antibacterial and antibiotic agents. On the other hand preventive medicine is applied to healthy people. Its prime objective is to prevent disease and promote health. For example, the beneficial effects of washing the eyes early in the morning with strained water of *Triphala* soaked overnight. It helps in combating any eye ailment and also ensures a good sight. It is also empirically believed that no glasses need to be worn even after 40 years of age by a regular user of this herb.

Social Organization of Health System

The health system can be broadly defined as the coherent whole of many interrelated component parts, both sectoral and intersectoral as well as the community itself, which produces a combined effect on the health of a population. The idea may be to have one unified health system encompassing promotive, preventive, curative and rehabilitative measures. Whether unified or not, a health system should consist of coordinated parts and extend to the home, the workplace, the school and the community [5]. The health system is usually organized in levels, primary health care pays particular attention to the point of initial contact between members of the community and health services. Expensive and specialized needs should be referred to secondary (intermediate) and tertiary (regional or national) levels, it is at the local level that the health care will be most effective within the context of the areas needs and limitations, duly recognizing the users of health systems as social beings in a particular environment.

The role of primary health care in the social organization of health system is significant. Before going into this aspect of health system let us first make a note of the basic characteristics of primary health care. It is essential health care based on practical, scientifically sound and socially acceptable methods and technology made universally accessible to individuals and families in the community through their full participation and at a cost that the community and country can afford to maintain at every stage of their development in the spirit of self-reliance and self-determination.

Thus, the primary health care forms an integral part of the country's health system and of the overall social and economic development of the community. Herein lies its relationship to the social organization of the health system. It is the first level of contact of individuals, the family and community with the national health system bringing health care as close as possible to where people live and work. This establishes the link between the basic unit of health system and society. Since primary health care is an integral part of the overall social and economic development of the community, it gives a new direction to the health system and goes beyond the more limited approach based on a system of health services alone. Some specific services and activities must be provided to individuals and communities at the local level. These essential elements are:

1. education concerning prevailing health problems and methods of preventing and controlling them.
2. maternal and child health care.
3. immunization against major infectious diseases.
4. promotion of food supply and adequate nutrition.
5. provision of essential drugs.
6. adequate supply of safe water and basic sanitation.
7. prevention and control of local endemic diseases.
8. appropriate treatment of common diseases and injuries.

Important Social Sciences Concepts and Application of their Relationship to Health Care Organizations and Health Systems

Norms are defined as the behaviors and thought patterns that members of group are expected to exhibit. Whereas norm is defined as that which we may think and do, values can be defined as that which members of a group want to do. Beliefs are ideas about the truth or falseness, right or wrongness, of some thought or action. Norms, values and beliefs constitute non-material aspects of culture about what behavior and thought are expected, what persons want to do, and about what is believed to be right or wrong to do. These can be examined within any group. People learn the norms, values and beliefs of any social group through the process of socialization. Norms, values, beliefs, socialization constitute primary elements in the non-material culture of group [6]. People's perception of sickness and health is influenced by their cultural definitions. There are sick roles in every society and to a large extent these are sociologically determined.

According to Talcott Parson's role theory of sickness in modern society, when someone is labeled 'sick' they are expected to behave in certain culturally appropriate ways and to receive culturally appropriate response from others.

Parson drew the following conclusions regarding the social construction of illness:

(a) Being healthy is a value in modern society, being ill is to be avoided.
(b) The role of sick person includes the right to be excused from social responsibility and other normal social roles as well as responsibility for the illness itself.

The role of sick person also includes a normative obligation to seek to get well, and to seek competent medical help in order to do so. The norms of modern society include the idea that everyone has a right to medical care if they are sick [4]. Parson's model helps us to understand sickness and health in modern society for it underscores the fact that the sick role is to a large extent sociologically determined [4]. There are examples of some illnesses to be culturally defined as legitimate enabling those who suffer from the particular illness to take on the role of sick person. For example, compare a person who has terminal cancer pain with that suffering from any of the complications of chronic alcoholism. Imagine the differences in the culturally accepted response in both the cases. The person with cancer expects to be treated with sympathy and patience. Such an expectation would be contained in the role of 'sick person'. Whereas, an alcoholic would also receive an appropriate treatment but the sympathy is lacking. He will be warned repeatedly not to drink in future, failing which he does not get the same response from the society.

Appelbaum and Chambliss [4] have highlighted another aspect of social construction of illness. This is manifested in the doctor-patient relationship. In modern society the doctor has assumed the role of authority in all matters of health and medicine. Their patients treat them with great respect because they have the technical expertise to make the difference between life and death. Talcot Parson viewed the unequal power between doctor and patient as functional for proper health care. It has been argued that doctors may be more effective in enforcing social norms and reproducing the domination of experts and professionals than any other social group [4].

Culture is the shared values and behavior that knit a community together. Culture provides meaning, direction and mobilization—a social energy that moves the health service organization into action [7]. Culture manifests itself through shared values, beliefs, expectations and assumptions but it is most controllable through norms. In the management of pain, culture has a definite place. Several such practices have now been scientifically proven, for example, acupressure, ingestion of sweet substances, counter irritation, reflexology, use of several herbal and yoga practices. Besides, yoga is a boon to the population at large by the rich Hindu culture as a curative and preventive management strategy in the identified or not yet identified disease conditions.

Key Terms

Health: A state of mental, physical and social well-being.

Medicine: An institutionalized system for the scientific diagnosis, treatment and prevention of disease, illness, and other damage to the mind or body.

De-biologization: Changes in the concept of health from restricting health of absence of death, chronic disease and physical disabilities to a holistic, multisectoral approach which integrates medicine with health, economic, political processes and socio-cultural factors.

Euthanasia: The act of putting a severely ill person to death as an act of mercy. It involves a belief dilemma.

Health system: The coherent whole of many interrelated component parts, both sectoral and intersectoral, as well as the community itself, which produces a combined effect on the health of a population.

Primary health care: This is essential health care based on practical, scientifically sound and socially acceptable methods and technology made universally accessible to individuals and families in the community through their full participation and at a cost that the community and country can afford to maintain at every stage of their development in the spirit of self-reliance.

Curative medicine: The primary objective is the removal of disease from the patient rather than from the mass.

Preventive medicine: It emphasizes a healthy lifestyle to prevent poor health before it actually occurs.

Social medicine: Study of man as a social being in his total environment. It is an expression of the humanitarian tradition in medicine. Society stands on two pillars, viz. medicine and sociology.

References

1. Rodriguez-Garcia, R. and Goldman, A. The Health Development Link, Washington, D.C. (PAHO/WHO), 1994.
2. Park, K. Park's Textbook of Preventive and Social Medicine, Banarsidas Bhanot Publishers, 18th Ed., 2005.
3. Erdman, L. Laughter Therapy for Patients with Cancer, *Journal of Psychosocial Oncology*, Vol. II, No. 4, New York, The Hawprth Medical Press, 1983.
4. Appelbaum, R.P. and Chambliss, W.J. Sociology, Harper Collins College Publishers, New York, 1995.
5. Kleezkowski, B.M. Health System Support for Primary Health Care, WHO Publication, 1984.
6. Denton, M.D. Medical Sociology, Haughton Mifflin Company, 1978.
7. Fotler, M.D., Hernandez, R. and Joiner, C.L. Strategic Management of Human Resources in Health Services Organizations. John Wiley & Sons, 1988.

Index